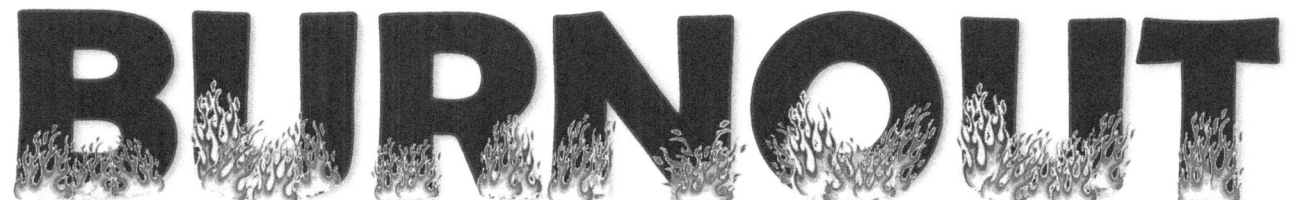

PREVENTION AND RECOVERY

RESILIENCE AND RETENTION

A white paper (that grew into a book) providing:

Evidence-based, experience-informed,

root cause solutions

Provided by Happiness 1ˢᵗ Institute, a *Thrive More Now Company*

Providing Education, Training, Research, Motivational Speaking, and Consulting Services

Jeanine Joy, Ph.D.

Phil Geissinger, FHFMA, CMPE

This book began with the intention of being a White Paper but as the available research was reviewed it became apparent that it would need to be a book.

Part I provides background on the problem of burnout in general and as it applies to healthcare professionals in particular.

Part II provides new evidence-based, experience-informed research that points the way to healthier responses to stressors that will help decrease chronic stress that causes burnout and that will help individuals experiencing symptoms of burnout recover.

Part III provides advanced and transformative coping skills that help you reduce stress, burnout, and suicide risk.

Part IV This section focuses on actions healthcare organizations can take, individually and collectively, to reduce burnout.

Appendices The appendices provide resources including questionnaires that can be used to determine if an individual is experiencing burnout, depression, anxiety, symptoms of stress, low self-esteem, and the types of coping skills he or she has available to deal with stressors.

HAPPINESS 1ST INSTITUTE, *A THRIVE MORE NOW COMPANY*

Happiness 1st Institute was founded in 2011 to share the results of Dr. Joy's two decades long pursuit of the answer to one question, "What makes humans thrive in spite of adversity?"

Her search for an answer to this big question led to the conclusion that the root cause of human thriving is the same in every area of life including physical, mental, emotional, behavioral health, relationships, and success in career or sports. The answer she found is strongly supported by research, ancient wisdom, and the texts of six major religious.

Happiness 1st Institute provides training, motivational speeches, and consulting focused on sharing the solution to human thriving with individuals and organizations. They have provided services to diverse groups from bank presidents, teenagers, entrepreneurs, employees, and homeless recovering addicts.

Dr. Joy is the sole author of seven books and has contributed to two books that were a combined effort including a peer-reviewed textbook on coping and resilience.

Phil Geissinger, FHFMA, CMPE has spent his career in healthcare with physician organizations, hospitals, health systems and other related patient care delivery organizations.

A joint effort between Phil and Jeanine provides actionable steps healthcare organizations and individuals can apply to prevent and recover from burnout. Most of the individual steps will provide the fastest relief because it takes longer to change the regulatory and employer environment. Burnout must be approached from both perspectives for the long-term health of our nation's healthcare providers.

Increasing resilience is not an excuse to ignore the wounds inflicted on healthcare workers by a system that largely ignores the humanity of healthcare providers. This is not to lay blame on employers. It is the collective accumulation of government mandates, regulatory agencies, insurance companies, legal risk management, and employer requirements that has created an untenable situation. Taken individually, the requirements would not be nearly as onerous. Much like an individual will surely recover from a single shallow knife wound but die from a hundred such wounds; physicians and other healthcare providers have been subjected to repeated blows.

To a large degree, new regulations and mandates have not taken into consideration psychology related to self-esteem, motivation, employee engagement, resilience and other factors that could have and should have been considered. It is possible to introduce the same requirements in ways that support mental health or in ways that diminish mental health. The way things are perceived matters more than their actual structure when it comes to our emotional response, motivation, engagement, and resilience.

We seek to empower physicians to adjust their perceptions to more empowered stances and help employers understand significant factors that should be considered when responding to outside mandates and developing internal policies. We also make recommendations about collective actions focused on the business of medicine that will improve outcomes for patients, providers, healthcare organizations, and their employees.

Although the focus of this book is healthcare workers, with a leaning toward providers, the skills and knowledge presented will help anyone in any occupation increase their level of resilience and prevent or recover from burnout. The same techniques will benefit 1st responders, LEO's, teachers, call center employees, social workers, or any other profession that experiences high levels of burnout.

Thrive More, Now Publishing

Burnout: Prevention and Recovery, Resilience and Retention:
Evidence-based, experience-informed, root cause solutions

All rights reserved

Copyright © 2017 Jeanine Joy and Phil Geissinger

All rights reserved, including the right to reproduce this book or portions thereof in any form whatsoever. For information address: Thrive More Now, P.O. Box 6888, Concord NC 28027

For information about special discounts for bulk purchases or speaking engagements, please contact Thrive More Now.

ISBN-13: 978-1545501313

ISBN-10: 1545501319

ACKNOWLEDGEMENTS

We would be remiss if we failed to acknowledge the thousands of researchers whose work has informed our expertise in understanding the cause of and cure for burnout. We greatly appreciate the work they put into conducting the research and the often more arduous task of getting it through peer review. We also appreciate the business leaders who shared their views with us and the physicians we talked with for sharing their angst and struggles dealing with the onslaught of new regulations that have continually been thrust upon them.
More personally, the value of the feedback from those we have taught skills that increase their resilience and sense of empowerment cannot be quantified. They have helped us refine our explanations and methods so that we can communicate more effectively with our readers.

DEDICATION

This book is dedicated to all those who serve others and especially to healthcare providers without whom this book would have never been written. Thank you for your service, dedication, and persistent focus on delivering the best care you can provide.

Contents

Happiness 1st Institute, *a Thrive More Now Company* 3
Acknowledgements 6
Dedication 7
Contents 8
Preface 13
Introduction 14
Part I – Definition of problem and its breadth 15
    Statistics About Burnout 19
        Suicide 21
    Contributing Causes 24
    Bureaucratic Tasks 25
        Difficult work relationships 25
        Lack of Purpose and Meaning 26
        High Demands 26
        Compassion Fatigue 27
        The Business of Medicine 28
        Personality 30
        Individual Perception 31
Part II – Evidence-based Progress 33
    Understand how Your brain Processes Data 42
        Rational Thought 44
    New Definition of the Purpose and Use of Emotions 45
    Emotional Guidance Scale 50
    Coping vs Thriving 52
    Meta-cognition 58
        Meta-cognitive Processes 60
    High-Level Factors That Contribute to Positive Outcomes 62
    Resilience 63
    Psychological Capital (PsyCap) 66
    Personality 66
    What Humans do and why They Do It 68

- Long-term vs. Short-term Goals.. 68
  - Dark Side Personality Traits 70
- Develop Psychological Flexibility.. 71
- Energy 75
- Purpose and Find Meaning.. 77

Part III – Advanced and Transformative Coping.. 79
- Transformative and Advanced Coping Skills 79
  - Emotion Regulation Process: Overview 80
- Unhealthy Habits of Thought 83
  - Catastrophizing/Awfulizing 84
  - Self-Criticism 85
  - Negative rumination 87
  - Low Self-esteem 87
  - Suppressing Emotions 88
  - Pessimism 90
  - Low Self-Efficacy 90
  - Willingness to seek support 91
  - Surface-Thinking 91
  - Maladaptive Detachment (Disengagement) 91
  - High Neuroticism 92
  - Denial 92
  - Cautious (overly) 92
  - Cynicism 92
  - Addictions 93
- Distractions 93
- Humor 93
- Don't give Up Pleasurable Activities 93
- Develop Healthy Habits of Thought... 94
  - Respond proactively to emotions... 96
  - Optimism 97
  - Cognitive restructuring 98
  - Positive affirmations 101
  - Reappraisal (Right Response) 102
  - Planning 104
  - Re-define Your Best 104
  - Positive Reframing 107

- Savoring 109
- Core Self-Evaluations (CSE) 110
- Healthy self-esteem 110
- Meta-cognition 117
- Open to new experiences 117
- Growth mindset 118
- Internal Locus of Control 119
- Positive Thinking 121
- Supportive, Empowering Beliefs 123
- Diversity Appreciation 124
- Human Dignity 126
- Compare CBT to The Smart Way 127
- Expectant Questions 136
- Appreciation 137
- Social Support 138
- Make Happiness a Priority 139
- Set Limits: Say No 140
- Mindfulness 142
- Meditation 143
- Religion/Spirituality 143
- Volunteerism 144
- Practice Is Important 144

Adaptive Coping 145
Anticipated Changes 146
Physician's Power 147
Core Concepts 148
Part IV - Retention Strategies 150
- Measurement 151
- Thoughts on the Business of Medicine 152
- Psychological Contracts 153
- Stop the Silence 155
- Workload 155
- Work/Life Balance 155
- Time Management 156
- Autonomy 158
- Intrinsic Motivation 160

Emotional Labor	160
Administrative Burdens	160
Flexibility	165
On-site Psychologist	167
Coaching Environment	167
Teamwork	171
Environment	172
Supportive Management	173
Physician Well-Being Committees	175
Perception of Physicians	177
Workplace Justice	178
Home-Work Interference aka Work-Family Conflict (WFC)	181
Death and Dying	181
Secondary Trauma and Compassion Fatigue	182
Workplace Bullying	183
ROI: Burnout Prevention and Retention	184
Health Consequences	185
Risk Management	186
Human Thriving	187
WIN-WIN-WIN-WIN	188
Final Thoughts for Healthcare Providers	188
Reviews	188
Dr. Joy's Books	188
About the Authors	190
Jeanine Joy, Phd	190
Phil Geissinger, *FHFMA, CMPE*	191
Appendix I – EGSc	192
Appendix II – Burnout Questionnaire (Clinical Subtypes)	193
Appendix III – Burnout Questionnaire	194
Appendix IV - Depression Questionnaire (PHQ-9)	195
Appendix V - General Anxiety Questionnaire (GAD-7)	196
Appendix VI - Questionnaire Scoring (BCSQ-12)	197
Appendix VII - Depression Questionnaire Scoring (PHQ-9)	200
Appendix VIII - General Anxiety Questionnaire (GAD-7) Scoring	203
Appendix IX – Burnout Questionnaires	204
Appendix X – Burnout Questionnaire Scoring	205

Appendix XI - Stress Symptom chart...205
Appendix XII – COPE Questionnaire 206
Appendix XIII - Brief COPE 209
Appendix XIV - COPE Scoring 211
Appendix XV - Brief Cope Scoring 212
Appendix XVI – High Level factor Chart Biblio..213
Appendix XVII - Effects of a Positive Mindset 214
Appendix XVIII: Self-Esteem Questionnaire..215
Appendix IXX: Self-Esteem Questionnaire scoring 217
Appendix XX: Thriving Questionnaire 219
Appendix XXI – State of Burnout Research and Future Directions 220
Appendix XXII – Thriving Questionnaire Scoring 221
Bibliography 223
Citations 236

PREFACE

This book covers burnout prevention and recovery through two distinct lenses:

1. What an individual can do to protect themselves and/or recover from burnout, and
2. What healthcare organizations can do, individually and collectively, to prevent burnout and help employees recover from burnout syndrome.

We recognize that physicians and healthcare organization executives are busy and may not have time to read the entire book. If you want to know what you can do to protect yourself against burnout and/or recover from burnout, you can cover the applicable material by reading the following Pages 32-149.

If you are a healthcare executive who wants to know what you can do as an organization, or in collaboration with other organizations, you can cover the applicable material by focusing on the solutions presented on Pages 149-187.

Executives may want to review the section for individuals because training your staff to understand the knowledge and skills presented will increase resilience, emotional intelligence, and create a more positively focused workforce. It will also help you deal with daily stressors in your role including workplace politics.

The Appendix has questionnaires for burnout, depression, coping, and anxiety. You can use them or not. You may find it interesting to do a self-test before you read the book then again after you finish. We expect you will find an appreciable gain from your expanded knowledge. Some results may indicate you should obtain professional help and we encourage you to do so if your test results indicate it is advised.

Scientific support for our approach is included throughout the book but we've made an effort to make the material readable and not too textbook-ish. Dr. Joy's first five books had deep dives into the science so for those who love the background research we recommend you take a look at her earlier books.

The strategies shared in this book will help you prevent or recover from burnout but that's not what has us the most excited. What is really exciting is that the same strategies that help you prevent and/or recover from burnout will help you thrive. Through years of primary research and experimentation we've learned that a salutogenic approach to wellness increases human thriving beyond what the majority of people achieve with a pathogenic approach to health.

Throughout the book, when I, me, and my, are used, it is Dr. Joy's voice.

INTRODUCTION

It is tempting to conclude that excessive workload and absence of support are directly caused by poor working conditions. However, such an interpretation is not straightforward. It is particularly difficult for the doctors in our study because the study is longitudinal, and workload and lack of support correlate with stress and burnout reported five or six years earlier, when the doctors were carrying out entirely different jobs.
– McManus, Keeling, and Paice, BMC Medicine (paraphrased)

Although there is no doubt that the medical profession has more potential stress from administrative burdens and close scrutiny than was common in the past, the primary focus of this book is on activities, elements and thinking which the worker can control. There have always been individuals who thrive under difficult circumstances. By studying them and teaching ordinary people about the habits of thought that fuel extraordinary success, their level of thriving increases. This is not about thriving because of greater sacrifice. More is accomplished but less is sacrificed when healthy habits of thought support us. This is where individual empowerment comes into focus.

- A physician, nurse and other healthcare providers can control these factors whereas they have a limited ability to dictate organizational changes;
- Applying the skills and knowledge shared in these pages increases personal resilience which is a protective factor against burnout;
- Transformative and Advanced coping skills reduce stress. Chronic stress is the most significant pre-burnout symptom, so reducing the influencers of stress provides additional protection against burnout;
- Increased self-efficacy is another protective factor against burnout;[1]
- Maladaptive coping is associated with higher incidence of burnout and the skills presented in these pages provide methods to change from unhealthy coping styles to healthier coping behaviors.[2]

Organizations will receive substantial returns on any investments they make to train workers in these skills.

The section on Retention Strategies is devoted to actions organizations should consider for their own employees and things they could collectively attempt to change relating to administrative burdens from outside sources. Consideration is given to factors that are known to increase the sense of autonomy because lack of autonomy increases the risk of burnout in all professions. Consideration is also given to motivation theory because individuals who feel motivated feel more energized about their work.

We named the collection of advanced and transformative coping skills we teach *The Smart Way*™ because it amplifies the "salutogenic model" which promotes well-being. Reading and applying the strategies outlined in this book provides you with a good understanding of *The Smart Way*™. The processes are designed to explore the limits of human wellness and thriving. *The Smart Way*™ is the only training program we are aware of that incorporates current scientific findings about the purpose and meaning of emotions and overturns common false premises about the purpose of emotions that contribute to adverse outcomes.[3,4,5,6,7,8,9,10]

PART I – DEFINITION OF PROBLEM AND ITS BREADTH

Burnout syndrome is often described as resulting from prolonged exposure to chronic stressors in the workplace. This definition is myopic because it fails to consider the fact that not all individuals who are exposed to the same stressors experience burnout which would be the case if it was a simple stimulus-response process. Omitting individual differences makes the best path to prevent and recover from burnout less obvious.

I suggest a modified definition:

> *Burnout is the result of chronic stress, largely from one's work, when an individual has inadequate stress management and coping skills for the stress they're experiencing.*

This modified definition is supported by the following:

- An individual with adequate stress management and/or coping skills would not become burned out under the same circumstances,

- Although burnout is highly associated with workplace stress, research shows that home-work conflicts contribute to the development of burnout which makes sense because stress loads are cumulative.
    - The negative health effects of chronic stress are cumulative. Adults with stressful childhoods who continue to experience high stress during adulthood suffer more ill-health (all else being equal) than adults who have similar adult stress but not the childhood stress.
    - Epigenetic changes and pre-term delivery are associated with cumulative chronic stress.
    - Chronic stress is associated with shorter telomeres which indicate more rapid aging.

Solutions that focus solely on changing the environment are common. While there are many environmental changes that would benefit healthcare workers and patients, the problems with focusing solely on reducing stress and not on building resilience are worth noting.

- It is not usually within the individual's power to bring environmental changes about without requiring the person to give up their job. It is likely that another position will come with its own stressors.
    - ➢ Focusing on things an individual cannot control increases their sense of not having control and disempowerment, which increases the level of stress further.
    - ➢ Focusing on what an individual can do increases their sense of empowerment lowers the stress they experience.
- Building resilience helps in every area of life; not just at work.
- Changing the work environment does not address work-home conflicts.

- Environmental changes may not be fully within the employer's power. Government mandates, insurance company requirements, and certifying boards contribute significantly to administrative hoops healthcare workers face on a daily basis.
- Individual resilience can be built much faster than the healthcare environment can be changed.

The healthcare environment will always have some inherent stressors that cannot be removed including dealing with death, patients who suffer from trauma, working with patients who are uncooperative or uncivil, government intervention, economic directives, and other inherent stressors healer's face on a daily basis.

The DSM does not recognize burnout as a psychological disorder but it is listed in the ICD-10 as 'Problems related to life-management difficulty."[11] It is interesting that this definition ignores the environmental factors that contribute to burnout and puts the onus solely on a lack of life management skills.

Burnout is a war that should be won on two fronts by building individual resilience and by working to make the healthcare work environment less stressful.

In 2015, for all industries, the "global burden of burnout cost is in excess of $300 billion annually."[12] Historically, burnout was identified using the Maslach Burnout Inventory (MBI) and "defined as a syndrome, which is caused mainly by stress, especially among occupations with humanitarian and social contribution."[13] Historically, burnout symptoms were generally described as:

- Emotional exhaustion – indicated by low emotional and physical energy toward one's work
- Depersonalization – evidenced by increasing levels of cynicism
- Low sense of personal accomplishment or meaning found in the work

Recent research has led to changes in the way burnout is measured and discussed.[14] Depersonalization is now considered a maladaptive coping strategy as opposed to a symptom of burnout.

Burnout co-exists with a lower than desired emotional state. Like all lower emotional states, it is associated with less than ideal behaviors and professional outcomes including:

- Lower quality of care[15,16,17]
- Increased likelihood of errors[18,19]
  The estimate of preventable deaths attributed to medical errors was recently revised to "nearly one-sixth of the deaths in the country each year."[20]
- Increased likelihood of leaving the profession
- Increased likelihood of turnover in search of greener pastures[21]
- Worse patient safety outcomes[22]
- Worsening relationships both at work and outside work, including increased divorce and relationship turmoil[23]
- Problematic behaviors including excessive alcohol and drug use[24]
- Suicide ideation and attempted suicide[25]
- Lower customer service scores[26,27]
- Worse response to workplace changes[28]
- Increased absenteeism due to increased susceptibility to colds, headaches, fevers, and chronic fatigue.[29]
- Decreased patient compliance with prescribed medications and follow-up appointments[30,31]

- Higher levels of general psychological distress[32, 33]
- Decreased patient success in drug rehabilitation programs[34]

The pathway from a stressful work environment to burnout varies by individual. Individual differences in cognition are being recognized for their contributory and protective factors. Additionally, three subtypes of burnout have been suggested:[35]

- Frenetic
- Under challenged
- Worn-out

A self-test for burnout and these three clinical subtypes is provided in Appendix II – Burnout Questionnaire (clinical subtypes).

Physicians experience burnout at higher rates than the general population[36] but the numbers for the general population are also significant. In a study that received survey responses from 7,288 physicians and 3,442 working adults, 45.8% of physicians were experiencing at least one symptom of burnout with 37.9% reporting they felt emotionally exhausted. 27.8% of the non-physician working adults reported at least one symptom of burnout. Although this number is 18% lower than physicians, nearly thirty percent feeling emotionally exhausted is still cause for concern and corrective action.

We haven't seen a study that attempted to determine whether patient emotional burnout has a negative effect on physician burnout but the correlation between burnout and physical and mental illness means it contributes to physician workloads and the struggles physicians often experience with low patient adherence to treatment plans.

While physician burnout is critical with over 50% experiencing at least one symptom of burnout, and physicians in some specialties experiencing burnout at rates as high as 68%,[37] it is clear that this is a public health problem that should be aggressively addressed for both physicians and other workers.

Some countries, such as the UK, mandate that employers manage and reduce stress in the workplace. US protections are lagging behind. The UK put their protections in place in 1974. Employers in the UK are required to:[38]

Identifying problems with stress

- Monitoring working conditions to spot signs of stress
- Be aware of working conditions that could cause ill-health
- Consult with employees to get their views on the workplace
- Giving consideration to employees with specific health needs or disabilities

Prevent harm

- Assess the potential impact of workplace stressors
- Identify measures that could prevent ill-health
- Ensure employees are aware of preventative measures

Protect individuals

- Take action where harm to individuals is foreseeable
- Consider the needs of individuals
- Make reasonable adjustments to meet specific health needs or disabilities

Managing the workplace

- Monitor the ongoing impact of work on vulnerable individuals
- Avoid discriminating against individuals because of their health needs or disability

Prevent workplace bullying and harassment

In order to better appreciate the impact of stress, we have constructed an illustration of how employee burnout and employee engagement exist along a continuum. Viewing engagement and burnout as a high-level factor, there are numerous lower-level factors that move along the same continuum in the same direction.

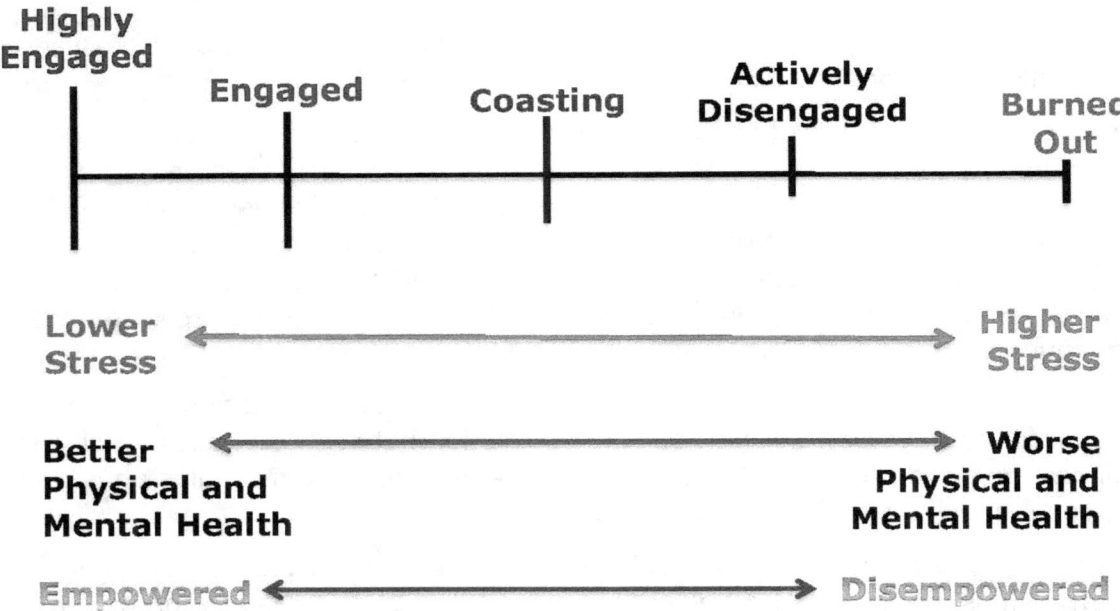

Highly Engaged: Performs like a business owner regardless of level in the organization; i.e. takes ownership, looks for solutions and opportunities to make improvements, exceeds expectations

Engaged: Is meeting expectations of the role but not going above and beyond frequently

Coasting: Does enough to get by, meets most of the expectations of the role.

Actively Disengaged: Does minimum amount of work, does not meet expectations and sabotages success of the organization (i.e. by spreading negativity, by undermining management, theft, dishonesty, etc.).

Burned Out: Unhealthy levels of stress lead to physical and mental exhaustion, likely to leave the job soon and is probably experiencing initial symptoms of both physical and mental illness.[39]

Although the above is a continuum, not all employees will exhibit unethical behaviors when their level of engagement declines but it is common when someone is actively disengaged. If an individual's personal ethics or morals are strongly established, their personal beliefs about how they should conduct themselves will override deliberately doing wrong. However, low emotional states narrow cognitive function which can lead to situations where individuals do not consciously recognize the ethical or moral ramifications of a situation in the same way they would when their level of stress is lower. People experiencing high stress have less cognitive access to as many solutions as they would be able to perceive if they were experiencing less stress.

STATISTICS ABOUT BURNOUT

Although burnout rates among physicians have been high for over a decade, there has been a recent alarming spike in reported rates of burnout. "In the Medscape Physician Lifestyle Report, 46% of all physicians responded that they had burnout, which is a substantial increase since the Medscape 2013 Lifestyle Report, in which burnout was reported at slightly under 40% of respondents."[40]

Physician burnout is not a new phenomenon. Sir William Osler, one of the four founders of Johns Hopkins Hospital, wrote about burnout in the 1800's. As the rapid introduction of HMO's in the 1990's changed modern medicine the Northwest Center for Physician Well-Being commented:[41]

> This shift in power has been disconcerting to the medical profession, and it has led to stress, burnout, change of jobs, change of specialty, and early retirement.

Physicians haven't caught a break since then. The rapid changes in regulations, insurance company practices, medical board mandates, and employment structure continually changed the landscape in which medicine is practiced.

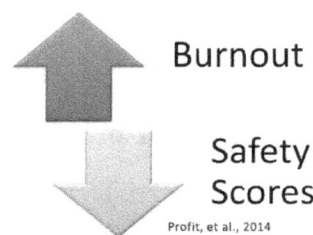

in a special edition of BMJ Careers devoted to "Doctors' Wellbeing", that excessive workload and absence of support are directly caused by poor working conditions; "the way in which the NHS is run generates stress of members of the workforce every day." However, such an interpretation is not straightforward in general. It is particularly difficult for the doctors in our study because the study is longitudinal, and workload and lack of support correlate with stress and burnout reported five or six years earlier, when the doctors were PRHOs[a] carrying out entirely different jobs."[42]

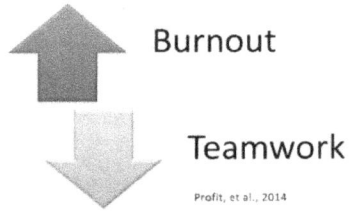
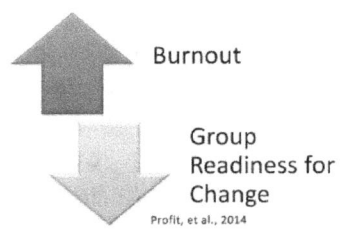

Physician burnout often begins before they leave medical school. In a study of Yale residents, burnout measured 4.3% at the beginning of the year and climbed to 55.3% at year-end.[43] An Australian and New Zealand study of radiation oncology trainees reports 49.% had high levels of emotional exhaustion.[44] Veterinary students also experience significant levels of burnout.[45] A literature review of 100 published journal articles reported burnout rates among medical students varying between 27% – 75% and found that high stress and burnout levels were associated with:[46]

- Decreased life satisfaction
- Serious consideration to dropping out of medical school
- Suicidal ideations
- Poorer performance
- Reduced commitment
- Increased stress

---

[a] PRHO's is an acronym used in the UK referencing Pre-Registration House Officers which is a physician trainee role.

There is a tendency for physicians to have an attitude about burnout that resembles learned helplessness:

> *Surgeons experiencing distress are unlikely to seek help on their own initiative. A belief that distress and burnout are a normal part of being a physician and lack of awareness of distress level relative to colleagues may contribute to this problem. . . Of 1,150 US surgeons tested, a majority (89.2%) believed that their well-being was at or above average, including 70.5% with scores in the bottom 30% relative to national norms.*[47]

In a study of 355 healthcare professional that compared burnout rates in intensive care to those in palliative care, "working in intensive care units more than doubled the likelihood of exhibiting burnout."[48] A 2015 systematic review reported burnout rates in ICU's from 0% to 70.1%.[49]

An Australian study of 5,897 physicians found 10.3% affected by major depression and 50.7% by symptoms of burnout.[50] Burnout significantly increases the risk of depression.

Dr. Schrijver summed up the reason physician burnout is such an important issue:[51]

> In order to *do* well, they must *be* well.

Dr. Catherine Rublee, an Ob/Gyn wisely commented:[52]

> *The problem is that the practice of medicine is not fun anymore. It used to be. Once upon a time Medicine was considered a calling, a vocation like the clergy, or the military. One with the privilege of a good mind and work ethic one used one's talent to serve humanity for a higher purpose as Osler said "To diagnose, to treat but always to comfort."*
>
> *I think we as doctors have lost our way we have become slaves to the agenda of pharmaceutical companies, government and institutional bureaucracies, victims of an adversarial legal system and victims to the demands of "consumers" not "patients.*
>
> *Our relationship with patients has shifted. With the emphasis on "patient autonomy" the patient has become a consumer of health rather than a vulnerable human being in an unequal relationship (which it is) because we have the knowledge, the health and the power.*
>
> *A professor once said to me "Doctors have no power anymore" I disagree. We have the ultimate power; the power of life and death. Think of this when you are faced with a patient that you have just discovered has a cancer, a terminal illness or someone who you are operating on.*
>
> *I have encountered colleagues who after making an error (we all do we are human) are devastated with what has happened to "them" their ego and not what has happened to the patient!*
>
> *I think when one loses perspective about what the job is about and what one defines what need to be done and draws the line about what we are able to accomplish perhaps burnout will be less of a problem."*

Multiple sources, including *Medscape's Physician Compensation Report*[53] and an editorial in the *Journal of General Internal Medicine* are reporting burnout rates that are beyond alarming. When we consider physician burnout we look first to the effect on the physician's wellbeing but we cannot stop there. Physician burnout affects patient outcomes and the health of our entire healthcare system which means the health of our nation is at stake. A physician or other healthcare worker who is experiencing burnout cannot deliver the level of care they were trained to provide.

Burnout is beyond epidemic rates according to a recent Medscape survey of over 15,000 physicians:

50% or higher burnout rate	**More than 40% burnout rate**	**More than 30% burnout rate**
Critical Care	Radiology	Pathology
Emergency Medicine	Ob/Gyn & Women's Health	Psychiatry & Mental Health
Family Medicine	Neurology	Dermatology
Internal Medicine	Pulmonary Medicine	
HIV/Infectious Diseases	Cardiology	
	Diabetes & Endocrinology	
	Orthopedics	
	Plastic Surgery	
	Pediatrics	
	Oncology	
	Anesthesiology	
	Rheumatology	
	Allergy & Clinical Immunology	
	Ophthalmology	
	Gastroenterology	

Our healthcare providers are at risk which means our healthcare system is at risk.

SUICIDE

Shocking physician suicides, attributed largely to burnout, have fueled attention to physician burnout. Burnout among physicians has been high for years but recent suicides have received more public attention than in the past. Suicide is never the result of a single cause but burnout is a significant contributing factor in many of the 400 physician suicides that occur in the United States each year. A 2012 study of 7,288 physicians revealed that 6.9% of them had experienced suicide ideation (thoughts of taking their own life) during the past year.[54]

A male physician who attempts suicide is 70% more likely to die than a non-physician male who attempts suicide and female physicians are 250-400% more likely to die than non-physicians which contributes to physician suicide rates being higher than in the general population.[55,56]

"Inadequate treatment [for mental illness] and increased problems related to job stress may be potentially modifiable risk factors to reduce suicidal death among physicians."[57]

A large study of medical students showed increased suicide ideation in association with burnout.[58] In a study of medical students experiencing burnout, 26.8% recovered.[59]

"Recovery from burnout was associated with markedly less suicidal ideation, which suggests that recovery from burnout decreased suicide risk."[60]

When several Suicide warning signs are present it is time to act without delay.

Suicide Warning Signs: Act Now

- Depression (prolonged)
- Feeling sad
- Feeling angry
- Pessimism
- Personality change(s)
- Self-criticism
- Talk of death
- Making a will
- Plan to hurt self
- Plan to hurt others
- Withdrawal: family
- Withdrawal: friends
- Neglect of appearance
- Desperation
- Anxiety
- Panic
- Agitation
- Rage
- Not self-supporting
- Feels shame
- Difficulties at school
- Difficulties in sports
- Difficulties at work
- Change in sleep patterns
- Change in eating patterns
- Setback viewed as a failure/sign of low worth
- Rejecting compliments
- Physical symptoms of emotional pain
- Feeling hopeless, "beyond help"
- Giving away possessions
- Increased drug/alcohol abuse
- Sudden improvement after lengthy sad withdrawal
- Lacks sense of purpose
- Reckless behavior/driving
- Sense of being trapped
- Uncontrolled anger
- Seeking/planning revenge
- Dramatic mood changes
- Believe they are a burden to others/society
- Suicidal thoughts (ideation)

When several warning signs are present it is time to act. Trust your read of the situation and save a life.

Risk factors do not indicate an imminent threat of suicide. Their presence only indicates an increased risk of suicide—it is far from a certain outcome.

It's important to point out that perfectionism and self-inflicted high demands are risk factors that are common in physicians. Perfectionism is an insidious risk factor because it 1) increases the likelihood an individual will hide their distress, and 2) increases the likelihood that a suicide attempt will result in death. Physicians have a much higher rate of deadly outcome from suicide than non-physicians because they have a greater understanding of how to end their life. This is unfortunate because the rate of completed suicides (suicide attempts that result in death) in the general population is 1 out of 25 attempts. Many people are grateful their attempt failed because it led to getting the help they needed and a turning point in their life. It would be so much simpler to ask for help without risking one's life and health in a suicide attempt.

Unfortunately, stigma and concerns about negative medical board actions prevent many physicians from seeking help. Medical boards should review their policies to determine if they may be inadvertently contributing to physician suicide and reluctance to seek care for burnout.

Until recently, North Carolina Medical Board's license renewal application, question 4, asked the applicant if he/she "was aware of any medical condition that impairs or limits your ability to practice medicine safely?" Medical conditions included "... psychological conditions or disorders ..."[61]

When weighed against the potential loss of the ability to work in their chosen occupation it is understandable that medical professionals would be hesitant to seek the help they would then be required to disclose. It seems mental health stigma was alive and well in North Carolina.

With the help of Dr. Bob Henderson and Miriam Schwarz and others, the North Carolina Medical Board has changed question 4 to one that mandates physician self-care. This is a favorable change.

Based on an article Dr. Henderson wrote, *A Change in Policy Regarding Physician Burnout*[62] the new language reads:

> *The Board voted in September to replace the current renewal question that asks licensees to state whether they are under treatment for a condition that may adversely affect their ability to practice with the following language:*
>
> *Important: The Board recognizes that licensees encounter health conditions, including those involving mental health and substance use disorders, just as their patients and other healthcare providers do. The Board expects its licensees to address their health concerns and ensure patient safety. Options include seeking medical care, self-limiting the licensee's medical practice, and anonymously self-referring to the NC Physicians Health Program (www.ncphp.org), a physician advocacy organization dedicated to improving the health and wellness of medical professionals in a confidential manner.*
>
> *The failure to adequately address a health condition, where the licensee is unable to practice medicine with reasonable skill and safety to patients, can result in the Board taking action against the license to practice medicine.*

I am very happy to see this policy change and hope that other states with policies that inhibit physicians from taking care of their own health needs, especially mental health, stress management, burnout prevention, depression, anxiety, and other highly preventable

Suicide Risk Factors

- Prior suicide attempt(s)
- Suicide plan
- Homicidal ideation
- Preoccupation with death
- Mental disorder
- Low self-esteem
- Stress related to LGBTQ
- Mood disorders
- Impulsiveness
- Aggressive tendencies
- Social isolation
- Alienation from family/friends
- New residence during last year
- Lack of social support network
- Family changes
- Relationship
- conflict
- Absentee parent
- Dysfunctional environment
- Suicide clusters
- Traumatic experience
- Bullied or Bully
- Smokes cigarettes
- Abused as a teenager
- Multiple tattoos
- Rx for mental disorder
- Personality disorder
- Schizophrenia
- Anxiety
- Psychosis
- Alcohol or drug abuse
- Physical illness with loss of activities
- Depression (especially longer than 2 weeks)
- Feels hopelessness
- Learning disabilities
- Self-harm behaviors
- Exposure to violence
- History of childhood abuse
- New school during last year
- Suicide of close friend or family member
- Loss of status
- Recent disappointment or rejection
- Feels mental/behavioral health stigmatizing
- Perfectionism
- Feeling disconnected: religious/spiritual
- Cultural acceptance of suicide
- Irresponsible portrayal of suicide by media
- Self-inflicted high demands
- Abused (especially before age 10)
- Multiple body piercings
- Raised in violent home

Risk factors do not mean suicide is likely-- they increase the risk but most people never attempt suicide

Suicide Prevention Help
If you are thinking you would be better off dead or that your loved ones would be better off if you were, call the toll-free 24-hour hotline of the **National Suicide Prevention Lifeline** now at 1-800-273-TALK (1-800-273-8255); TTY: 1-800-799=4TTY (4889) to talk with a trained counselor.
Or, **Call your doctor**
Dial 911 (or the local emergency number)
or go to an emergency room

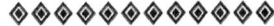

Media/Press: Save Lives. Please comply with suicide reporting guidelines.

and curable issues take note and follow their lead. The AMA *Principles of Medical Ethics* also mandate that physicians take care of their own health.[63]

One physician remarked, "I have to look after myself and I can't believe how much more productive and energetic I am if I pay attention to that piece."[64]

There are many actions that can be taken to reduce physician suicide including:

- Increase physician resilience
- Decrease stigma associated with seeking mental health treatment
- Remove barriers that put their license to practice medicine on the line when a physician seeks help with burnout prevention or recovery
- Decrease workplace stress
- Education (I hesitate to include this one because there is a tendency to educate people repeatedly on risks without providing effective solutions. We do it in wellness programs and many other areas where it is proven that the efficacy of education is small. Once is enough when it comes to risk factors and warning signs. Efforts to train people in techniques that lower risk will provide greater progress.)

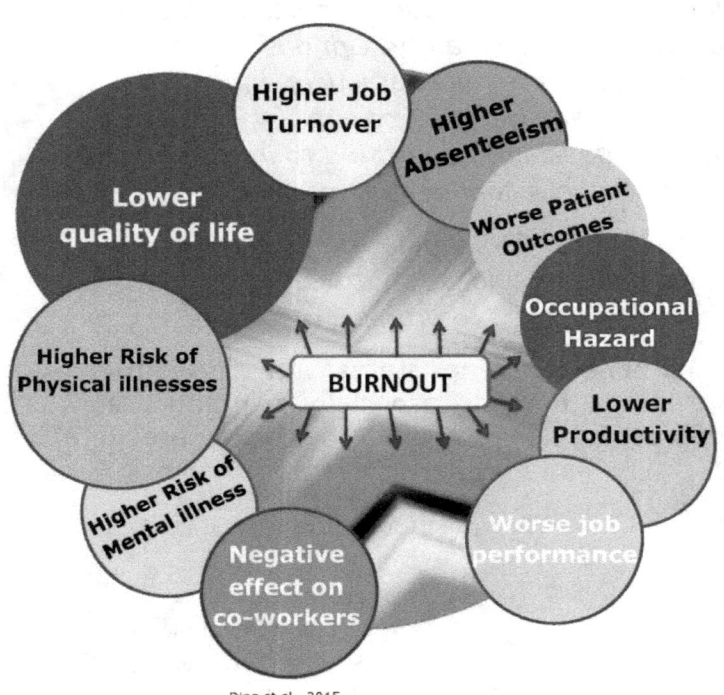

Ding et al., 2015

The cost of burnout extends from the individual to co-workers, family, community, and employer. This makes preventing and recovering from burnout an imperative. The good news is that preventing burnout prevents a lot of other problems. Organizations that choose to spend training resources on reducing burnout also improve patient outcomes, co-worker relationships, overall productivity, employee wellness, productivity and performance. When the true cost of burnout is understood, preventing burnout becomes an easy decision.

CONTRIBUTING CAUSES

The article, *The influence of health care organizations on well-being,* began with the following quote:[65]

> Human beings can be proactive and engaged or, alternatively, passive and alienated, largely as a function of the social conditions in which they develop and function.

This quote reflects a simple stimulus-response structure that fails to account for the human ability to think about what is being thought about and consider alternate thoughts about the situation (meta-cognition). While there are many people who do not utilize meta-cognition in their day-to-day lives, there is no reason they cannot do so. I've taught widely disparate groups, from CEOs to homeless recovering addicts to use meta-cognition to reduce stress and increase psychological well-being.

We can suffer or thrive, dependent upon our environment, or we can take greater conscious control of our thoughts and thought patterns, develop psychological flexibility become masters of our emotional state and not subject to the whims of the environment in which we find ourselves for our happiness. With mastery of skills that increase psychological health and resilience, our dependence on a pleasing environment is reduced. The choice is between suffering more or less. As soon as the choice is understood, the obvious choice is always the answer. My job is to help you understand how to make the choice.

A Medscape survey of over 19,000 physicians asked what contributed to burnout.[66] Their responses can be divided into two categories based on whether a physician can do anything to change the situation or not. They can also be identified by whether perceptions impact the level of stress through a variety of pathways that may include low-autonomy, lack of value, etc.

BUREAUCRATIC TASKS

The amount of time "Physicians spend 20% of their time on non-clinical paperwork"[67] varies. Some physicians report that they spend twice the amount of time documenting than they spend with patients. In a physician's own words, "I spend as much time on documenting a patient visit as I spend with the patient."[68]

Some organizations have found solutions that reduce the amount of time physicians spend documenting their work. At least one organization has recording devices that record their words for transcriptionists to record the written documentation.

TIME STRESS

- Difficulty keeping up with new developments
- Inadequate time with patients to develop relationships and deliver the quality of care desired
- Government continuing to build reporting and analysis processes around quality metrics, diagnostic and procedural claim details, and, requiring incremental reporting processes by a provider ("their practice or employer"), all of which demands more time and effort to complete.
- Continual reviews of claims and authorizations submitted to the commercial insurance companies requires time and effort from the staff and often times the provider in order to get called for clinical care "approved"

DIFFICULT WORK RELATIONSHIPS

In the solutions section of this book you'll learn information that will help you understand the negative relationship spiral that results when an individual experiences symptoms of burnout. A group of individuals who are experiencing various levels of burnout is a recipe for worsening teamwork and relationships in general. Burnout can increase quickness to anger and suspicion.[69] People associated with the provider will be adversely affected by the exhibited behaviors and caustic relationships which ensue, including:

- Patients
- Colleagues
- Staff

- Employer

Stereotype threats can create a work environment that feels hostile. Stereotype threats are associated with more negative emotions and higher rates of burnout.[70]

LACK OF PURPOSE AND MEANING

If you feel like just another cog in the wheels, remember your work and your life has great meaning. If you're not feeling this it isn't your life that is off track, it's the way you perceive your life that has taken a detour. The worse our emotional state becomes the less value we attribute to our life.

One way to regain the sense of purpose is to reconnect with why you went into medicine in the first place. Simply asking yourself the question, "Why did I choose medicine and am I fulfilling my purpose?" with an attitude that expects to receive an answer (not an attitude of plaintive complaint) will help your mind remember your why.

Pay attention to things you see and conversations you have after you ask this question. Asking questions with the expectation of receiving an answer is a new method of positive inquiry that is proving valuable. Connecting with your meaning will reduce your risk of burnout[71, 72] and increase your level of job satisfaction.[73]

Pay attention to your language, especially the way you explain what you do when someone asks you what you do for a living. For decades, regardless of the job title I held, my explanation always reflected helping people in some way. I didn't realize that my purpose was helping people until I was preparing to teach a class on finding purpose and meaning in your work and it dawned on me that long before I shifted to my passion career, I always described my role by how I helped others within that role.

Look for the stories and the human elements that correspond with your work. Think about your work in terms of stories. When I talk about my work I talk about helping people—not the processes I use to help them. Don't talk about doing an appendectomy, talk about helping a child improve their physical well-being and imagine that child doing whatever it is the child likes to do, healthy and enjoying life.

Use the processes in the solutions part of this book to feel better and your sense of purpose will return. When we're in a negative emotional state your mind automatically focuses on the negative. Perceiving your life as meaningful is inconsistent with a low emotional state. You don't have to withdraw from life and meditate on a mountain to regain your sense of purpose. Not that meditation is a bad practice. We meditate 15 minutes every day and life goes better.

HIGH DEMANDS

High psychological demands, effort and effort-reward ratios were associated with job related burnout among lawyers[74] and nurses.[75] If you've ever worked for more than one boss at the same time, you have a sense of how difficult it can be to satisfy more than one person at a time. It seems that physicians were viewed as a place where money is in motion and attracted many others who wanted to make money from the physicians work. There is some support for every "master" with a say in the mix, but the combination of them, all independently asking for more from physicians is creating too much of a burden. If the many masters would simply coordinate and use one source of information it could ease some of the burden. Each insurance company wants to use its own forms; the government wants to use its forms, and the employer wants to use its own systems. The government is not one entity; it is many different areas of government, from the 130,000 pages of Medicaid regulations to employment law and licensing mandates. The government also includes layers. Federal, State, and local laws all affect the practice of medicine. If a physician lives near a state border they have to jump through licensing hoops in more than one state (and pay for the privilege).

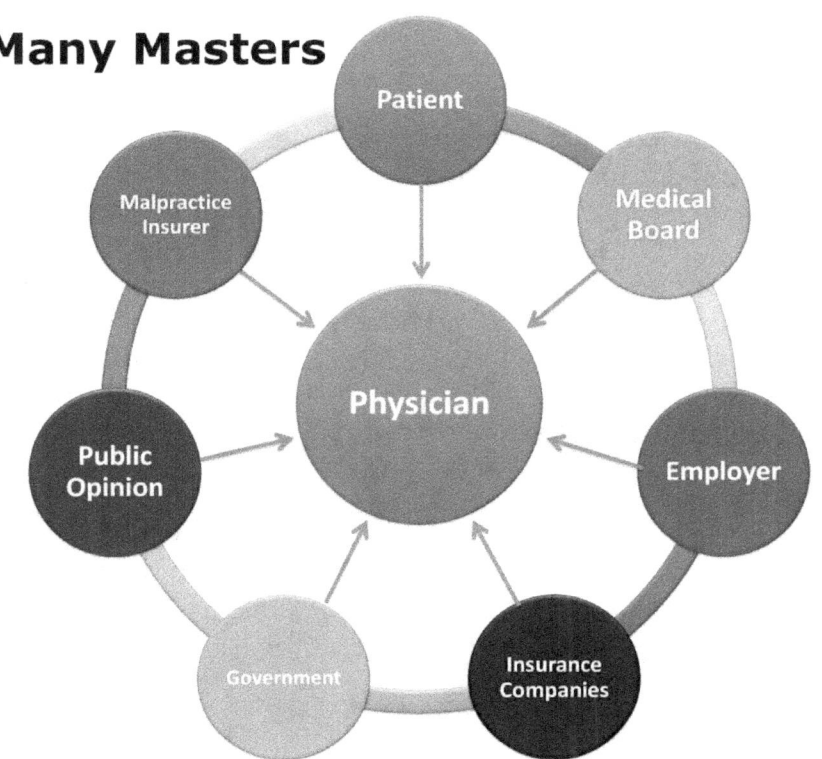

This diagram doesn't reflect the need to keep up with new research and continuing education requirements.

COMPASSION FATIGUE

Compassion fatigue is "a state of physical or psychological distress in caregivers, which occurs as a consequence of an ongoing and snowballing process in a demanding relationship with needy individuals."[76] Healthcare workers who experience frequent death and dying lean heavily on several ways of dealing with compassion fatigue:

1. **Become philosophical**

    I can't imagine dealing with death without having found a framework/worldview that soothes and comforts me. I don't think it matters what the viewpoint is nearly as much as it matters how it allows you to feel. I've met people with worldviews that are very different from my own who manage to think about and deal with death and dying without being swamped by stress.

    Too many people avoid thinking about death and forming their own belief system around it until they're faced with it. It's easier to consider your beliefs and find ones that soothe and comfort you before you're stressed.

2. **Focus on your successes**

    Everyone dies at the end of their physical life. Physicians and healthcare workers focus on delaying that time as much as they are able, consistent with the patients' wishes. There are more successes than failures. Celebrate success. If someone with "a year to live" survives two years that's a huge success.

3. **Re-define success**

    This is closely related to celebrating success but not identical. Find achievable, patient-specific ways of defining success. For one it might be helping the person stay alive long enough to meet a great grandchild. For another it might be keeping them alive long enough for a loved one to fly in to say goodbye. For another it might be recovery and remission. If success always means staying alive you're fighting the inevitable. Dying on one's own terms is achievable. Never dying is not, to my knowledge, an achievable goal. Be optimistic in your goal setting. Go as far as you can go and still feel hope. Remember that sometimes people are simply ready to go. In Native American traditions old people would sometimes simply decide they were ready to go, walk into the woods and sit down, close their eyes and drift away.

4. **Self-compassion and self-care**

   Don't pick up the weight of full responsibility for someone else's death. Do your best to help the person. When you lose a patient recognize the loss and be kind to yourself. Recognize that it is, in many ways, your loss. Reaffirm your goodness and positive self-concept. Celebrate life. Get a massage or relax in a hot tub. Connecting to self-compassion by caring for the body can help you heal secondary trauma. You are human and like all humans, you have value in this world. If you have any remorse or guilt focus your attention by asking what you'll do differently in the future and keep your attention on how you'll improve; not what you didn't do as well as you'd like (if anything) in this situation. If you find yourself struggling with this aspect, see "Re-define Your Best."

5. **Facilitate opportunities to share**

   A detailed look at how medical specialists dealing with death and dying deal with it revealed a need to have a balance between objectivity and connection with their patients. The thirty-three physicians interviewed had developed subjective individual methods of coping but thought sharing perspectives with and learning from colleagues could help them develop a well-rounded approach.[77]

Reported rates of compassion fatigue vary widely in published reports, ranging from 7.3% to 40%.[78]

THE BUSINESS OF MEDICINE

New physicians start their careers stressed about the business of medicine. Over 40% are concerned about their ability to deal with payers (insurance companies, Medicare, Medicaid), 40% are worried about malpractice which puts the emphasis in the wrong place (they should be concerned about doing the best job they can do), nearly 40% are worried about healthcare reform, and 22% are worried about their low level of knowledge about running a practice.[79] The last number would probably be higher if they knew what they don't know.

Physicians are either an employee, often in large health systems where their autonomy is lower, and they may not be able to be as aligned with the reasons they chose medicine in the first place or they are business owners. Medical school does not teach business, over half of first-year residents received no formal training about contracts, hiring, compensation arrangements, or interviewing techniques[80] which can leave physicians feeling overwhelmed by the business requirements of running a practice. 48% of first year residents feel unprepared for the business aspects of medicine and only 9% feel well prepared.[81] It isn't just the business of medicine that is being squeezed by increasing regulations, all of which take time away from the primary mission. Laws relating to hiring and payroll are complex and it is easy to make mistakes because they aren't based on logic. Interviews of 24 physicians indicated most of them found dealing with staffing issues stressful, partially because the practice management training they received was inadequate.[82] Running your business ("Medical practice") requires a functional understanding of much more than your clinical training. When confronted with business problems try not to "go it alone". Use the resources available and allow other experts to help.

Business ownership for a physician comes with the same hurdles all businesses face including access to capital, regulatory requirements, staffing, office space, facilities management, human resource policies, payroll taxes, and more. Most physicians feel unprepared for the business of medicine. In today's environment with the incursion of the Affordable Care Act, and now the ACHA or whatever version makes its way through the legislative process, the business of medicine is even more confusing and complex with ever-increasing regulations that directly affect physician compensation.

Quality of care and patient outcomes are now taken into consideration in compensation formulas which sounds fair and good on the surface, unless you're aware of the tremendous and well-documented research that shows that patients often do not adhere to the instructions they are given about following diet and medication regimes. In fact, lack of patient adherence has a huge impact on overall healthcare spending in the United States. The World Health Organization reported that about 50% of prescribed treatment plans are not followed and indicated that improving treatment compliance could be the best thing we could do to improve health outcomes.[83]

While physicians have some influence over compliance with treatment plans, such as ensuring patients understand the regime and minimizing the complexity to the extent possible, they do not have complete control. The patient has a responsibility to let the physician know if there is confusion and to follow the plan outlined. Giving patients choices about their treatment increases their sense of autonomy and buy-in but it is not always possible to make treatment plans more palatable to patients.

Burnout increases the risk of health problems.[84] I'm not sure why we spend so much money researching the connection between burnout and specific health problems when we already know burnout is an indicator of chronic stress and that stress has a negative impact on those same factors. Do they think changing the categorization of it from chronic stress to burnout will improve outcomes?

Burnout has specifically been associated with poor outcomes or increased risk in the following areas:

- Cardiovascular diseases[85, 86, 87]
- Type 2 diabetes[88]
- Sleep problems[89, 90]
- Musculoskeletal pain
- Impaired fertility
- Mortality
- Alcoholism and drug abuse/addiction
- Higher rates of suicide

If you want to take the leap (baby step) from chronic stress to outcomes, we can add established outcomes from current and/or chronic stress which include, but are not limited to:

Physical Health Outcomes:

- 50% more chance of developing cardiovascular disease compared to individuals experiencing low stress (Positively focused)[91]
- Increased pain

Mental Health Outcomes:
- Depression
- Anxiety

Behavioral Health Outcomes:
- Fewer pro-health behaviors[92]

Career and Academic Outcomes:
- Worse customer service ratings
- Lower levels of success even in advantaged situations
- Inherent competitiveness in achieving success as a provider
- Set lower goals

Relationships (Social Connections):
- Less likely to marry
- More likely to divorce
- Fewer social connections
- More discord in relationships

Non-health Behavioral Outcomes:
- Less ethical
- More likely to short-change the effort to care for patients
- More likely to commit a crime
- Not as kind or compassionate

The outcomes of chronic stress are documented more thoroughly in my earlier books.

PERSONALITY

Personality has to be mentioned because some of the burnout research points to personality factors. While personality can be correlated with burnout, the existing research does not take into consideration the latest research on personality or the trajectory of the most recent personality research.

It was once believed that our personality was just who we are and that we could not change our personality. That, in essence, our personality was who we are. That belief included the belief that personality did not change much across the lifespan. New research reveals that personality does change more than earlier believed.

Personality is more a function of our beliefs than of who we are. It appeared stable because the function of our brain is to support our beliefs and interpret reality as if our beliefs are true.[93] In my work, I teach people how to change their beliefs and have witnessed many personality changes in others and in myself as the result of changed beliefs.

Many people are afraid they will lose themselves if their personality changes. In all the years I've been helping people change their beliefs I have not had one person who did not like themselves better after they changed unsupportive beliefs. When their personality changed, they felt more comfortable as the new person than they ever did before the changes. They commonly remark that they have become who they always wanted to be or they feel they are finally being the outwardly reflecting the person they were on the inside.

Sometimes people in their lives didn't like the changes as much because it was uncomfortable for them but more new people liked them more than new people had liked them in the past. In other words, positive changes to personality increase likability. If your grumpy friend is unhappy that you no longer see the world through the same bitter lens they use, well, they can choose to change their beliefs at any time. You should not have to be miserable just because someone else makes that choice.

In most cases, the people closest to the person recognized the positive changes and wanted to have some for themselves so they became willing to use the same techniques.

Some personality traits (i.e. neuroticism) correlate with increases in the risk of becoming burned out while others correlate with lower stress (i.e. agreeableness). Just remember that your personality is not you and that even if those traits are currently present in your personality, you have the ability to reduce your risk by changing the underlying cause of the personality traits.

INDIVIDUAL PERCEPTION

The tendency to perceive one's situation as highly stressed shows consistency across time (in different work environments). Physicians who perceived their earlier environment as having "a high workload, a less supportive-receptive environment, and less choice-independence" [autonomy] five to twelve years later reported higher stress, burnout and less satisfaction with medicine at the later date.[94]

Physicians who perceived their earlier environments as less stressful perceived their roles as physicians as less stressful.

These differences are logical. When an individual has advanced coping skills stressors do not feel as stressful because they are dealt with and don't create the same cumulative effect as they do when coping skills are not advanced. We often attribute an individual's ability to withstand high levels of stress to personal fortitude and while there may be some of that, the most common difference is the presence or absence of good coping skills.

Researchers concluded ". . .Stress is not a characteristic of jobs but of doctors, different doctors working in the same job being no more similar in their stress and burnout than different doctors in different jobs."[95]

We would separate it by different levels of coping skills, not different doctors.

EMOTION REGULATION: AUTOMATIC AND CONSCIOUS

We've all noticed that the amount of stress we experience in response to events is not the same as the stress others in like circumstances experience. Our level of stress may be higher or lower than other people experience. Our perception of stress is influenced by several significant factors including automatic emotion regulation which is influenced by our:
- ◈ Beliefs ◈
  - Includes self-efficacy beliefs
  - Includes worldview
  - Includes any beliefs that are relevant to the topic
- ◈ Expectations ◈
- ◈ Emotional State ◈
- ◈ Habits of thought ◈
- ◈ Focus ◈

- ◇ Goals and desires ◇
- Conscious emotion regulation
    - Influenced by our:
        - ◇ Awareness of emotion regulation strategies ◇
        - ◇ Level of skill in regulating emotion ◇
        - ◇ Accurate interpretation of the emotion we are feeling ◇
        - ◇ Accurate interpretation of the meaning of the emotion we feel ◇
        - Time available
        - Resources in that moment including:
            - Hunger
            - Thirst
            - Illness
            - Pain
            - ◇ Emotional state (stress level) ◇
            - Sleep/Fatigue
            - Drugs
            - Alcohol

This book will help you achieve mastery over the factors marked with ◇'s.

PART II – EVIDENCE-BASED PROGRESS

Most of the published articles about easing physician burnout blame factors that are beyond the control of physicians who are employees.

> *How stress is processed determines how much stress is felt and how close a person is to burnout. An individual can experience stressors but be unable to process the stress well and thus experience burnout. Another person can experience a significant number of stressors, but process each well, and avoid burnout.* – Gandi, et al., 2011

The focus of this section is to increase the ability of individual physicians to process the stress they experience on a daily basis. "Individuals' personality traits and psychological function are the most important factors in stress management and preventing burnout."[96]

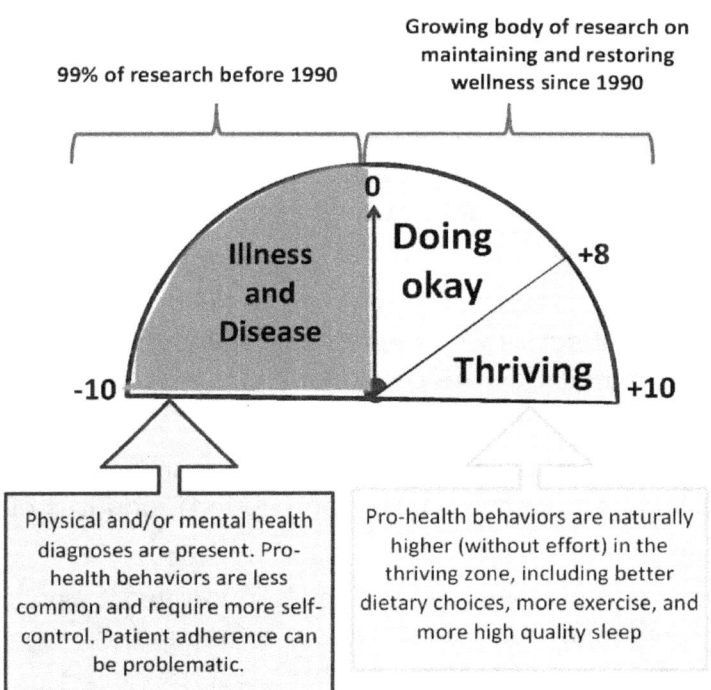

The medical paradigm tends to look at broken things, things that are ill or diseased, and ask "How can we fix this?" You won't cure burnout from that perspective.

You have to look at those who are doing well, those who are not suffering, the physicians who are thriving and ask "What are they doing and can those who are suffering do what they do?"

The answer is yes. Those who are thriving are resilient and they are resilient because of a combination of factors that are all learnable skills. Children can be taught to be resilient. You've made it through medical school. You can learn anything a child can learn, including skills that increase resilience.

What is resilience? Is it the ability to just keep going no matter how much pain (emotional or physical) you're experiencing? Absolutely not. Resilience comes from developing skills that reduce the pain without requiring the situation to change. Resilient people don't experience the same level of stress as non-resilient people do in like circumstances. Since they experience less stress they have less to recover from so they expend fewer resources recovering from adverse experiences.

How are you doing? Are you one of more than 50% of physicians who are experiencing at least one symptom of burnout?

During the past month:

1. Have you felt burned out from your work?

2. Have you worried that your work is hardening you emotionally or felt cynical toward your work or patients?

3. Have you often felt down, depressed, hopeless, or wondered about the point of it all?

4. Have you fallen asleep unexpectedly or when you didn't want to such as when you were driving?

5. Have you felt overwhelmed, as if there is too much to do and that completing all the tasks is impossible?

6. Have you felt anxious, depressed, irritable, or easily angered?

7. Has your physical health declined or have you been ill more frequently?

8. Do you feel your work is important and that it matters?

9. Do you find yourself simply wanting to escape your reality such as by reading a lot of fiction, binge watching shows, surfing the web, alcohol or drugs or other addictive behaviors?

See Appendix X for scoring.

If you would like to check your before-and-after burnout, depression, coping, or anxiety scores, the Appendices provide questionnaires and scoring instructions you can use to self-test. Burnout and depression often develop in tandem.[97]

Stress appears to be caused by circumstances but it actually begins in the mind. The way we process our experience determines the amount of stress we experience. That is good news because it is far easier to change our minds than change the people and circumstances around us.

Your work is valuable. It can be a source of satisfaction to you, security for your family (yes, even in this environment—whether it feels secure depends on your perception), and it is of great value to the larger community.

Medical school did not train you to use your mind in ways that are self-supportive. It's not part of the curriculum. Resilient mindsets feel empowered. Resilience is a function of optimism, healthy self-esteem, and an internal locus of control. All three factors can be increased and when they are, your energy returns. Your relationships are smoother. You sleep better. Your brain works better because your level of stress is lower. Stress focuses our attention on problems instead of solutions. When you lower your level of stress you have cognitive access to solutions that were not perceptible when you were stressed.

How well you feel and how well your life goes begins in your mind. If you believe you can the thoughts you think will reflect that belief. If you think it is too difficult to deal with the stress of medicine, with the uncertainty, with the lower sense of autonomy and the increasing economic pressures you will suffer far more than another physician in the same circumstances who believes he or she is capable of finding solutions to each of those problems.

Our minds are very powerful but we haven't been taught to use them. We've been taught to memorize things but we haven't been taught to program our minds for success and wellbeing. Everyone's mind is programmed. Most of the programming was established by age 10. The good news is that we can re-program our mind at any time by consciously making decisions and using techniques that will change the programming. Life gets much better when you upgrade from the default programming.

We've also all been taught to misinterpret the purpose and meaning of our emotions. Research that is now a decade old and supported by a growing body of journal articles, teaches us that our emotions are far more useful than most people believe; we just have to interpret them accurately. Burnout and even depression can be cured simply by learning the new evidence-based, experience-informed purpose of emotions.

There are ways for you to feel better soon:

- Develop skills that increase your level of resilience
    - Learn and use the new definition of the purpose and use of emotions together with meta-cognitve techniques that reduce your stress.
- Practice self-compassion.
- Since most healthcare providers are self-sacrificing, remember that everything you learn about how to help yourself has the potential to help your patients who are also experiencing stress.

If you are experiencing symptoms of burnout it took a long time for them to develop. The road to recovery is much shorter. As you learn to apply meta-cognitive skills to the way you perceive your life you can begin feeling better right away and become sustainably less stressed in just a few months.

There are many stressors in healthcare, all the traditional ones and new ones created by uncertainty in healthcare laws and regulatory policy, the non-stop demands of recording and reporting your work (e.g., EMR, quality metrics, customer expectations, and demands, etc.), and loss of autonomy as the government, health systems and insurance companies interject their priorities into the practice of medicine (your practice). You can deal with all of these issues and more from an empowered mindset that sets you free to once again enjoy the practice of medicine.

Treat yourself well, not just today, but every day. You deserve it.

Recent government interventions, from the Affordable Care Act to Medicaid program to MACRA (e.g., MIPS, AAPMs, etc.) legislation has encroached on the practice of medicine.

Some physicians have established concierge medicine practices, Direct Pay Clients (DPC), where clients pay a monthly fee regardless of whether or not they need services and the physicians don't contract with insurers which removes some of the headaches and hoops doctors routinely jump through. Some patients don't see the value of such an arrangement and change doctors. I interviewed a woman with a single pre-puberty child whose pediatrician had changed to this model and although she sang the doctor's virtues, she chose to find another pediatrician instead of paying a monthly fee. Obviously many people would be without physicians if they all chose to exit the insurance based payment world and because not everyone is willing to participate, it's not likely all the doctors would have enough patients to sustain themselves.

While researching this book I was pleased to learn that the US Surgeon General agrees with me, "It is critical," he said, "to first understand what causes burnout. And that is not necessarily a large workload."[98] Workloads are one of many factors that contribute to chronic stress but an individual's ability to change the workload without sacrificing other important priorities is negligible.

Telling an employee that the solution is something they know they have no control over increases their sense of powerlessness which adds to their stress and eventual symptoms of burnout. It is healthier to focus on what a person can control. For most physicians, the most controllable factor is their own perception of the situation. Even physicians who are running their own practices can't escape all the legislated rules and regulations designed to legally manage patient care provided by physicians.

At the AMA's Medical Student Advocacy and Region Conference, the US Surgeon General, Dr. Murthy, commented: "It is critical to first understand what causes burnout. And that is not necessarily a large workload. What causes burnout is when people feel a lack of self-efficacy, when they feel like they're working hard and it's not meaning as much as it should, when they feel like they aren't valued in the community they're practicing in. . . Those things will accelerate burnout even with a reasonable workload."[99]

The transformative and advanced coping skills provided in this book are presented to empower you with skills that allow you to regulate your emotions in ways that are beneficial to your physical and mental well-being.

> *It is now widely appreciated that emotion regulation plays a crucial role in healthy adaptation and that difficulties with emotion regulation are associated with psychological and physical health problems.*[100]

Developing resilience and transformative and advanced coping skills reduces the stress load at work and at home. This is important because conflicts between home and work increase stress and eventual burnout.

The following chart, reflecting the result of research with 422 healthcare providers working with fragile NICU patients reveals that the mental habits of the healthcare worker contribute significantly to the outcome (burnout or no burnout). Beneficial mental habits include:

- Self-efficacy, a combination of healthy self-esteem and belief that one is capable and confident
- Adaptive coping (covered later)
- Mindfulness
- Resilience

You'll note that maladaptive coping increases resilience but also increases burnout. This suggests to me that it might be beneficial in some circumstances to use some forms of maladaptive coping initially if you quickly (as soon as possible) turn to more adaptive forms of coping.

For example, yesterday one of my friends unexpectedly passed away and later I learned that my mom's cancer had returned. Not a great day in anyone's book. I used a variety of methods to manage my emotions including distraction and withdrawal (foregoing some planned activities) during the day. At the end of the day, I drank two glasses of wine knowing they would help me sleep. Over the course of a year, I drink about a dozen bottles of wine and rarely drink more than one glass at a time so this maladaptive coping method is rare for me. If I used this method on a daily basis, it would not be healthy. Given the circumstances and the emotional state I was in, it was the best I could do at the time.

After a good night's sleep, I was able to effectively use advanced coping skills to restore my equilibrium. I'm of no use to Mom if I'm upset. For example, about six years ago Mom had a long hospitalization during which I was able to maintain my emotional balance in a relatively good state. While spending time at her bedside I noticed that she had coughing fits after she ate or drank. This wasn't something they had been looking at but after I pointed it out to her doctor and some testing they discovered that a valve that should close when she was eating or drinking to keep food debris out of her lungs wasn't closing all the way. They were able to improve this problem with physical therapy.

A little wine so I could have a good nights' sleep, which is restorative, was adaptive given the circumstances. Alcohol is maladaptive when it becomes habitual or a regular crutch and also when it is drunk in excess. When it is the only coping method an individual has in their tool box, it can easily become habitual.

For individuals in healthcare settings where there are frequent loses of life and secondary trauma is common, a toolbox full of advanced and transformative coping skills is essential to avoid developing symptoms of burnout.

We are not stuck with our initial emotional response or our initial stress level. We have the ability to choose different perspectives that reduce stress and increase emotional state. If you bought a car for college and its reliability in the ensuing years has decreased, you're not stuck with it because it was your first choice. You can make a decision to change it. In the same way, you are not stuck with your initial thoughts and resultant emotions about any situation you are currently experiencing or any situation from your past.

Just as you'll make a better decision about the next vehicle you purchase if you acquire some knowledge of safety features, cost, gas mileage, insurance rates, etc., you'll make better decisions about the perspectives you accept if you understand your choices.

This chart demonstrates that resilience decreases burnout as well as factors that increase resilience. Maladaptive coping can increase resilience but it increases burnout substantially. Think of this in terms of the limited use of wine to facilitate sleep after an especially bad day so that you're better able to apply advanced coping skills the next day vs maladaptive skills being the only ones in the toolbox.

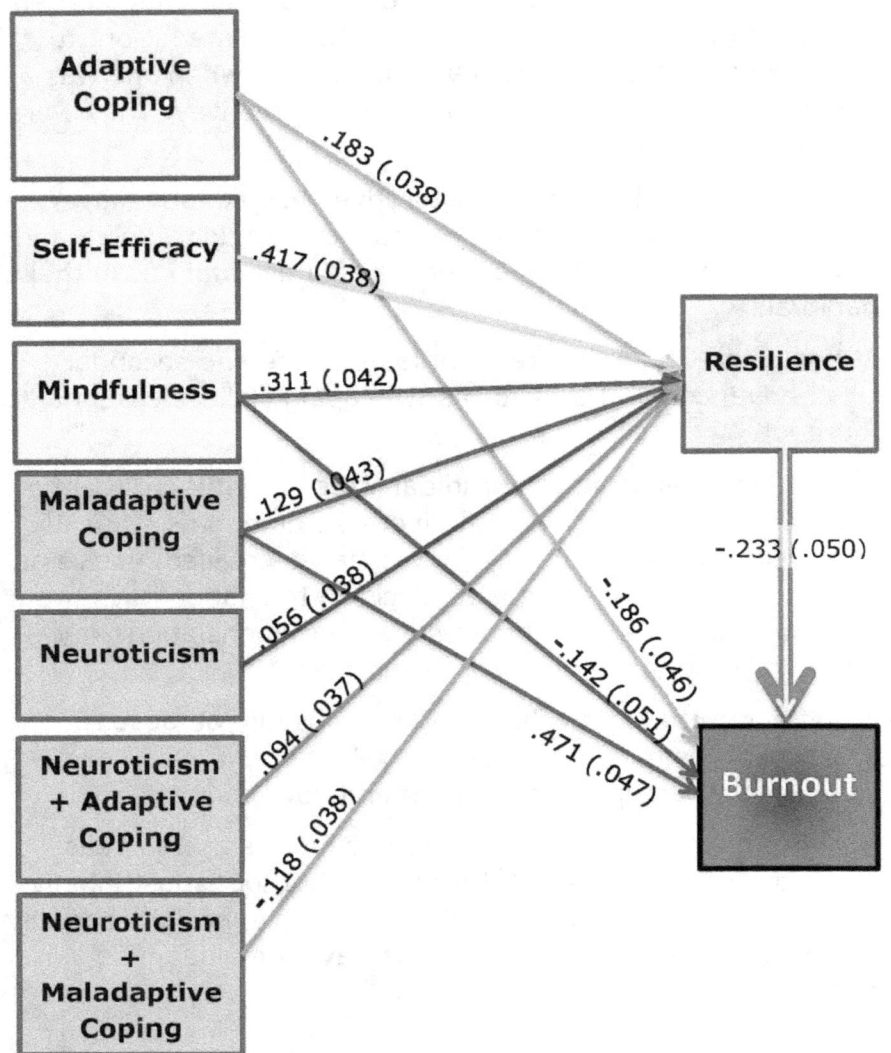

Adapted from: Rees, C. S., Heritage, B., Osseriran-Moisson, R., Chamberlain, D., Cusack, L., Anderson, J., et al. (2016, July 19). *Can We Predict Burnout among Student Nurses? An Exploration of the ICWR-1 Model of Individual Psychological Resilience.* Frontiers in Psychology, 7(1072), 1-11.

As you probably know, neuroticism is one of the Big Five higher-order personality traits. Individuals who score high on neuroticism are more likely than average to be moody and to experience such feelings as anxiety, worry, fear, anger, frustration, envy, jealousy, guilt, depressed mood, and loneliness. Personality is the outcome of the habits of thought we've developed, not an inborn and unavoidable outcome. You will learn how to adjust your habits of thought and how to change any habits of thought you don't find beneficial to you.

Note that neuroticism reduces the benefit of adaptive coping by about 50%. Many of the strategies provided herein will help individuals change their neuroticism levels by giving them greater conscious control over anxiety, worry, fear, anger, frustration, envy, jealousy, guilt, depressed mood, and even loneliness.

Mindfulness is defined as:

1. The quality or state of being conscious or aware of something.

2. A mental state achieved by focusing one's awareness on the present moment, while calmly acknowledging and accepting one's feelings, thoughts, and bodily sensations, used as a therapeutic technique.

The Smart Way™ differs from mindfulness in several important respects that lead to improved outcomes. It meets the definition of the 1st definition above but not the second.

The Smart Way™	Mindfulness
Doesn't restrict thought to the present moment, but consciously chooses (as often as possible) subjects to think about based on how they feel. Leaves room for savoring pleasant or delicious memories. Leaves room for eagerly anticipating future events.	Requires focusing on the present moment.
Applies the most recent research on the purpose and use of emotions to create a framework for a flexible adaptive coping style that improves outcomes, reduces stress, and increases resilience and emotional intelligence.	Acceptance is contraindicated by the new research on the purpose and use of emotions that concludes that emotions are designed to guide our behavior. By simply accepting emotions they cannot serve as the guidance they are designed to be.
Awareness of thoughts and feelings but not just accepting them, the individual using The Smart Way™ consciously thinks about what is being thought about and evaluates how they feel when thinking a specific thought compared to how they prefer to feel and finds perspectives that elicit better-feeling emotions. It is a conscious, adaptive, pro-active approach that understands our thoughts have an emotional response and while we can't directly change our emotions, we can change our perception which will change our emotional response to the thoughts we think.	Requires calmly accepting one's feelings, thoughts, and bodily sensations.

Being mindful is a good thing and acceptance is better than suppression and numerous other maladaptive methods of dealing with emotions. It is not a best practice now that researchers[101, 102, 103, and 104] have discovered that the reason humans can't directly change their emotions is because the purpose of emotions is to guide us toward self-actualization and away from danger. Maslow defined self-actualization as the desire for self-fulfillment and the tendency to become everything that one is capable of becoming.[105] Our definition is slightly different because our potential expands as we grow so we never become fully self-actualized. We can, however, continually move toward self-actualization.

The new definition of emotions indicates their purpose is to provide guidance. It is helpful to think of them as road signs. Thriving feels energized and often involves learning.[106]

When you're driving down the road and you see a Dangerous Curve Ahead sign you don't just accept the presence of dangerous curves. You check your speed and slow down if your speed is too fast for the coming road conditions. You pay more attention. It's not the time you reach for you iPod to change your music selection or call your spouse. When you feel overwhelmed, you don't just accept how you're feeling, you look for solutions. If you're angry about something you will be better off if you check for baggage that may be contributing to your anger that is more about your past than your present situation.

You'll learn more about the new, evidence-based, experience-informed purpose and use of emotions in a later chapter.

An example will help:

The Smart Way™	Mindfulness
A young patient is severely beaten and is paralyzed by his injuries. You initially feel horrified by what was done to him and worried about his future. While recognizing your emotions are normal in this situation you also acknowledge that you'd like to feel better. You begin evaluating your thoughts about this patient. You recognize that medicine has advanced significantly since you began your career and progress helping people with paralysis is significant. You consciously recognize that he is young and his strong body has a better chance than an older person does to recover from the injury. You also consciously recognize that if the paralysis is permanent, the rate of progress being made may allow the young boy to live a far better life than he would have (given the same injuries) just a decade earlier. You feel grateful for all the work done in this field and for the researchers who have made progress possible. You decide to learn more about it if the young boy's body doesn't recover quickly. Your feelings have changed from feeling awful to feeling guarded optimism that one way or another his life is not completely ruined.	A young patient is severely beaten and is paralyzed by his injuries. You feel horrified by what was done to him and worried about his future. You accept these emotions as a normal response to the situation. You don't make evaluative judgments about the emotions as good or bad.
During each of the above steps you paid attention to how your thoughts felt and leaned toward the ones that felt better. As thoughts of his life being ruined forever crossed your mind, you reject the thoughts (not the emotions) because you	

recognize you have access to better-feeling thoughts and know that better-feeling thoughts are better for you and for your patient (because your cognitive abilities will be better).

Another example:

The Smart Way™	Mindfulness
Your co-worker has been calling in sick frequently and you've had to take additional, undesired, shifts to make up for your co-worker's absences. It just happened again and you're emotions are fluctuating between anger and frustration. You begin evaluating how you feel and realize that although you pride yourself on being compassionate you're not feeling very compassionate here—you're departing from the person you want to be.	Your co-worker has been calling in sick frequently and you've had to take additional, undesired, shifts to make up for your co-worker's absences. It just happened again and you're emotions are fluctuating between anger and frustration. You accept your emotions and work the extra shift.
Then you realize that although you've worked with this person for a few years you've never had personal conversations and you don't know the situation. You don't know if there are elderly sick parents, a sick child or if the co-worker is ill. You decide the situation is one you'd probably feel a lot of compassion for if you knew the details of what was going on in your co-workers life and it's really the not knowing more than the absences that led to your initial emotions.	
You consciously decide to give your co-worker the benefit of the doubt and decide that just because you don't know the reason doesn't mean it isn't a good one. You begin feeling like you're helping a co-worker in need by taking the shift rather than one who is taking advantage of you. Your anger dissipates. When the co-worker returns to work you're supportive and welcoming. You let the co-worker know they've been in your thoughts and you hope all is okay with them.	

These examples reveal that the responses to undesired emotions by an individual applying The Smart Way™ are informed by the specific emotional message, consciously applied and preserve or restore more desirable emotional states through "open, approach behavior, adaptive development and social cooperation."[107]

It may sound as if I am saying mindfulness isn't a good practice. That's not my intention. I'm saying mindfulness is not a *best practice*. Mindfulness does a lot of good but it also leaves a lot of potential for thriving unrealized. Before we had access to an accurate understanding of the purpose and use of emotions mindfulness was a best practice.

In the same way that other knowledge is expanded upon and improved, The Smart Way™ replaces mindfulness as a best practice for achieving optimal results. We readily accept new ways of doing things when their benefits are easily quantifiable. The Smart Way™ is best understood through visceral experience. The old commercial, "Try it, you'll like it" comes to mind. An intellectual understanding is minuscule in comparison to an understanding that comes from experience.

> Dial-up > Cable > Wi-Fi >

Knowledge of something new and better does not make the less effective method bad. It simply means it is no longer the best practice. Best practices are superior to other methods because they achieve better results.

> Early Coping Skills > Mindfulness > The Smart Way™ >

For example, one of my earliest clients was a Vietnam veteran with PTSD who used mindfulness. Despite being trained to use mindfulness and being consistent in his practice, he had retired because being around a lot of other people had become too much for him. His life was shrinking. He was under the care of a psychiatrist, receiving counseling, and medicated for his condition but nothing had done much good for him beyond slowing his decline. After teaching him The Smart Way™ his condition began improving. Soon he was becoming more involved in the outside world. He began traveling and his psychiatrist took him off meds because he was doing so well. He was very sensitive to loud noises when we first met and now they don't startle him or create anxiety. The first year I knew him he stayed home on the 4th of July because the potential of fireworks was too much for him. Now he goes to view fireworks on the 4th.

UNDERSTAND HOW YOUR BRAIN PROCESSES DATA

Everyone's brain does not process the same inputs in the same way. The conclusions two individuals given the same data reach may be very different. The main reason for the differences is the way their brain is programmed to process the data.

Our *rational minds* are far from rational. We all have cognitive biases that affect how we view the world. In a 2016 Medscape study, 40% of physicians surveyed admit to being biased with emotional problems topping their list of reasons they felt bias and weight coming in second.[108] This survey did not measure implicit biases.

Most of the programming our brains use to process data was programmed when our age was still in the single digits. Fortunately, we can take conscious control and re-program our brains with programming that helps us achieve our goals and that reduces both implicit and conscious biases.

Although there are well over 180 documented cognitive biases, conscious control of only four filters the brain uses to determine the tiny portion of the big data recorded by our senses to pass on to our conscious mind makes a tremendous difference in the level of stress we experience every day.

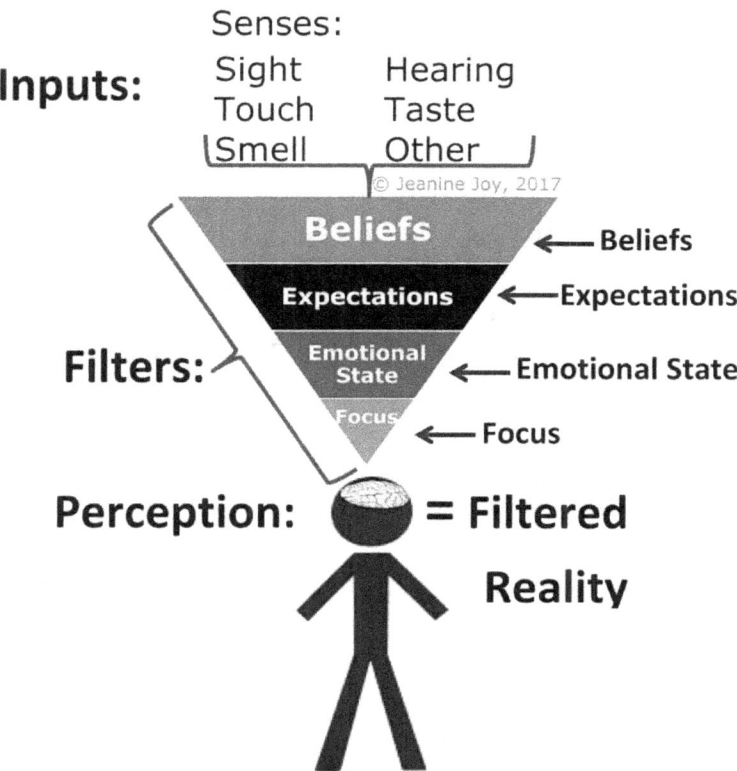

Our brain works to maintain our existing beliefs. Below our conscious awareness the brain makes up *back stories* to explain why things happen the way they do.[109] The *back stories* our brain makes up may or may not be true. *Back stories* are different from lies because they are created by our unconscious mind to help us interpret reality according to our existing beliefs.

For example, the brain of an employee who believes they are excellent at a task that is counseled or corrected about that task will be given a *back story* by his unconscious mind that explains the contradiction between being good and being corrected. The *back story* will strive to maintain the employee's belief about her level of skill. Examples could include:

- The boss is making up things because the boss doesn't like the employee,
- A co-worker sabotaged the employee's work,
- The boss doesn't know what they are talking about,
- The boss is joking.

Remember, the employee doesn't even realize their mind made up a *back story*. To the employee, the *back story* seems like reality. Events are experienced (felt emotionally) as if the *back story* is true.[110] The mind doesn't try to create a story that will serve the

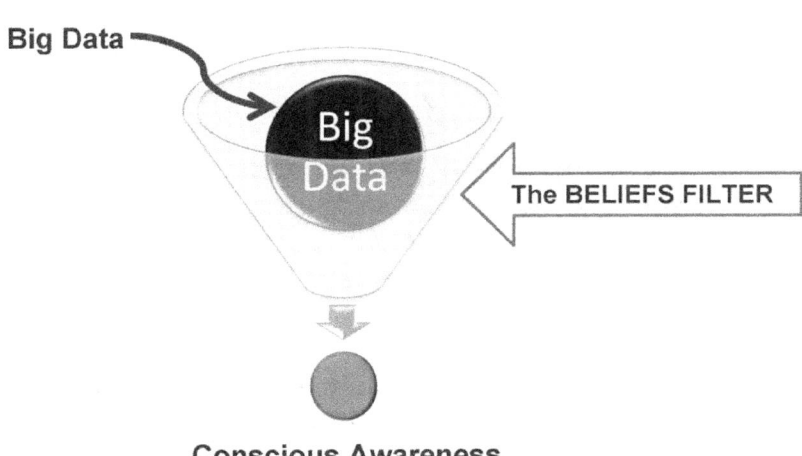

employee's highest good and doesn't lean toward creating stories that feel good over stories that feel bad. The main job of the *back story* is to protect existing beliefs, even if those beliefs are making it more difficult for the employee to achieve desired goals.

An individual who understands their mind makes up stories to protect existing beliefs will be more flexible in reaching conclusions. The person who understands this won't automatically believe every thought he or she thinks and won't defend their thoughts without considering whether they could be wrong because of an inaccurate *back story*.

Fortunately, the new definition of the purpose and use of emotions that you'll learn about later in this section allows us to recognize when our mind is making up back stories that are detrimental to the outcomes we desire.

RATIONAL THOUGHT

Rational thought is an oxymoron. We believe we are rational but if you had a time machine and transplanted most of us back 100-200 years in the past we would be considered insane by the standards used at those times. We create schema's through which we perceive the world. Those schemas are assumptions based on experience and they are often not wholly accurate. Most communication is at a superficial surface level where the distortions are not evident. When deeper communication occurs, differences in schemas become more apparent.

If we believe the world is made up of mostly good people our perception is vastly different from someone else who is convinced the world is made up of mostly bad people who would do horrific things if they weren't forced to be good by laws and law enforcers. Both individuals will be sure their schema is right and that people with other beliefs are wrong. In truth, both are right from the perspectives from which they are viewing the situation. It is the perspectives, not the conclusions, where change is productive.

Before anyone can benefit from advanced and transformational coping strategies they have to realize that there are 1,000 (or more) perspectives about any given situation and the viewpoint we choose determines how empowered or disempowered we feel. It also determines how we feel emotionally.

These statements will make some people want to argue against situational ethics. We don't have to go there. Most cognition isn't about ethical issues. They are more along the lines of the room is too hot, too cold, or just right. They are a matter of perspective. The room may be too cold for me when I am wearing shorts and a tank top but if I put long pants and a sweater on it may be too hot.

Do what feels best to you. If you have absolutes when it comes to right and wrong ethical or moral choices you can retain them while expanding your ability to see multiple perspectives about situations that don't involve ethics or morals.

CONFABULATION

According to Psychpedia, confabulation is:

> *"The memory disturbance might be the creation of a memory that never occurred, the gross distortion of an actual event, or the insistence that something that did happen actually did not occur. Confabulations are heavily influenced by emotion. Most people confabulate sometimes, and mundane examples occur regularly."*

Pay particular attention to the last sentence. As you learn how truly flexible our minds are and their ability to see one situation from a multitude of perspectives you will begin to realize how fluid 'facts' can be.

Researchers found that when students defended a position the student did not support on an emotional topic like immigration or violence, 69% had a higher preference for the choice they did not support a week later.[111]

NEW DEFINITION OF THE PURPOSE AND USE OF EMOTIONS

Historically, emotions were viewed as determinants of the rightness or wrongness of what we perceive and as the beginning of a cascade of biochemical responses in our body that prepare us for fight, flight, or freeze responses situations. However, there is a distinct difference between the fear that makes our hair stand up on the back of our necks and the fear we experience for our children when the nightly news continuously pumps stories designed to scare us into our homes.

Physical, hair standing up on the back of the neck fear indicates we may need to fight, flight, freeze, or take evasive action to avoid a dangerous situation.

The old paradigm about emotions theorized:

> *From an evolutionary perspective, emotions are induced to prepare the organism and to produce responses that will be advantageous to the organism or to its relations. Specifically, emotions are generated when an organism attends to a certain situation that is given a valenced meaning, and this evaluation gives rise to a coordinated set of experiential, behavioral, and physiological responses.*[112]

The new definition of the purpose and use of emotions overturns this viewpoint. The following example demonstrates the difference between the old paradigm and the outcomes it would create and the potential outcomes from the new paradigm.

A friend telephones you upset and afraid because they've been let go from their job. They've been working at the company for six years and a new boss came in who wanted to bring his own people with him. Your friend stood in the way of his desire to hire people he knew and he's been making your friends work life difficult for months.

The Old Way to Use Emotions

You become angry on your friend's behalf. You see how unfair and unjust the situation is and you feel powerless that you can't fix it for your friend. Both of you speak about the unfairness and injustice of the situation, reinforcing your righteous anger. You consider your anger a confirmation that his new boss was wrong in his actions. The worse you feel for your friend, the more wrong his being let go feels to you.

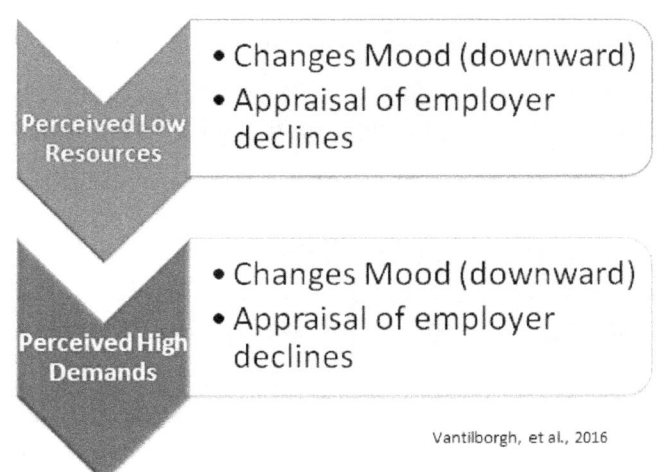

Vantilborgh, et al., 2016

Before your friend called, you were in a pretty good mood but now your day has been ruined. You'll continue stewing about this situation and worrying about your friend for the rest of the day and continue doing the same to a lesser degree tomorrow.

Because communication is interpreted in a mood congruent fashion, when you go to work your trust in your employer is lower even though it is not the same company that fired your friend. Your interpretation of comments managers make is more cynical than it would have been before your friend was fired.

Your friend is struggling to come to terms with the situation and reaches out to you again. The two of you meet for drinks and spend the evening talking about how unfair life is while drinking enough to make driving home illegal. Your conversation focuses on the problem and does not consider viable solutions that you would talk about if your cognitive functions weren't narrowed by negative emotion.

New Way to Use Emotions

At first, feel angry on your friend's behalf. But you have well-developed emotion regulation skills and when you feel anger you immediately begin looking for other perspectives about the situation. You know that anger means that there is a better way for you to perceive the situation.

This particular friend is a dedicated worker who continually upgrades his skills. He is also a very loyal person who tends to remain in a job long after his skills would qualify him for a better job. Remembering this about your friend, you have the thought that the loss of this job may be a blessing in disguise. It's too soon to say this directly to your friend, but you can easily reassure him about the level of his skills and the demand for people with those skills in the job market.

As you reassure your friend you sense that he would now be open to considering potential benefits of his situation. You mention the time you were laid off and got a substantial raise in the new job you quickly found and suggest he could experience the same type of outcome. This perspective is supported by the facts. His salary did not keep up with his increased skills. The market value for his skills is more than he has been making. He begins feeling enthusiastic about finding a new job that matches the skills he developed and making more money.

The next day when you think about your friend you feel hopeful about his prospects in the current job market. You don't focus on who fired him or why because that is not something you can change. All that sort of focus would do is make you feel bad. During the day you hear that a co-worker is moving to follow his wife to a new job and you call your friend to encourage him to apply for the open position. He's been researching the market value for his skills and working on updating his resume. He's pumped because his market value is substantially higher than what he was making at his old job.

It's clear the new way to use emotions does a better job of producing responses that will be advantageous to the organism or to its relations, which was a stated goal of the old way.

To many people, the second example will feel unrealistically optimistic. They will deny that it is possible to feel optimism after losing your job. I have lived that experience personally as a single parent with two children. The first time it happened after I had begun being more deliberate about maintaining positive emotions I wasn't completely stable, I had moments of doubt and concern but for the most part I was able to confidently move forward without losing sleep.

The second time I had to down regulate my expressed emotions during the meeting where our entire company was told that we were closing out of sensitivity to my co-workers. In my mind I was thinking thoughts like, "Every time I am laid off I get a better job making more money without any days of unemployment. I know something good is coming. I wonder what it is?" Outwardly I expressed appreciation to my boss for keeping the company alive during the worst of the downturn in the economy and offered reassurance to co-workers by relaying that I was seeing increased recruiter activity.

I had a few minutes during which I felt unsure as I contemplated two upcoming vacations, one to Australia and New Zealand for nearly a month and another one to Panama and Florida for two weeks. I felt a small voice of doubt about the wisdom of continuing with those plans but when I thought, "I'll find a way to make it all work" the positive emotion I felt reassured me that going forward with my plans was the right path for me to take.

Within thirty hours the parent company of the firm I worked for notified me that they had decided they wanted me to work for them and to be on the Board of Directors. The decision was based somewhat on my skills but mostly on my positive reaction and helpful attitude in letting them know regulatory issues they needed to deal with as the result of closing the subsidiary. If I had been angry it is doubtful I would have shared that information so readily.

You've been trained to respond to emotions using the old paradigm. The shift to the new paradigm can cause uncertainty. I used both methods in the beginning and evaluated which would bring the better result. I encourage you to heed the bard's words and doubt the veracity of the old paradigm but also approach the new paradigm with critical thinking skills.

Modest doubt is called the beacon of the wise.
William Shakespeare

I always tell my classes not to take my word for the information I share. Try the techniques. Feel the difference in your own stress level. If you want to doubt that they work that's fine, but try them anyway. It won't hurt and they've helped thousands of people—many of them significantly. Feeling an unpleasant feeling in your gut along with doubt may be more about unease at learning that something you thought you knew isn't as you thought it to be than about the truth of the new information you're receiving. You can interpret that feeling in multiple ways.

Defending what you previously believed to be true is not the path with the lowest risk. Exploring the new idea with healthy skepticism, trying it out to see how things go, and then making up your own mind once you have personally experienced it is the lower risk choice. This wouldn't be good advice if you were being offered an unknown drug, but you're only being asked to explore alternate viewpoints in the privacy of your own mind.

Recent research overturns the earlier theory about the purpose and use of emotions that stood for nearly a hundred years. The new, validated theory is that our emotions are a sensory feedback system designed to guide our behavior toward self-actualization.[113, 114, 115, 116, 117] Self-actualization is fulfilling our best potential. It should be noted that we never become fully self-actualized because as our skills and knowledge increase, our potential also increases.

We can't decide how we want to feel and feel that way just because we want to but it can be almost that easy. We have to think thoughts that elicit the emotions we want to experience. The reason we cannot directly change our emotions is because emotions would lose their ability to guide us if we could change them at will. Our emotions are a response to our thoughts which we can change. Learning how to change our thoughts is the key to attaining and sustaining positive emotions more frequently. Positive emotion indicates you are experiencing low stress levels.

Our sense of sight, touch, taste, smell, and hearing are all sensory feedback systems. Researchers believe that our emotional guidance feedback system is the earliest sensory feedback system every organism develops.[118] Even one-celled amoebas have a sensory feedback system. The difference between the one-celled amoeba and humans is that the amoeba always heeds the guidance it receives. Humans often override their guidance with irrational thought because they believe their brains are rational.

The new definition of the purpose and use of emotion states:

1. The purpose of positive emotion is to guide us toward *self-actualization*.[b]

2. The most productive response to negative emotion in modern life is a Right Response (RR), which is:

   "...to affect the internal environment in the personal mindscape, in conscious knowledge acquisition, in an act of deliberate learning and personal mental tactic to invoke optimal belief structures to reappraise."[119]

   In other words, reach for a different perspective about the situation, one that feels better, and adopt that perspective as your own because it serves your highest good to do so. In the paper where Katherine Peil coined the phrase, Right Response (RR), she elaborates and clarifies the difference between a RR and suppressing emotions,

   "There is a vast difference between a RR and suppressive emotion regulation, as the corrective action itself is informed by the specific emotional message, is consciously undertaken and it self-preserves through open, approach behavior, adaptive development and social cooperation. In short, the RR is a self-developmental response more indicative of the neurally well-endowed, culturally creative human being."[120]

In the example above where the friend was fired, looking for and finding a potential silver lining (blessing in disguise) is a Right Response.

Katherine Peil and I first met when we were both presenting at a Health Promotion conference in 2012. I presented in the morning and was shocked when she began her presentation by stating that I'd made it easier for her because my presentation had taught them how to use the Emotional Guidance she was going to tell us about. It was a beautiful synchronicity in the purest sense of Carl Jung's meaning.[c] Our work fit together perfectly.

Emotions as guidance toward self-actualization is supported by a growing body of modern science, ancient wisdom, and the texts of six major religions.

Emotional Guidance is simple to understand. Children tend to master it faster than adults because we were actually born using it. Modern society trains us to ignore it in favor of our irrational minds and the preferences of others.

One of the first arguments people make against following emotional guidance is that it seems selfish to do what feels best to us regardless of what others want. It definitely sounds selfish but when you dig deeper you find that people selfishly want a lot of things that counteract that objection including:

- We want good relationships with others,

---

[b] Self-actualization is the realization or fulfillment of one's talents and potentialities, considered a drive or need present in everyone.
[c] Synchronicity is a concept, first explained by analytical psychologist Carl Jung, which holds that events are "meaningful coincidences" if they occur with no causal relationship yet seem to be meaningfully related. (Wiki)

- If we're happy, we want others around us to be happy and we're far more likely to be happy if we follow our emotional guidance,
- We enjoy doing nice things for other people, even strangers, when we feel good, and
- When we feel good we are far more likely to behave in socially acceptable ways.

Our Emotional Guidance considers everything we want and is excellent for finding paths that allow us to maintain great relationships without having to give up things that are important to us. Our guidance also tells us that it is not our job to attempt to control others' behaviors so we stop trying to make others behave the way we want them to so that we will be happy. We choose to be happy even when those around us do not do what we would prefer they do.

The way emotional guidance works bears a strong resemblance to the children's game where an object is hidden and the child is given clues such as *You're getting warmer* or *hot* or *You're getting colder* or *cold* to help the child find the hidden object. Katherine Peil and I both used the children's game to illustrate how emotional guidance works in our presentations the day we met. Positive emotions mean you're moving toward self-actualization and negative emotions mean you're moving in opposition to self-actualization.

Once the purpose and use of emotions is understood the value of developing skill at identifying alternate perspectives about situations that don't feel good becomes self-evident. Eventually, individuals can train their minds so that their initial, automatic thoughts about situations are less stressful than they were in the past because the first thought they think is more supportive of self-actualization. The cumulative effect of less stress throughout the day becomes significant to health, relationships, and quality of life. The sections on aligning with your purpose, reprograming unhealthy habits of thought, and developing healthy habits of thought all describe methods of finding more positive perspectives.

Studies about increasing resilience and social and emotional learning skills often mention that the increased skills require boosters to be maintained. When emotions are understood as providing guidance, they provide guidance in response to every thought we think which works as a natural booster that maintains the gains made.

> EMOTIONAL GUIDANCE IS AN INNATE BOOSTER SYSTEM THAT SUSTAINS INCREASES IN RESILIENCE AND SUPPORTS ONGOING INCREASES IN RESILIENCE ONCE EMOTIONAL GUIDANCE IS UNDERSTOOD.

When something happens, an unconscious appraisal of the situation, person, or event occurs that leads to a conscious thought about the situation. The conscious thought we experience is based on an appraisal of the situation that can vary significantly from person to person and even in the same person depending on the individual's current emotional state.

Factors that go into the unconscious appraisal include our beliefs about our locus of control, self-efficacy, value and worth (deservedness), the future (positive or negative), and our current emotional state. The unconscious appraisal is only one of many potential perspectives a person could take about the situation. Multiple people experiencing the same circumstances will not all arrive at the same unconscious appraisal of the situation. Our beliefs lead directly to our automatic thoughts[121] and directly affect the way we appraise every situation.

The appraisal of the situation compared with our self-actualized self then determines our emotional response. For example, someone who wants to go to college to become a teacher would feel ecstatic to be accepted to a college that will give her reduced tuition because of her chosen profession. Someone else, who only applied to college to please her parents will not be ecstatic to be accepted.

Our responses differ because we appraise the situation differently[122] and because our goals are unique.

We do not have to accept the unconscious appraisal as the only possible appraisal. Most situations have many ways to accurately perceive them. Emotional Guidance helps us identify appraisals that serve our highest good.

EMOTIONAL GUIDANCE SCALE

This scale is a continuation of/expanded version of several scales used by earlier writers.[123] The zones are my addition and separate emotions by the level of empowerment/disempowerment individuals experiencing those emotions feel. The Sweet Zone feels the most empowered. The sense of empowerment decreases in each level until the Powerless Zone where people feel disempowered.

Sweet Zone	Hopeful Zone	Blah Zone	Drama Zone ↓↑↓↑↓	Give Away Zone	Red (Hot) Zone	Powerless Zone
Joy	Hope	Contentment	Ornery	Blame	Anger	Hatred
Appreciation	Gratitude	Boredom	Irritation	Resentful	Revenge	Powerless
Enthusiasm	Upbeat	Pessimism	Frustration	Doubt	Rage	Jealous
Happiness		Apathy	Impatience	Guilt	Provoked	Grief
Optimism		Uninspired	Impatient	Worry	Outraged	Fear
Belief			Disappointment	Discouraged	Furious	Despair
Freedom			Overwhelmed			Hopeless
Eager						Lethargic
Love						Depressed

The scale shown above is abbreviated. It does not attempt to show all possible emotions in the scale. Any emotion you feel can be accurately placed into the correct zone by paying attention to how empowered or disempowered you feel when you feel the emotion.

This next chart shows the relationship between engagement and burnout as it relates to the Emotional Guidance Scale. The Zone refers to the chronic emotion the employee feels in relationship to work. It doesn't mean the employee does not experience other emotional states. It means the predominant emotions they feel are in the Zone(s) indicated for their level of engagement.

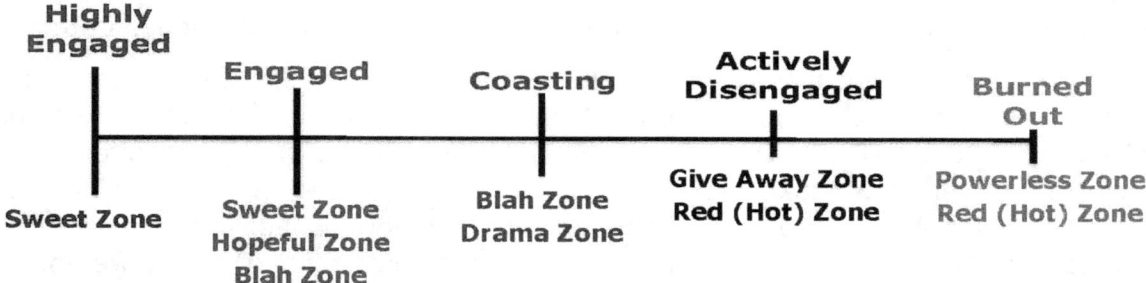

For example, an engaged employee may enjoy aspects of the job enough to spend part of the day in the Sweet Zone but finds parts of the job boring and experiences the Blah Zone when performing those tasks.

The following illustration demonstrates how emotional state and stress level are related to our perceptions and focus. There are three places/times we can focus on:

- Where we are
- Where we want to be
- Where we don't want to be

There are three important aspects of our relationship with where we want to be and where we don't want to be:

- How far we perceive ourselves to be (near or far)
- Our perception of the possibility of achieving the desired or undesired state (achievable vs. not achievable)
- The speed at which we believe we will arrive at the desired or undesired state and how long we think it should take

For example, at the beginning of medical school, a student who believes he or she will graduate will feel positive emotion even though graduation is a lot of work and years in the future. In this example, the student perceives the possibility of achieving the desired state as achievable and believes it will take a reasonable amount of time.

A similarly situated student who fears he or she will flunk out of medical school will feel negative emotion. This student is focused on where he or she doesn't want to go instead of the desired destination. Instead of working towards what is desired the student's focus is to fight against failure. This student will experience a higher level of stress which reduces cognitive capabilities and increases the likelihood of failure.

Use the diagram to help you identify how you are perceiving situations and events that are of concern to you.

Potential examples could include:

- A malpractice suit
- Malpractice insurance increases
- Patient outcomes
- Leisure time available to you
- Insurance company dictates about patient care and treatment
- Regulations that adversely impact your income
- Ability to keep up with new procedures and medications

What is your pattern? Do you tend to focus on what you want or what you don't want? Deliberately shift your focus between what you want and what you don't want and feel the emotional difference that occurs. Do you doubt yourself or your skills? Do you accept responsibility for outcomes that you cannot control? Do you worry about things you cannot control?

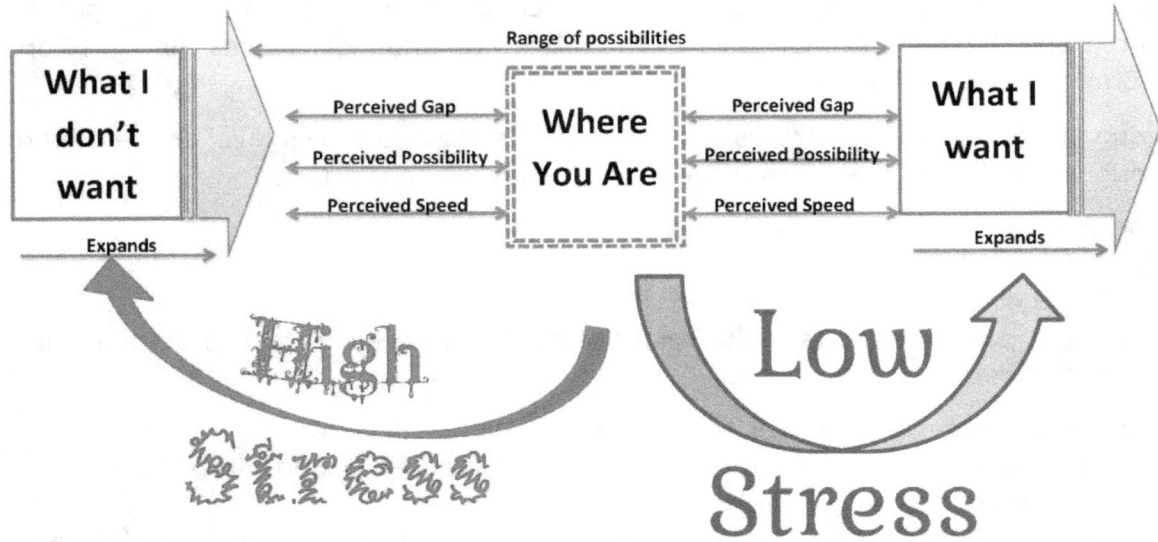

As we move through time the three categories of what is desired, not desired, and where we are change. As we accomplish more, our desired accomplishments increase. Things that were once wanted can become unwanted things. My first apartment is a perfect example. I was thrilled to move into that small apartment with no dishwasher and a wonky air conditioner when I was 18 years-old. I would be decidedly unhappy to find myself back there today when my desired home has shifted dramatically.

This diagram makes it easy to see that we can be in the same situation and depending on what we are focused upon and our perceptions, feel very different levels of stress. Learning to change our perspectives to ones that are less stressful provides many advantages. A diagram in Appendix XVII illustrates many of the benefits of lower stress and improved emotional states.

COPING VS THRIVING

There is a difference between coping and thriving. The coping style used affects burnout.[124] "A person will be psychologically vulnerable to a particular situation if he or she does not possess sufficient coping resources to handle it adequately and places considerable importance on the threat implicit in the consequences of this inadequate handling."[125] For example, my husband is watching a golf tournament at TPC Sawgrass and commented that the 17th hole would be stressful. It has a small green on the opposite side of a pond. I looked up at the situation and said, "It wouldn't be stressful to me because I would have no expectation of getting the ball where it needed to go and I wouldn't care that I couldn't do it." My husband, on the other hand, would care about getting the ball on the green so he would appraise the situation as stressful if his golf skills were as nonexistent as my own.

Attempting to handle stressors without advanced coping skills resembles walking along a gravel road barefoot. We step gingerly and often become bruised. We can't travel fast or far. We have to focus on ourself in order to ensure our own wellbeing but even with focused effort we can't avoid bumps and bruises from the rough ground.

Thriving is walking along the same gravel road in sturdy, light-weight hiking boots. We feel confident traveling as fast as we want to go and can travel significant distances without injury. We can enjoy the journey and view because we don't have to pay as much attention to every step we take.

"Proactive approaches to managing health and aging can be taught, with sustained gains in both proactive competence and health outcomes."[126] There are five broad categories of coping.

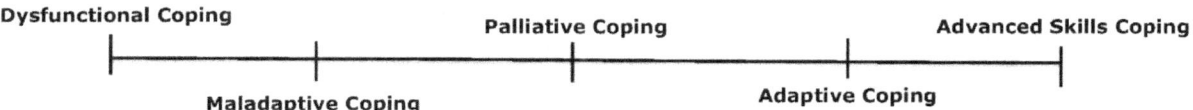

Palliative Coping functions primarily by distracting you from the source of stress. Some forms, such as exercise, can positively change the biochemistry of your body which provides additional assistance. The most commonly recommended strategies are Palliative Coping strategies. There are two detriments to Palliative Coping methods:

1. Palliative Coping methods are dose-dependent meaning that, like a headache pill, they have to be applied each time in order to be effective. A headache pill you took last week isn't going to help you with the headache you developed this afternoon. Also, research has shown that even people who use palliative coping strategies such as exercise don't exercise when they feel "too stressed" even though they know it would help.[127]
2. Palliative Coping doesn't change the underlying cause of stress. In most cases, it distracts you from it.

A third potential downside exists and that is that dysfunctional or maladaptive coping styles will be combined with palliative coping strategies. For example, adult coloring is currently a popular form of palliative coping. On its own, adult coloring is a distraction. If the person coloring simultaneously ruminates about the source of stress it can be maladaptive. If the person coloring drinks a bottle of wine while coloring it can be dysfunctional. If the person coloring applies advanced coping skills such as meta-cognitive strategies while coloring it can be very helpful. If the person coloring applies problem-solving strategies, it would be adaptive coping.

There are millions of sources for palliative coping techniques but almost none of them provide any information about how to avoid maladaptive and dysfunctional combinations or how to increase adaptive or advanced coping skills. Your emotional guidance will let you know what you are accomplishing with the coping techniques you employ.

Dose-dependent strategies are useful but they are not a solution and they do not change the initial hit someone experiences from stress.

Dose-dependent stress reduction methods are ways to cope with stress but they are like driving over a spike strip in your driveway every morning, changing your tire, and going on with your day but leaving the spike strip in your driveway. Permanent stress reduction methods remove the spike

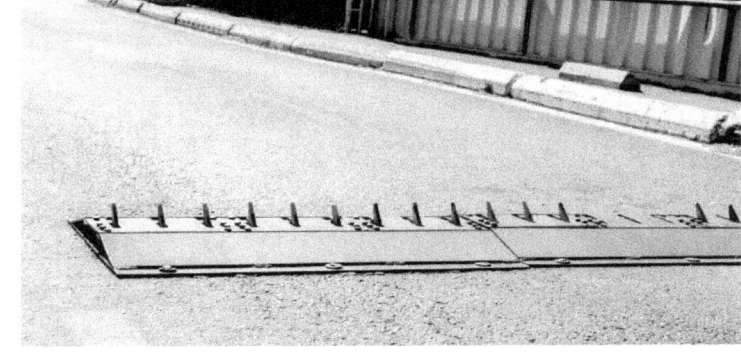

strip.

The Smart Way™ was designed to reduce the stress an individual experiences from the very beginning of a potentially stressful situation and assist in returning quickly to the pre-stress emotional state.

Most people attempt to manage stress with the same strategies over and over again. Developing competence with coping skills is suggested as a way to prevent burnout.[128] Some use a variety while others use just one or two main styles. The style used is generally the one(s) that have the least risk and the best effect of the strategies the individual knows how to use. When new strategies are learned they have to be practiced enough that they will come to mind when they are needed instead of reverting to old, default responses.

This is easier than it seems because practicing feels good. There is no pain during this gain. Well, unless you beat yourself up for not having known what you're learning now sooner. Don't do that. It's far better to simply appreciate that you know now. Self-flagellation is an unhealthy habit of thought.

Maladaptive coping is associated with higher burnout.[129] Many detrimental outcomes associated with dysfunctional coping are well-known.

Dysfunctional Coping	**Maladaptive Coping**
Makes matters worse	*Increases stress, allows problem to fester*
Use alcohol or drugs to suppress emotions, self-harm, violence	Unsuccessful attempts to decrease stress without attempting to solve the problem that is creating the stress.
Self-mutilation	Denial
Ignoring or storing hurt feelings	Wishful Thinking
Sedatives	Displaying anger
Stimulants	Withdrawal[130]
Acting out	Workaholic behaviors
Projection	Humor (depends on how it is used)
Suicide	Passive communication (makes it easy for others to ignore your thoughts and feelings)
Violence	Dissociation (dysfunctional when extreme)
Retribution	Compartmentalization
Smoking	Suppress or ignore emotions
Drugs	Cynicism
Alcohol	Eating
	Self-criticism
	Whining

In a study of 558 teachers, individuals using palliative coping styles had higher levels of burnout.[131] Adaptive coping is associated with lower burnout.[132]

I would use "religious practice" to describe the level of commitment to Yoga, Meditation, or Tai Chi required to move it from Palliative to Adaptive but that could lead to confusion about whether I am referring to commitment or perceiving the practices as religious in nature. All three practices may be perceived as religious, or not religious, depending on the perception of the perceiver. Both ways can be categorized as Palliative or Adaptive depending on the frequency and consistency of practice.

Palliative Coping	**Adaptive Coping**
Decreases anxiety but does not solve the problem	*Changes situation*

Palliative Coping	Adaptive Coping
Visualization	Problem-solving
Deep breathing	Assertiveness
Relaxation training	Positive self-talk
Adopting healthy lifestyle	Self-acceptance
Reducing competing activities and commitments	Stress management
Social connections (talking)	Anger Management
Exercise	Increasing skills
Going outside	Conflict resolution
Helping others	Time management
Adult coloring	Goal Setting
Meditation/Mindfulness (not rigorous practice)	Asking for help
Yoga (not rigorous practice)	Social Connections (Asking for help)
Tai Chi (not rigorous practice)	Social and emotional learning skills
Laughter Yoga	Community living skills
Humor	Meditation/Mindfulness (rigorous practice)
Watching television	Yoga (rigorous practice)
Surfing the internet	Tai Chi (rigorous practice)
Music	Plan to avoid temptations
Golfing	
Massage	
Sleeping	
Petting a pet	
Bubble baths	

Journaling is not listed because the category it falls into depends on what is written and thoughts a person thinks about while journaling. If the writing is complaining or documenting ways you were wronged, it is maladaptive. If it is plotting revenge, it is dysfunctional. If it is brainstorming for solutions it is adaptive. If it is writing about things that feel good and creating neuropathways of appreciation it can be transformative.

An example of Adaptive Coping skills is when a young physician observed an older physician's practice and commented, "When I went there. . . I saw how he took these big, long lunches and he'd go to the gym. I thought, gee that's a good idea, because I used to always go after work. You're tired after work and you don't want to go. All of a sudden you sort of fall out of routine. It's a great idea to keep me going to the gym because it's that time set during the day and I can, and you're not having any responsibilities to see anybody (like) your family at that time of the day."[133]

Advanced and Transformative Coping Skills

1. *Belief change to improve automatic emotion regulation*
2. *Proactive advance mitigation of potential stressors, and*
3. *Quick, proactive reduction of experienced stressors*
4. *Change Perspective*

Meta-cognition

Critical Thinking Skills

Emotional Guidance

Change of perspective

Use "the pause" before reacting

Apply knowledge of factors that influence behavior (available resources)

Develop healthy habits of thought

Develop and apply mental strength and resilience

Psychological Flexibility

Psychological Capital (PsyCap)

Growth Mindset

Pay attention to early signs in order to be proactive

Re-program negative habits of thought

Give others the benefit of the doubt

Learn realistic optimism

Self-supporting thoughts

Internal Locus of Control

Once someone has learned advanced and transformative coping skills they will use them if they are being aware of what they are doing. If they are following habitual habits of thought they may temporarily resort to established habits. Awareness that they have new and better skills will return and when it does they will switch their tactics. It takes time to develop new neuropathways to make new skills the default strategy. It can be helpful to keep visible reminders that help you remember. Positive quotes are one way to do this. When I was developing new skills I ordered notepads and mouse pads with positive quotes and I even made a few t-shirts. In time, the new methods became a part of who I am and I no longer felt the need for frequent reminders that there were better ways to deal with stress.

Developing the habit of asking yourself, "What is the best way for me to deal with this stressor?" can help you be conscious of your choice of coping style.

Emotional guidance should not be confused with emotion-based coping or emotion-focused coping as described by Lazarus and Folkman in the 1980's. Their emotional coping methods contained a combination of coping styles that are included in the dysfunctional, maladaptive, and palliative charts. Only one of the elements of their emotion-based coping fits into the advanced chart. The names may be similar, but the concepts and processes are not similar.[134]

META-COGNITION

Meta-cognition is thinking about what you're thinking and why you're thinking what you're thinking. Humans think an average of 60,000 thoughts a day. Obviously, every thought we think is not thoughtful. Most of our thoughts are the result of habits of thought we developed many years ago. We don't have to attempt to think about every thought we think. If the thoughts feel good when we think them they are serving us. The positive emotion is letting us know those thoughts are leading toward self-actualization. Negative thoughts can be manipulated using a combination of techniques and Emotional Guidance to find perspectives that will serve us better.

For example, if a new required task affects your job responsibilities an initial thought may resent being forced to do something someone else decided you should do. Through the use of meta-cognition combined with Emotional Guidance you could manipulate this disempowering (bad-feeling) thought to a completely different stance.

When they first began requiring me to report data every time I encountered a patient who was struggling with Opioid addiction, I resented it. It felt invasive of my patients' privacy and pointless. Now I know that the data collected has focused national attention on the problem and that resources that would not have been made available to help people with Opioid addiction are now reaching those who need them the most because of that data. I am glad I live in an era where we have the ability to gather data that leads to real changes in the way we do things and to better outcomes for patients.

This perspective in this example moved from resentment to appreciation. The shift is not something you would expect to be able to do in one step. It is best to shift one level of empowerment at a time. (Remember, each Zone on the EGSc is separated by how empowered emotions in that Zone feel.) Once someone has become adept at changing their perspectives and developed a tendency to lean toward the positive they will notice two changes:

1. Their initial assessment of situations will be more positive than it would have been in the past, and
2. They are able to move to more empowered emotional states faster.

When it comes to #2, it becomes possible to be a few minutes into a situation that would have previously been a significant stressor that led to months of feeling low (such as being laid off or the end of an important relationship) and find positive perspectives (i.e. silver linings or new knowledge/insights) that eliminate the stress of the situation. This is not suppression. It is, as Peil stated, "conscious knowledge acquisition, in an act of deliberate learning and personal mental tactic to invoke optimal belief structures."[135]

One person may look at a situation and see a problem while another sees the same situation as an opportunity to be of benefit. By choosing positive perspectives Using meta-cognition where we think about why we are thinking the way we are thinking about the subject we're thinking about and choose the thought (consciously) that feels the best to us instead of going with our first thought about the subject we can feel better. Our first thoughts are often suboptimal, especially if we haven't deliberately cultivated beliefs that lead to self-supporting automatic thoughts.

The thoughts we think are influenced by the mood we are in when we think them. If we're in positive mood we are more likely to appraise something in our environment as positive. If we're frustrated we are more likely to appraise something in our environment as frustrating. In other words, our cognitions are related to our mood (mood congruent).[136] Our mind appears to interpret our environment in ways that support the continuation of our emotional state. It makes sense to deliberately cultivate the emotional state we want to experience.

If your initial thoughts are to reject positive thinking you'll want to keep reading. Later, a significant amount of scientific support for realistic optimism will be provided. The following chart provides an overview of employee behaviors related to the emotional Zone an employee is experiencing.

Emotional State

Emotional Guidance Scale (EGSc)

Sweet Zone
Joy	Appreciation	Wonder
Appreciation	Love	Awe
Passion	Enthusiasm	Eagerness
Happy	Flow	Belief
Inspired	Trust	Faith
Optimistic	Serene	Satisfied
Fulfilled	Secure	At ease

Hopeful Zone
Hopefulness   Gratitude

Blah Zone
Contentment	Boredom	Pessimism
Apathy	Dispirited	Empty

Drama Zone
Frustration	Irritation	Impatience
Overwhelmed	Disappointment	Indignant

Give Away Zone
Doubt	Worry	Blame
Guilt	Discouragement	Offended

Hot (Red) Zone
Anger	Revenge	Rage
Outraged	Provoked	Furious

Powerless Zone
Hatred	Bullied	Jealousy
Insecurity	Depression	Unworthiness
Learned Helplessness	Fear	Despair
Powerless	Grief	Guarded
Hopeless	Melancholy	Unwanted
Suicidal	Unimportant	Exploited

Engagement and Behavior

Empowered
- More time 'In Flow'
- Higher productivity
- Higher employee engagement & alignment with corporate mission
- Associated with better corporate citizenship
- Associated with better customer service
- Associated with pro-health behaviors and pro-social behaviors
- Associated with resilience (optimism, internal locus of control, healthy self-esteem)
- Associated with better relationships, less discord at work & fewer divorces
- Associated with problem-solving
- Rarely associated with crime; Low association with alcohol and drug abuse
- Increased cognitive abilities

Disempowered
Associated with decreasing engagement and other undesirable outcomes
- Higher levels of dissatisfaction with job and organization, lower engagement
- Increasing intrusion of non-work problems into work time
- Increasing discord with co-workers and managers; lower pro-social behaviors
- Lower Core Self-evaluations
- Potential for alcohol and drug abuse increases
- Less regard for established rules and procedures
- Less likely to accept responsibility for errors and missed goals
- Crimes of opportunity become more likely
- Crimes of retaliation for perceived wrongs
- Increasing crimes due to financial needs and fear
- Increasing depression, anxiety, risk of suicide
- Increasing absenteeism
- Increasing turnover
- Increasingly poor health and chronic illnesses; fewer pro-health behaviors
- As emotional state declines, clarity of thinking declines
- The phrase *Going Postal* is usually the result of someone who has been in the Powerless Zone for a long time and it's a last ditch effort to regain a sense of power

META-COGNITIVE PROCESSES

The first step in using meta-cognitve processes is knowing which thoughts to think about. Thoughts that are stressful can be changed to less stressful thoughts. That's the target for most of your meta-cognitve work. Remember, thinking a thought does not make it right or good. Thinking a thought that isn't right or good doesn't make you bad. We're designed to consider many thoughts on a subject.

When your emotional guidance helps you identify a thought that is stressful, ask yourself questions about the thought.

Is this thought true?

Is it only true for me or is it true for everyone?

How do other people look at this situation?

Have people been in this situation and found silver linings?

Have people been in this situation and later been grateful for the experience?

Am I being specific? If yes, can I think more generally about this subject?

Do I have to solve this today?

Is this subject important?

What is the silver lining?

Are there opportunities hidden within this problem?

Have I successfully handled similar issues in the past?

What skills do I have available that will help me deal with this?

Am I comparing my bloopers to someone else's highlight reel?

What were my resources when I did something I now regret?

What resources can I draw upon?

Am I giving myself enough credit for my ability to handle this situation?

What thoughts feel better than the thought I'm thinking?

As you explore the answers you receive to these questions, pay attention to how they feel. When an answer brings a sense of relief stay with it and decide if you can adopt the perspective it represents about the situation. You may benefit from writing the new perspective down.

Keep your focus on how things feel rather than what you believe is true. As long as you remain aware of the difference between fantasy and reality there are situations where fantasizing about doing things you wouldn't, or couldn't, actually do will relieve stress.

One nursing manager whose boss wanted her to quit because he wanted to bring in his own person imagined her boss's bald head was the golf ball she was hitting. It led to the best game of golf she ever played but more importantly, from then on she was able to relieve some of the stress she experienced at his underhanded maneuverings by imaging his head as a golf ball. She would have never hit his head with a golf club, but the thought of doing so felt more empowered than being at the whims of his game playing.

If you choose to use a technique similar to this to reduce stress, make sure it is one where you cannot follow through.

Your emotional response to a thought lets you know if your thought is moving you toward (or away from) the accomplishment of what you want to achieve. When you use a long-term perspective, thoughts that feel good indicate they are helping you and thoughts that feel bad indicate they are hindering you. With advanced coping skills you can navigate between the emotional Zones as easily as you can drive a car or ride a bicycle. It just takes a little practice.

HIGH-LEVEL FACTORS THAT CONTRIBUTE TO POSITIVE OUTCOMES

High-level factors is a name for groups of lower level factors. For example, the high level factor "resilience" consists of three lower level factors: Optimism, healthy self-esteem, and an internal locus of control. At first glance, it seems like all the high-level factors recommended to support positive outcomes (physical, mental behavioral health, good relationships and success in academia and career) are nearly impossible to attain. There are just so many different ones and they continually seem to be coming up with new ones.

Fortunately, it isn't that complicated. The following chart reflects the overlap between the most commonly recommended high-level factors.

High-Level Factor	Lower Level Factors								
High Core Self-Evaluations	Internal Locus of Control	Healthy Self-esteem	Self-efficacy				Emotional stability		
Resilience	Internal Locus of Control	Healthy Self-esteem				Optimism			Self-Compassion[1]
Psychological Capital (PsyCap)	Internal Locus of Control	Healthy Self-esteem	Self-efficacy	Resilience	Hope	Optimism			
Growth Mindset	Internal Locus of Control								
Happiness	Internal Locus of Control	Healthy Self-esteem			Hope or better	Optimism		Metacognitive Skills	Self-Awareness
Psychological Flexibility	Internal Locus of Control							Metacognitive Skills	
Burnout Prevention	Internal Locus of Control	Healthy Self-esteem	Self-efficacy	Resilience		Optimism		Self-Awareness	Self-Compassion
Salutogenesis Health Promotion Physical and Mental	Internal Locus of Control	Healthy Self-esteem		Resilience				Metacognitive Skills	Self-Awareness

---

[1] Self-Compassion is not traditionally included in the definition of resilience but when I was researching burnout prevention I saw research alluding to its inclusion. It makes sense. I'm going to explore this relationship further. (JJ-5/.

When we look at the lower level factors that make up the higher level factor, it becomes clear that an internal locus of control is a critical success factor. Healthy self-esteem and optimism are also important success factors. Resilience is more important than it looks because resilience is:

Internal Locus of Control + Healthy Self-esteem + Optimism = Resilience

I'm not sure why the creators of PsyCap included resilience in PsyCap since it was already covered by the three lower level factors that create resilience.[137] When I developed the lower level factors for Happiness I didn't include resilience because it is included in the lower level factors. Happiness has three additional low level factors which are detailed in a more complex high-level factor chart (page 120). I don't include emotional stability in Happiness because emotional stability is not the goal. My definition of True Happiness is:

> *"The state of True Happiness does not require a constant state of bliss. It is a deep sense of inner stability, peace, well-being, and vitality that is consistent and sustainable. Awareness that one possesses the knowledge and skills to return to a happy state, even when not in that state, is a critical component of sustainable happiness. True Happiness is sustainable because the individual deliberately and consciously chooses perspectives that create positive emotions and has cultivated this habit of thought until the natural and habitual response focuses on the positive aspects of any situation."*

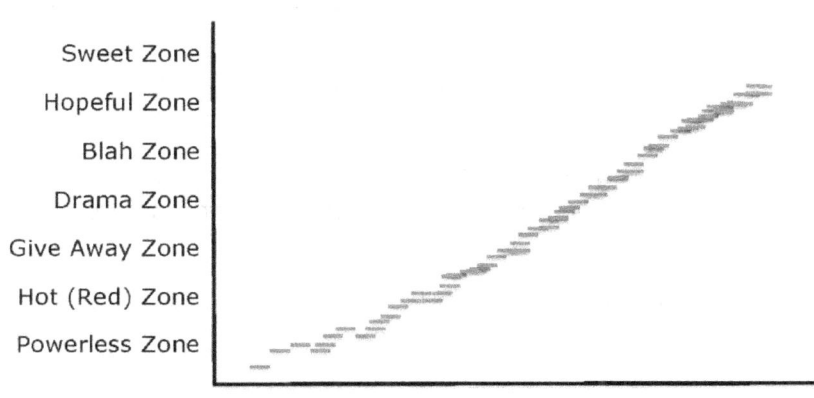

Trajectory of Emotional State across time

The lines on the chart illustrate the general trajectory of the emotional state of a person who is in the initial stages of applying *The Smart Way*™ and began in a low emotional state. The thicker areas indicate the person spent more time in that emotional state. They do not represent mandatory slowdowns. They are meant to illustrate that life events may temporarily decrease emotional state or stop progress.

Someone who is new to learning *The Smart Way*™ could take 3 – 12 months to move from the Powerless Zone to the Sweet Zone with each step along the way feeling better than the prior one. Someone who is experienced using *The Smart Way*™ could experience an emotional setback (loss of job, friend, etc.) and easily move the entire distance from the Powerless Zone to the Sweet Zone in a weekend.

RESILIENCE

The importance of psychological resilience is frequently cited as a critical skill in the future workplace and the future is here. Resilience provides protection against burnout and makes life better all-around because it lowers stress.[138, 139] Resilience is a significant negative predictor of burnout.[140] Practitioners who were more resilient tolerated uncertainty better.[141] A literature review covering a decade of resilience research concluded:[142]

> *Our findings suggest that nurses can actively participate in the development and strengthening of their own personal resilience to reduce their vulnerability to workplace adversity and thus improve the overall healthcare setting. We recommend that resilience-building be incorporated into nursing education and that professional support should be encouraged through mentorship programs outside nurses' immediate working environments.*

A 2014 study published in the *British Medical Journal Quality and Safety Journal* that included 44 NICUs and 2,073 healthcare providers,[143] and contributing authors coming from well-respected institutions such as Stanford University School of Medicine and Duke University School of Medicine reported:

> "The 'climate-like' nature of burnout suggests that in a clinical area where healthcare workers are resilient, the care context for delivering safe and high quality care may be more favourable. . . Ultimately, a resilient workforce may strengthen patient safety and quality of care."

Resilience is a high-level factor supported by three lower level factors:

- Optimism/Positivity
- An Internal Locus of Control
- Healthy Self-Esteem
  - Practice self-compassion

Using techniques to find more positive perspectives and using your Emotional Guidance to help you identify productive thoughts leads to natural increases in optimism and positivity. Optimists experience more positive emotions than pessimists and optimists perceive they receive more support from their partners.[144]

When the thoughts you work on with advanced coping skills are about yourself, the same process leads to natural increases in healthy self-esteem and decreases in defensive self-esteem.

As soon as you begin consciously using your Emotional Guidance to feel better and experience the fact that you have the ability to feel better without first having to change the situation, your locus of control becomes more internal.

An internal locus of control is the beliefs that your thoughts, words, and actions affect the outcome of your life. An external locus of control (see unhealthy habits of thought) is the belief that external factors control the outcome of your life.

The way a resilient person perceives and thinks about the situations they experience is different from the way a person with lower resilience perceives and thinks about the same situations. A person with lower resilience can increase resilience by shifting their perspectives to ones that increase resilience. They will feel better (less stressed) and be more resilient. The following chart highlights some of the differences.

> *Higher levels of resilience were found to have beneficial effects on worker's perceptions of stress, psychological responses to stress, and job-related behaviors related to stress regardless of difficult environments. Faced with especially difficult work environments, workers with higher levels of resilience seem able to avoid absences and be more productive than workers with low resilience.[145]*

Less **Resilient Habits of Thought**	More **Resilient Habits of Thought**
Obstacles are enemies	Obstacles are challenges
Feels disempowered	Feels empowered
Sees problems as permanent	Sees problems as temporary
Sees self as a victim	Sees self as survivor or thriver
Blames others	Accepts responsibility
Sees problems as unsolvable	Believes solutions exist & can be identified
Feels fearful/helpless	Feels confidence/capable
Responds reactively	Consciously chooses perspective
Rigid thinking	Feels curiosity
Holds onto anger	Forgives easily
Resistance to new ideas	Welcomes new ideas & experiences
Feels hopeless	Feels hopeful
Expects the worse	Faith
Tendency to attack oneself	Belief in Self & Ability to learn
Holds onto guilt	Characterizes failure as learning
Feelings of shame	Self-Acceptance and Approval
Negative emotional bias	Positive emotional bias
Long-term worry and anxiety	Trust
Feels life "just happens"	Feels Personal Control
Sees obstacles as enemies	Obstacles are challenges (opportunities)
Being "right" is highest goal	Places higher goals above "being right"
Feels despair	Looks for the silver lining
Feels out of control	Feels a sense of control over the response
Very specific thoughts	Zooms out to less specific thoughts

"Four main aspects of physician resilience were identified:[146]

1) Attitudes and perspectives, which include valuing the physician role, maintaining interest, developing self-awareness, and accepting personal limitations;
2) Balance and prioritization, which include setting limits, taking effective approaches to continuing professional development, and honoring the self;

3) Practice management style, which includes sound business management, having good staff, and using effective practice arrangements; and

4) Supportive relations, which include positive personal relationships, effective professional relationships, and good communication.

CONCLUSION: Resilience is a dynamic, evolving process of positive attitudes and effective strategies"

Valuing the physician's role includes putting more emphasis on what you think. Reconnecting with your why helps you maintain interest in your work.

PSYCHOLOGICAL CAPITAL (PSYCAP)

Psychological Capitol is:

> *A positive state of mind exhibited during the growth and development of an individual.*[147]

Hope is the only low level factor supporting PsyCap that is not included in the other high-level factors. *The Smart Way*™ doesn't include hope because trust, faith, or what I refer to as KNOWing are stronger than hope and supported by emotional guidance. With practice using emotional guidance, you begin KNOWing that you're helping yourself by shifting to more positive thoughts even before any aspect of your situation changes. If you use *The Smart Way*™ to increase resilience and happiness, you will develop PsyCap simultaneously.

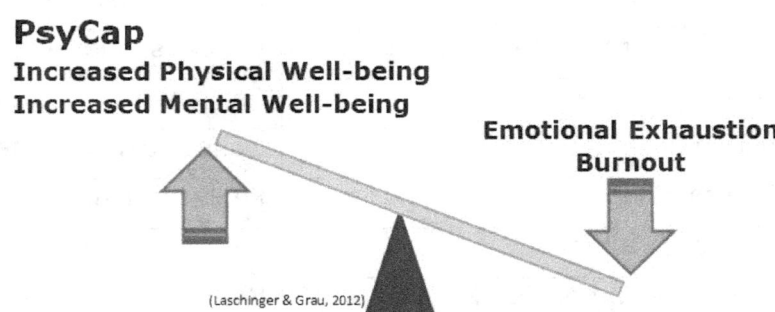

(Laschinger & Grau, 2012)

The main purpose for including PsyCap here is because it is one of several strategies for increasing quality of life that are currently being heavily promoted. It is important for the reader to know what PsyCap is in relationship to other high-level factors. In a study of 1,496 nurses, "all dimensions of PsyCap of nurses were negatively related to" all aspects of burnout.[148] In a smaller study, PsyCap was associated with reduced bullying exposure and improved physical and mental health.[149]

PERSONALITY

A theme that is woven throughout my work is a challenge to old ideas about personality traits. I differ from many other researchers and writers:

- Our personality does not define us
- Our personalities are not fixed
- The personality traits we demonstrate are the result of our habits of thought
- When we change our habits of thought our personality changes
- Everyone I know who has consciously chosen to change their habits of thought with the goal of feeling better emotionally likes their new personality better than their old one even if they were afraid they would lose themselves in the process before they changed their habits of thought.

I read a great synopsis of many of the personality models by Carver.[150] What was most obvious to me, however, was the lack of consideration given to emotional state and chronic emotional state.

The researchers describe personality as if it is fixed and unchangeable, without regard to the emotional state of the individual. But we all know that is ridiculous. Our behavior changes with our mood. In better-feeling moods we are nicer, kinder, and even more likely to help strangers. In bad moods, we are not as nice, even to those we love. Sustained low emotional states can lead to the most egregious behaviors.[151]

Better accuracy and completeness of personality models can be obtained by including mood/emotional state in the data collected when research is done. Existing personality models seem to explain behavior because most individuals maintain a relatively consistent chronic emotional state throughout life.

Emotional State (ES) is a way of referring to the emotion someone is feeling in-the-moment. (i.e. happy, sad, depressed, hopeful, hopeless, frustrated, angry, anxious, eager, etc.)

Chronic Emotional State (CES) is the set point, or emotional state a specific individual tends to return to repeatedly in the absence of a reason to feel otherwise.

The behavior individuals exhibit is tied most closely with the current Emotional State. The personality model research I've reviewed looks at behavior, but not emotional state at the time the behavior is observed. Self-reports of behavior also do not gather data on emotional state at the time of the behavior.

An individual whose Chronic Emotional State is happy exhibits behaviors consistent with that Emotional State. There will be variances due to occasional lower Emotional States and during times of resource depletion (i.e. illness and sleep deprivation). High stress will cause temporary changes in Emotional State.

The consistency of Emotional State is well documented in the scientific literature. Lottery winners, newlyweds, and newly disabled individuals typically return to their Chronic Emotional State within two years after these significant life changes. The reason for the stability of Chronic Emotional States is not because it is genetic or a fixed human trait.

Chronic Emotional State is the result of habits of thought.

Why isn't this commonly recognized? First, it is because researchers do not tend to explore individual differences at the level of thought. The work would be extremely time-consuming and would lack consistency because at the level of thought the uniqueness of each one of us becomes very apparent. Even two people who make identical choices follow very different thought processes to reach the decision.

Secondly, because habits of thought are habits--but not recognized as such and we are taught our personalities are who we are, few people change their thought patterns. Many people have a fear that if they change their personality they will no longer be the same person. Some fear they will no longer know their self. The truth is, those who deliberately change their habits of thought know their self better than they ever did before they experienced the liberating power of changing habits of thought.

Like any habit, changing habits of thought takes commitment and does not happen overnight.

Patience with oneself is required. Understanding and being realistic about how long it takes to create new habits of thought is necessary. While we can think, and can even believe, new thoughts immediately, when we believe something that opposes our former habits of thought, the old habitual thoughts will continue coming to mind until the thought-paths that supported the beliefs are allowed to diminish and new thought-paths that support the new belief are developed. Until this process is completed, you may find yourself thinking (and in the early stages) even speaking things you no longer believe. It's just old programming that is still stronger than the new programming you're creating. It's natural and it does not mean you can't change the habit of thought, just that the process is not yet complete.

Personality factors do affect the risk of burnout,[152] but if those factors are considered fixed traits they will be perceived as unchangeable when they are areas where changes can be very effective and individually satisfying.

WHAT HUMANS DO AND WHY THEY DO IT

The answer is short and sweet:

We do what we believe will make us feel better, via approach or avoidance.[153, 154, 155]

The examples are endless. We do things we don't want to do because they serve the purpose of something we do want. We may go to a job we no longer enjoy because we want to provide for our family. We are civil to in-laws we don't like because we want a good relationship with our spouse. We treat our boss with respect even if we don't respect him because we want to keep our job.

It often doesn't look like this is the reason we do things but if you dig deeper into the motivations, the belief that we will feel better if we do something (or better if we do not do something) is the motivation.

This was one of the conclusions Baumeister, et al. reached in the literature review that developed the new definition of the purpose and use of emotions.[156]

LONG-TERM VS. SHORT-TERM GOALS

Whether we look long-term or short-term when we make decisions about what will feel best depends on a variety of factors, but mostly on which ones we've focused on more. If long-term goals aren't given a lot of airtime in our mind, short-term goals will steer our decision-making.

Focusing on long-term goals increases the consideration we give to the long-term consequences of our words and actions. However, it is important that the goals be our own-- not goals others attempt to impose upon us.

By deliberately choosing a different perspective, our thoughts change and better-feeling emotions can be deliberately cultivated.[157] Thoughts create meaning for events in life.[158] For example, if someone cancels an appointment the individual who is told the meeting will not occur is free to assign meaning to the event. Even when a reason is given, the reason may or may not be accepted by the receiver. If the reason is not accepted, the individual will create a reason to explain the event to himself. That explanation may be one that feels good or one that feels bad. Whichever is chosen, the event will be experienced (felt emotionally) by the individual as if the assigned reason is true.

It is really as simple as understanding that better feeling thoughts are guiding us toward our desires and thoughts that feel worse are advising us that we are moving away from our desires. Some clarity regarding desires is required. There is a difference between short-term and long-term desires. Although all desires contain the characteristic that we believe we will feel better in the attaining of them, some desires relate to immediate gratification; a response to current conditions without consideration for the long-term. Desires for some foods, drugs, alcohol, and other addictions are fueled by these types of desires. Short-term desires are often accompanied by conflicting emotions caused by conflicts with longer term desires. For example, a desire to feel better right now may be satisfied by enjoyment of a piece of chocolate cake but the desire to maintain a comfortable weight in the long-term may be in direct conflict with that desire.

There is an inherent desire to feel better. Many desires are not beneficial in the long-term. Without knowledge of techniques to change thoughts, endless loops can result—sugary foods, alcohol, drugs, shopping and more can temporarily improve mood, but do not build long-term resilience. To build long-term resilience one must reach for better feeling thoughts. The more attention that is given to long-term goals, the more they will be considered in the emotional response you receive when a short-term goal conflicts with long-term goals.

For example, in an upsetting situation it is not uncommon for individuals to reach for alcohol to provide relief from their negative emotions. Unfortunately, alcohol provides only a temporary dulling of the pain (or lessening of the focus on the painful thoughts) and can lead to even greater problems. Remember alcohol is a depressant. A more permanent method of approaching an upsetting situation is to reframe your perception of the event in a way that feels better.[159] With practice, finding better feeling thoughts becomes easier.

A more permanent and healthier method of approaching an upsetting situation is to reframe your perception of the event in a way that feels better. Memories can be retrospectively constructed from your present perspective to change the meaning of the past experiences. With practice, finding better-feeling thoughts becomes easier and it eventually becomes automatic. It is really as simple as understanding that better-feeling thoughts are guiding us toward our desires. Thoughts that feel worse indicate we are moving away from our desires. All desires contain the characteristic that we believe we will feel better by attaining them.

Generally, the desire that feels better in the moment will win. If there is little belief that a comfortable weight will be achieved or maintained, the desire for the chocolate cake will usually win over the long-term but unbelievable desire to achieve a comfortable weight. On the other hand, an individual with a high degree of confidence (which might be interpreted as determination or will power) may forgo the chocolate cake now because she is able to achieve the same (or higher) degree of positive emotion by focusing on her belief in achieving the long-term goal. Note that the greater belief in the ability to succeed in this (or anything) is the better feeling thought.

She could change her focus away from the chocolate cake and onto achieving the long-term goal and feel good without the chocolate cake. Set long-term goals to make them more relevant.

It's possible to maintain a positive bias about life when circumstances are not ideal. This has been proven by many in very adverse circumstances. Viktor Frankl discovered the importance of finding meaning in all forms of existence while he was in a concentration camp. Finally, the perspective made his current circumstances, even though unchanged and reprehensible, feel better and provided a reason to continue living. This is an example of a Advanced Stress Management Strategy, where the individual found better-feeling thoughts. Although the thoughts he found were philosophical in nature, any thoughts that felt better and thus made the situation more tolerable are an Advanced Stress Management Stragegy.

Science has tended to study various aspects of humanity in isolation (Psychology, biochemistry, medical, neurological, consciousness, behavioral, sociology, criminology, genetics, physics, etc.). These areas of science are often subdivided into specialties, such as addiction, immunology, cardiovascular disease, beliefs, epigenetics, and more.

It is all interrelated. Root cause solutions require an understanding of the larger picture. We receive emotional feedback in response to our thoughts. Our emotional stance affects body chemistry, bodily processes, behaviors/actions, and ultimate outcomes. Positive emotions improve positive outcomes in every area of life.

Circumstances do not create the emotion. Individuals who live lives that are far from advantageous circumstances can be happy with their lives and receive the benefits of positivity. Research into disparate outcomes in situations with homogenous incomes vs. situations with greater differences reflects that it is not actual circumstances, but perception thereof that matters.[160]

DARK SIDE PERSONALITY TRAITS

Much the way emotions are referred to as positive and negative, researchers have labeled personality traits as 'bright' and 'dark' side personality traits. A recent research study explored whether dark side personality traits might increase resilience. Four of the dark side traits did increase resilience including Bold, Diligent, Colorful, and Imaginative.[161] When considering personality traits and whether they will increase or decrease resilience, consider whether they feel more empowering or less. Basically, the more empowered you feel the more resilient you will be. This is the same as saying the better you feel, the more resilient you will be and it is the same as saying that the less stress you feel, the more resilient you will be.

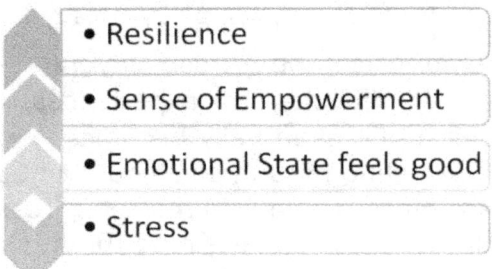

- Resilience
- Sense of Empowerment
- Emotional State feels good
- Stress

Bold personality traits include self-confidence, a sense of entitlement, and an over-evaluation of one's capability.

There is nothing at all wrong with confidence if:
- We don't beat ourself up if we don't meet expectations
- We don't win a Darwin award because of it
- My mom has white coat syndrome so as a child I placed doctors on a pedestal. I had fleeting thoughts of becoming a doctor but nearly as soon as the thought would cross my mind it was destroyed by my lack of confidence that I could do it. In fact, I was convinced I wouldn't be able to do it.
- Confidence will lead to attempting more than we otherwise would attempt

A sense of entitlement
- A sense of entitlement exists on the same continuum as self-esteem.

- The second from the right feels entitled to a good life but also perceives that everyone else deserves a good life. This entitlement isn't based on works,

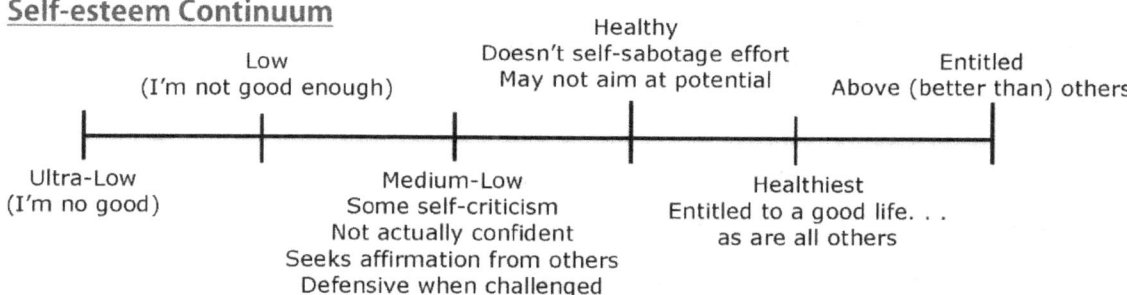

intelligence, education, etc. and it isn't about someone handing it to you without working for it. It's about perceiving that you're as deserving as anyone else of rewards and a good life (marriage, career, friends, money, etc.)

The greater danger for most of us lies not in setting our aim too high and falling short; but in setting our aim too low, and achieving our mark.

Michelangelo

- The belief that one is entitled to a good life protects against learned helplessness and increase resilience. It aids in efforts to frame failures as stepping stones on the way to success instead of as a sign that you don't deserve success or simply aren't good enough.
- Your emotional guidance will help you decide which belief would be best for you and help you find thoughts and develop beliefs that support healthy self-esteem.

An over evaluation of one's capability

I'll just leave this one with the father of modern psychology:

Most people live, whether physically, intellectually or morally, in a very restricted circle of their potential being. They make very small use of their possible consciousness, and of their soul's resources in general, much like a man who, out of his whole bodily organism, should get into a habit of using and moving only his little finger.

William James

On the other side of Bold is a Cautious personality, which is associated with increased burnout.[162] People with cautious personalities "fear being rejected" and this reduces their positive social interactions and their willingness to risk rejection.[163] Essentially, they reject themselves by taking themselves out of the running so that someone else can't reject them. If you consider the Cautious personality type on the self-esteem continuum it's easy to see how it correlates with low self-esteem.

DEVELOP PSYCHOLOGICAL FLEXIBILITY

How you explain your situation to yourself and others matters. The same situation can be perceived and explained as a challenge from which you'll learn and grow or as an experience that is ruining your life. It's all in how you perceive the situation.

Let's look at explanatory styles as they relate to emotional guidance. Categories of explanatory style include:

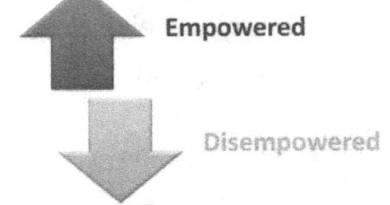

Personal: Whether the situation was caused by external forces (external locus of control) or internal causes (internal locus of control).

Permanent or Temporary: Is the situation perceived as stable (will it persist) or temporary (expected to change).

Pervasive: Are the factors that caused the situation global, local, or isolated?

Personality: Optimism and Pessimism are considered personality traits. There are two issues here:

- Most people believe personality traits are stable
- Many people believe their personality is who they are

Personality traits are simply indicators of the habits of thought a person has developed. Newer research is refuting the older belief that personalities are stable across the lifespan. Some people's personalities are stable because they don't change their habits of thought but others do change their habits of thought and their personalities change when they do.

Many people are afraid that they will lose themselves if they change their personality. If they try to be someone they aren't (i.e. extrovert when they feel more comfortable being introverted) this is a valid concern because that represents a situation where they are not being authentic. The difference is that when you change your habits of thought you actually change from the inside out. You're not being inauthentic—you're merely being more of the person you can be.

What I know is that everyone I have ever spoken with or worked with who changed their habits of thought so that they were more empowered loves the way they have changed. They find it easier to appreciate themselves and easier to live with themselves. They have a better relationship with themselves which makes their relationships with others better, too.

The idea that your personality is you is a false premise. Giving up that idea helps you become more of your potential best self.

Someone with optimistic tendencies tends to believe they can have an influence over the outcome of their lives and that negative events are temporary. Individuals with pessimistic tendencies tend to believe that negative events are permanent and pervasive and that there is little they can do to change the outcome.

Pessimism plus stress is a recipe for depression.

The same person's explanatory style can be different in different situations depending on their beliefs. For example, if someone sees themselves as having significant influence over their personal relationships and even who they have personal relationships with that person would have an internal locus of control relative to relationships. If this same person believes that his career depends on others (bosses or companies) he will have a more external locus of control for work situations.

In the quad graph we have whether thoughts we have about the situation are moving from where we are toward our highest potential or further away from our highest potential. Toward feels better and away feels worse. Thoughts that move toward our highest potential feel more empowered and thoughts that move away from our highest potential feel

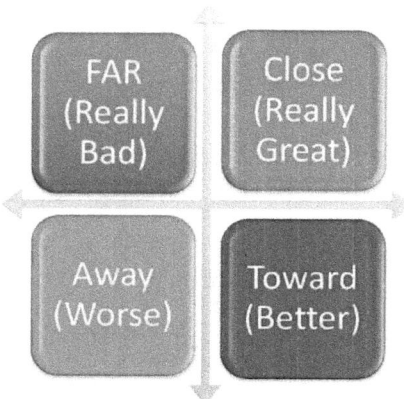

disempowered. The further away we are from our potential, the worse we feel. The closer we are to our potential, the better we feel. Let's look at a few scenarios where someone has been fired and compare explanatory style to their highest potential self by applying emotional guidance as a basis of comparison.

Imagine being fired from a job for failure to perform. Identify which thoughts are moving toward or away from your best potential self in this situation.

Here are some potential explanations:

I'm a screw-up. I'll never be able to get ahead because I can't keep a job.

This represents a disempowered perspective about the situation which means it is moving away from his best potential self. This is an internal attribution for the problem (*I'm a screw-up.*) but it isn't necessarily an internal locus of control because the person sees the situation as permanent (**I'll never be able to get ahead because I can't keep a job.**) If the person saw being a screw-up as something he or she could change the inability to get ahead wouldn't be perceived as permanent. It might be reflected in thoughts like this:

I haven't been doing my best. I need to stop being a screw-up so I can get ahead. (This is more empowered and moving toward his best potential self.)

The next statement reflects a different perspective:

They didn't recognize talent when it was right in front of them.

This is a disempowered perspective because it requires others to recognize one's talent but empowered because it indicates the person believes they have talent. This is a good example of what I refer to as **split energy**. Split energy is two steps forward and two back, repeated indefinitely. The number of steps doesn't matter. Some people take thousands of steps forward before they retrace their steps. You see them get a new job or a new romantic partner and everything seems fantastic, for a while, then it seems as if their new situation has become a repeat of an old scenario.

Seeking validation from external sources places all the blame on outside factors which mean the person has no ability to change the situation (external locus of control—disempowered).

Maybe I was in the wrong field and this is a chance for me to find something I'll be good at.

This is an empowered perspective. The focus is on the hope of something better coming. That something better is, by definition, moving toward the best potential self. This person sees the situation as temporary (*there is something I'll be good at I just wasn't doing that this time*) and an internal locus of control (*this is a chance for me to find*). This attitude will lead to thoughts, words, or actions that support finding a new job in a field where the person will perform better.

I'm not smart enough to keep a job.

This is a disempowered perspective and moving away from her best potential self. This looks like an internal locus of control because self-blame is involved (I'm not smart enough) but the situation isn't seen as temporary so it isn't an internal locus of control with respect to the level of intelligence. This person doesn't know that intelligence is something that can change with effort. Intelligence as a fixed characteristic is a common but now refuted understanding of intelligence. There is a great book by David Shenk, *The Genius in All of Us: New Insights into Genetics, Talent, and IQ* that I recommend to people who aren't happy with their level of intelligence and think there is nothing they can do about it. Because this person doesn't know they can change their level of intelligence, the situation is perceived as permanent.

Lots of people have been fired and found success in a new job.

This is an empowered perspective and leans toward becoming more of this person's best potential self. This is an internal locus of control because it reflects a belief that it is possible for her to find success in a new job. It is seen as a temporary situation with a better future (optimistic).

My boss was a jerk. I'm glad to be gone.

This person's best potential self would see the bosses' positive attributes. (i.e. *Working for that jerk helped me learn how to deal effectively with people who are negatively focused.*) Even though this person expresses positive emotions about losing the job (*I'm glad to be gone.*) the boss being a jerk seems like an external and uncontrollable factor. An internal locus of control might consider things such as whether they can gain skills in getting along with people even if those people aren't as pleasant as we'd like them to be.

How am I going to tell my spouse?

This one is subtle but it contains many nuances:

I don't trust my spouse to trust me to get another job.

I don't trust my spouse to be resilient.

Maybe: My spouses' opinion of me is how I determine my self-worth.

This perspective is not seeing the relationship with the spouse as the relationship their best possible self could have.

Remember that the stance (attitude) you'd take isn't a right/wrong. It is about whether your stance helps you or not and if it doesn't help, you can change it.

Before we complete this discussion of explanatory style I want you to reaffirm your competence and worth at work to offset any negatives that contemplating being fired might have stirred up. You can come up with your own or use the following affirmations.

Don't just read them. Read them, think them, and feel how they feel.

I make valuable contributions through my work.

I am a skilled employee/business owner.

My work is valued.

I am good at what I do.

While I am good at my work I am also always becoming better.

I deliver a service which heals, gives hope, and allows people to feel positive.

Many of the published peer reviewed journal articles cited in the bibliography mentioned that the uncertainty being experienced by physicians because of constant changes and unknown future changes contributes to burnout. Psychological flexibility and conscious resilience are the solution, not certainty. Certainty is an illusion. We can feel certain about where we are going and what we are going to do but we cannot be certain that our plans will work even when there aren't a lot of variables. An attitude of "Whatever the future holds, I am capable of surviving and thriving" will serve you better. Psychological flexibility is one of the top ten job skills cited as necessary for workers in 2020.

The novel, *Lucifer's Hammer*, demonstrates the difference between certainty and psychological flexibility. The main characters have psychological flexibility and resilience, the banker does not possess those skills.

ENERGY

Physicians know that there is something that animates the body and that when it is absent the person occupying the body is no longer alive. In Western medicine we can't really define what this energy is, we simply know that when it is present a person lives and when a person dies it is no longer present.

We can name a cause of death but not why some people die from things that other people manage to survive. In the ones who die, the energy that sustains life leaves. In the ones who live it grows stronger after they come close to death.

We may recognize that those who are the most afraid more often die when others who are hopeful survive in similar circumstances. We will say that some fight for life while others surrender or let go.

Webster Dictionary refers to Qi or chi as it is sometimes called as:
> *Vital energy that is held to animate the body internally*

Throughout this book, if you will consider whether actions, thoughts, or decisions increase one's energy or decrease the energy, the same energy which is ultimately present when we are alive and absent when we are not, you will see that we can understand the path we are on by paying attention to our energy levels long before a diagnosis is possible.

What am I trying to say? We feel more energized when we feel positive emotions than we do when we feel negative emotions. We can feel negative emotions and feel more energized than we did before if we are moving from a lower negative emotion to a higher one. For example, moving from depression to anger increases the energy that a person feels even though anger is still a negative emotion.

We don't notice subtle changes in our own energy level as much as we do the difference between our energy level and that of someone at a significantly different energy level. If we are in a high positive emotional state and encounter someone who is cynical and negatively focused the difference is immediately apparent. If we pay attention to subtle signals we may feel the urge to distance ourself from the person who feels much more negative than we do.

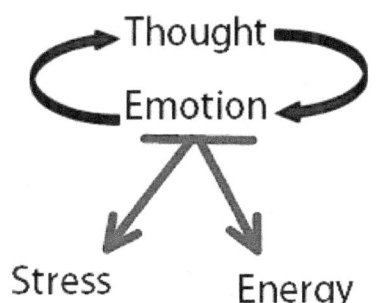

Over the long-term you'll discover that thoughts that lead to emotions that lead to burnout decrease the energy we feel coursing through us. If we can change our thoughts around to ones that elicit positive emotions our energy increases.

Getting out of bed in the morning isn't difficult when we're excited about what we're getting up to do.

Think about a time when you felt highly intrinsically motivated. Can you remember the energy available to you when you felt that motivated?

Remember a time when someone made you do something you didn't want to do. You may have to return to your childhood to remember this depending on your life experiences. One experience many people related in response to this is being forced to apologize when you felt wrongly accused or justified in what you were made to apologize for. Can you remember how the energy felt stuck?

Now remember a time when you sincerely wanted to apologize for something and your apology was accepted. Do you feel how the energy of a sincere apology is cleansing like the rain?

With emotional guidance you are asked to pay attention to how your feel and recognize your emotions as sign posts letting you know if you're moving toward or away from self-actualization. Your energy level does much the same thing. Awareness of your energy may be easier for individuals who were trained to suppress their emotions.

Energy

↑ Eustress

↓ Stress

Changing your thoughts changes your emotional response, stress level, and the amount of energy available to you.

This model helps to explain why lower emotional states such as burnout, depression, and anger are associated with both chronic and life-threatening illnesses and diseases. It helps explain why two 70+ year longitudinal studies show that positive emotions are associated with 10.7 additional years of life and about 18 healthier years of life.[164, 165]

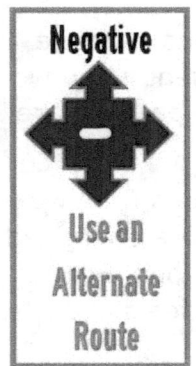

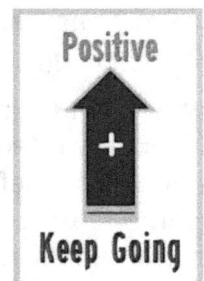

When an individual has the ability to accurately self-monitor the results of his or her thoughts with an early detection system that is accurate and knows where you want to be (your self-actualized self), it is easier to know what to do. Instead of feeling lost, wandering around an unmarked desert trying to find your way, you have road signs (emotions or energy) that let you know if you are moving in the desired direction in every moment of every day. All you have to do is read the signs. The core of burnout has been described as, "the reduction of energetic resources."[166]

Even if you forget and feel as if you've become lost, the signs are still there and they still know how to get where you want to go from wherever you happen to be. All you have to do is remember that there are signs and that you understand their language.

The process of preventing burnout is reading the signs and making course adjustments. The process of recovering from burnout is reading the signs and making course adjustments, each one of which will lead you to a slightly better state. Even though the most successful adjustments are small, they add up. Think of it in terms of climbing the steps at St. Paul's Cathedral in London. You begin at the bottom but when you're on the 3rd step you're closer to the top than you were when you were at the bottom. One step at a time is all it takes to find your way to a far better emotional state.

Your emotions will guide you to understand your purpose. When your work puts you in the Sweet Zone often, examine it for your purpose. Listen to how you describe the work you do. For decades before I realized that my purpose was helping people I described every job I had by describing how I helped people when I did my job.

- What do you look forward to doing?
- Why did you choose your career?
- What is your why?
- What aspects of your work energize you?

Spend time each day remembering what you love about your work, even if you haven't enjoyed it for a long time. Remembering will help your mind re-focus on the aspects you enjoy.

Robert Assagioli wrote about this subject in *Psychosynthesis*:[167]

> *It is well to recognize and remember the value of each human being and of every activity of his, however humble it may be. This helps us to bring good will and cheerfulness to bear in doing anything, even if wearisome and boring. However apparently insignificant in itself, an activity is in reality, as necessary as actions of greater prominence which seem more important. This balanced appreciation and the resulting good inner disposition are well illustrated by the story of the three stonecutters.*
> *A visitor to the site of where one of the medieval cathedrals was being built asked a stonecutter what he was doing. "Don't you see," replied the latter sourly, "I'm cutting stones," thus showing his dislike of what he regarded as unpleasant and valueless work.*
> *The visitor passed on and put the same question to another stonecutter. "I'm earning a living for myself and my family," replied the workman in an even tempered way that reflected a certain satisfaction.*
> *Further on, the visitor stopped by a third stonecutter and asked him: "And what are you doing?". This third stonecutter replied joyously: "I am building a cathedral." He had grasped the significance and purpose of his labor; he was aware that his humble work was as necessary as the architect's, and in a certain sense it carried equal value. Therefore he was performing his work not only willingly, but with enthusiasm.*
> *Let us remember the example of the wise workman. This recognition will enable us to accept every situation, fulfill every task, willingly, and with cheerfulness.*

When you perceive you work as aligned with your purpose, it has more meaning and you will enjoy it more.

If you've been focusing on aspects of your job that you don't enjoy, your mind will focus on other things that feel the same way. When you deliberately re-focus on aspects of your work you enjoy, your mind will begin automatically thinking about positive aspects more frequently.

This will help more than your perception of your job. When your mind begins focusing on things that elicit negative emotions your perception of other things, such as your relationships, can become more negative as well. You will have noticed this tendency by observing that when you or someone you're in a relationship with is in a bad mood about something that isn't relevant to your relationship it can make communication within the relationship more likely to erupt in an argument or other disagreement.

Our minds seek to reinforce our emotional state; as if it is designed based on our deliberately attaining the emotional state we want to have.[168] For the first time in history, using transformative and advanced coping skills with emotional guidance, we can deliberately cultivate the emotional state we want to experience. Once we do that, our brain will help us sustain it by focusing on aspects of our environment that reinforce that emotional state.

PART III – ADVANCED AND TRANSFORMATIONAL COPING

TRANSFORMATIVE AND ADVANCED COPING SKILLS

> NOTE: IF YOU WANT TO TAKE THE COPING QUESTIONNAIRE, YOUR RESULTS WILL REFLECT YOUR USUAL BEHAVIORS IF YOU TAKE IT BEFORE YOU READ THIS CHAPTER. THE QUESTIONNAIRE IS IN APPENDIX XII AND A BRIEF VERSION IS IN APPENDIX XIII.

There are healthy and unhealthy methods of coping with stress. Many methods of coping that are modeled and encouraged in our society are not healthy. Coping styles can be divided by whether they usually lead to optimal (healthy) outcomes or suboptimal (unhealthy) outcomes.

The more healthy skills an individual has to help them respond to stress, the less impact they will experience from stress.

"Coping is defined as the set of cognitive and behavioral strategies used by an individual to manage the internal and external demands of stressful situations."[169] Unhealthy coping styles lead to undesirable outcomes and are usually not effective in reducing the amount of stress experienced. In the long-term, unhealthy coping styles can make problems worse and contribute significantly to downward spirals. Situations are more likely to be perceived as threatening, harmful or as causing a loss, which can be material or emotional (such as losing respect).[170]

Positive coping is proactive rather than reactive. In most situations, the best response to stress is a cognitive change that may or may not be followed by action. In many situations, finding a more empowered perspective is all the work that needs to be accomplished to reduce or eliminate stress. For example, the simple act of changing your thoughts about a subject from believing the task is too difficult to believing you are capable of success is all it takes to allow your mind to begin finding ideas that will make solving the problem easier. Action is still required to solve the problem but the stress has been reduced or removed.

Regular use of positive (healthy) coping skills increases resilience, self-efficacy, self-esteem, quality of life, emotional state, relationships with others and self (less self-criticism), and provides a foundation for a life that it feels good to live. Positive coping protects and fuels your energetic resources.

Positive (healthy) coping sees risks but evaluates them as something that can be managed or mitigated. Healthy coping includes active problem-solving but problems are considered surmountable or may be viewed as opportunities. Although individuals who are not well-versed in healthy and unhealthy coping styles often view positivity with distain, considering it Pollyannaish, this view reflects their lack of knowledge. Denial, avoidance, and wishful thinking are unhealthy (negative) coping styles as evinced by a significant body of research.

Mental Health

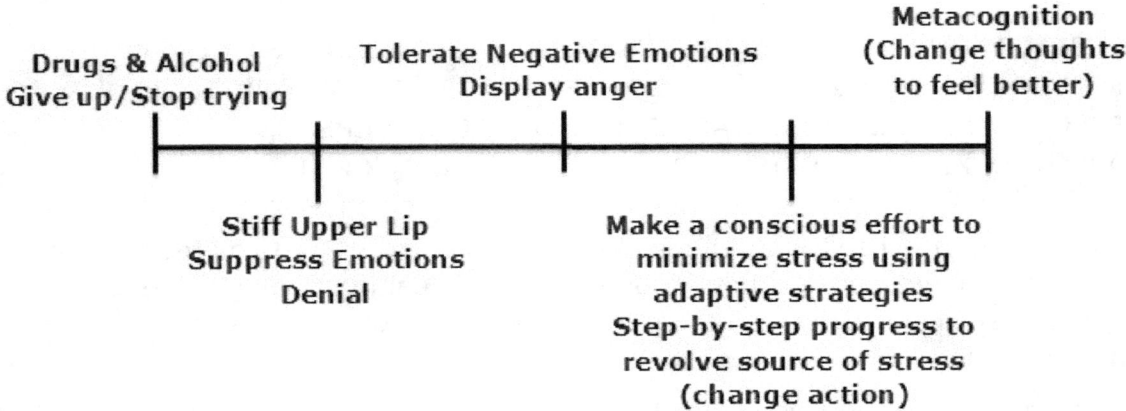

Emotional Intelligence (EI) and Emotion Regulation are not the same thing but the concepts are being integrated because they are complimentary.

Emotionally Intelligent individuals shape their emotions from the earliest possible point in the emotion trajectory and have many strategies at their disposal. Second, high EI individuals regulate their emotions successfully when necessary but they do so flexibly, thereby leaving room for emotions to emerge.[171]

EMOTION REGULATION PROCESS: OVERVIEW

Coping strategies are attempts to deal with emotions. Most coping strategies attempt to deal with negative emotions although some down regulate positive emotions because the emotions being experienced do not fit the social norm for the situation. We can also increase positive emotions and sustain them longer.

Advanced and Transformational Coping Skills reduce the level of stress. For example, changing beliefs about your ability to handle stress so that you feel more capable of dealing with stressful experiences reduces the level of stress you initially feel when you encounter a stressful situation. Your mind perceives the situation, deems you capable of handling it (based on your own beliefs about your capabilities) and then you feel the emotional response. Emotional Guidance helps us determine which beliefs will help us self-actualize.

Belief change is transformative.

If you find yourself thinking or saying, "I can't take any more" what you really mean, at the basis of the statement, is you can't handle any more stress. It is common to misinterpret the feeling and begin believing you're at the end of your rope and you can't take one more authoritarian demand from your employer, one more bad encounter, one more financial strain, etc. It isn't the situations; it is the perception of the situations that brings you to feel that you can't take any more.

Man's ability[d] to be resilient is unknown. We haven't reached the end of our potential resilience.

> I'M NOT SAYING THAT WE SHOULDN'T WORK TOWARD CHANGING THE FACTORS THAT CAUSE STRESS. I AM SAYING OUR GREATEST IMMEDIATE POWER IS IN CHANGING OUR PERCEPTION.

When you apply skilled emotion regulation to stressful situations, the amount of stress you experience decreases. When the stress you experience decreases your ability to deal with the situation improves.

Simply begin looking for examples of people who were able to handle what you're experiencing is helpful. Asking questions can be helpful.

Have others lived through an experience like this (or worse) and been okay?

What could I do to make this better?

Can I look at this from a broader perspective? Will it matter tomorrow or in a year?

What is good in my life?

What can I plan to look forward to?

The graphic illustrates important parts of our perception of the world. Our bodies are so good at translating inputs in ways that make our perception seem like a stable reality that it is easy to forget that our perceptions are the result of factors that vary between individuals.

---

[d] I wish we had an English pronoun that was genderless. This refers to humans; not just men.

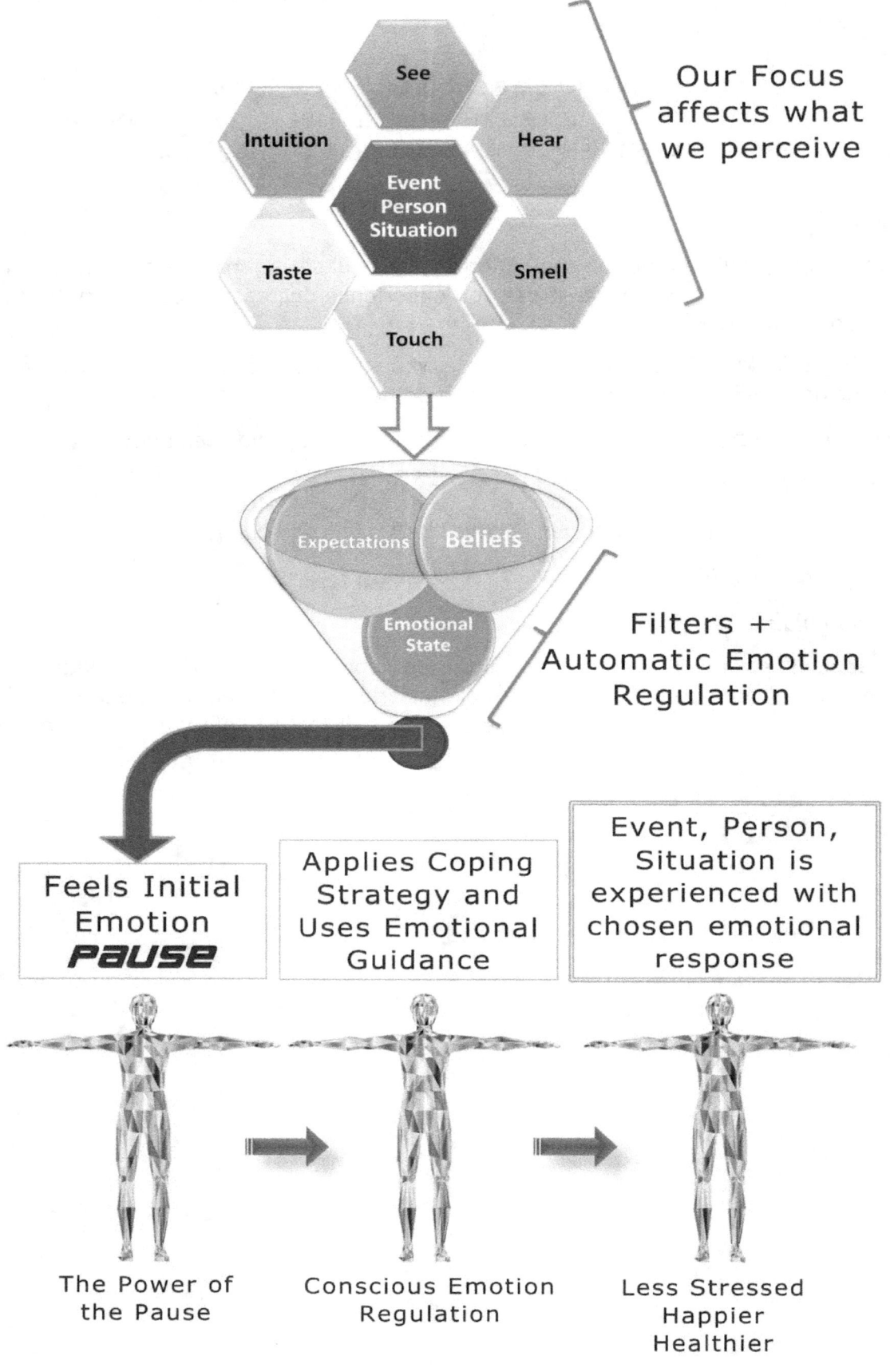

UNHEALTHY HABITS OF THOUGHT

We know that unhealthy habits of thought lead to undesired outcomes. Fortunately, habits of thought can be changed. Changing habits of thought is one of the fastest ways to improve outcomes.

The suppression of negative emotions is unhealthy.[172] Before the new paradigm of emotions as guidance was understood the fact that experiencing and suppressing negative emotion were both bad for our heart health perplexed researchers. When the new paradigm of emotions as guidance, much like road signs providing directions, it becomes clear that we are not designed to experience sustained negative emotion.

Given the preponderance of evidence that our minds, bodies, behavior, relationships, and careers are all better when we experience more positive emotions, the importance of using healthy strategies to regulate emotions becomes evident. The adverse outcome of negative emotions is not the result of experiencing them; it is the result of sustained negative emotions. The healthy way to live is to pay attention to negative emotions and use healthy strategies to find better feeling perspectives.

We have the capacity to regulate our emotions to "increase, maintain, or decrease positive and negative emotions."[173] Given the benefits of positive emotions and detriments of negative emotions detailed throughout this text, it makes sense to increase positive emotions and decrease negative emotions.

Conscious reappraisal of negative emotions is often not done "even though proactive regulation may have offered hedonic benefits."[174]

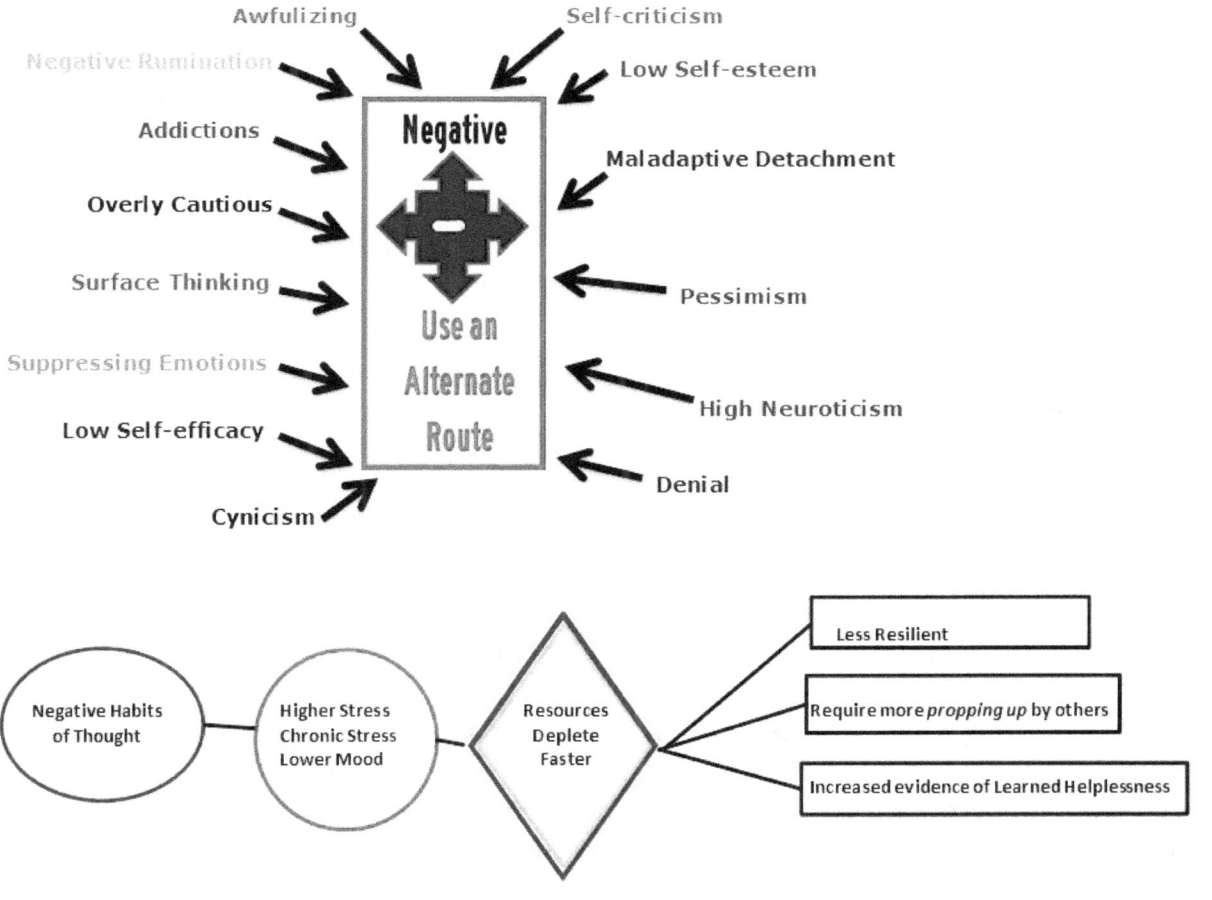

The coping strategies detailed in the next chapter indicate that we have a choice about how we cope with potentially stressful events in our lives. The choices we make are largely dependent upon the strategies we know how to use.

Learning and applying healthy coping strategies improves results. Although your emotional guidance will assist you in identifying what works and what doesn't work, it is useful to recognize unhealthy coping strategies and unhealthy habits of thought.

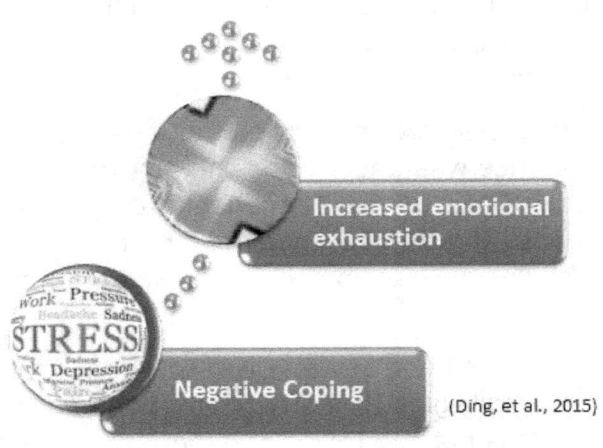

(Ding, et al., 2015)

CATASTROPHIZING/AWFULIZING

Catastrophizing or awfulizing reflect the presence of unhealthy habits of thought that lead to perceiving situations as:[175]

- Permanent
- Pervasive
- Personal

Do you have a tendency to see things as permanent and pervasive?

Do you think or talk in terms of always, never, only, or constantly? Do you take a single situation and apply it to the entire world or to your whole life or an entire relationship?

Don't worry if you do. It's just a habit of thought that isn't serving you well. In fact, if you're doing this it means there is an easy way to make your life feel better. When a person who awfulizes or castrophizes situations changes their habits of thought their life feels better even though the circumstances haven't changed at all. They're just happier (or less depressed). Their stress level declines and they feel more empowered to change things they don't like. They feel less beaten up by the things they don't like about their life or their world.

Set an intention to be aware of times when you or others use always, never, only, constantly, everyone, no one or any other words that have those meanings. Then active refute their truth.

Surgeons perceive surgery as both "an act that might save and an act that might kill."[176] While it is prudent to understand the risks, it is not necessary to stress over them in order to perform at one's peak. In fact, stressing about the potential to harm that "makes the threat of the complication omnipresent in surgeons' lives"[177] probably decreases effectiveness because stress decreases cognitive abilities.

> *Severe and/or prolonged stress causes over activation and dysregulation of the hypothalamic pituitary adrenal (HPA) axis thus inflicting detrimental changes in the brain structure and function. Therefore, chronic stress is often considered a negative modulator of the cognitive functions including the learning and memory processes. Exposure to long-lasting stress diminishes health and increases vulnerability to mental disorders. In addition, stress exacerbates*

functional changes associated with various brain disorders including Alzheimer's disease and Parkinson's disease.[178]

The evidence suggests it would be better for surgeons to focus on being their best and believing that their training has prepared them to be successful in the surgeries they are planning to perform. It takes training of one's mind to change one's outlook but given the potential immediate and long-term harm to patients and surgeons, it is work worth doing. Focus on being their best doesn't mean seeing themselves as infallible in ways that would make them careless. It means seeing themselves as experts who know how to manage the risks. In complex situations, rather than worry about one's effectiveness, asking "What is the best way to achieve this successfully?" will direct the brain to answer the question. Believing, "I can find the best solution" which can involve asking others to share their knowledge and experience is beneficial.

Challenging intrusive thoughts about potential failures can take away their power. There is a path between irrational confidence and irrational fear that can be found and followed. Make decisions to perform, or not perform surgery carefully but once made, align with the decision and don't second guess yourself unless something changes one of the criterion used in making the decision.

It might be easier to think of it relative to another subject. Suppose someone gets married and continually questions whether they made the right decision. Imagine the outcome of that scenario compared to someone who gets married and decides that they are going to do the best they can to make the best of the relationship.[e] The first person would be more stressed and continually second guessing their decision. The second person would be focused on making the marriage the best it can be.

Surgeons also attempt to "satisfy the cultural image of surgeons as strong, decisive and responsible for their patients"[179] which is contradicted when the surgeon frets about the potential risks of surgeries. Just manage the risk without worrying about it. What does that mean? It means that if you think of something else to do, do it, but if all you're doing is worrying if you made the right decision and imagining scenarios that don't turn out well, you're not helping yourself or the patient.

It's important to note that, together with self-criticism and blaming others, catastrophizing is associated with sub-clinical paranoia.[180] It is also correlated with depression and chronic depression.[181]

SELF-CRITICISM

Self-criticism is unnecessary. Many of us were taught to view ourselves critically. Research has revealed that self-criticism delays accomplishments. There are too many factors that go into it. Part of it is that self-criticism leaves us feeling inadequate for the goals we want to reach so we don't move forward.

Self-criticism is sometimes referred to as self-flagellation. When we recognize that something about ourselves is not as we would like it to be, the best path is to make a choice to change whatever that thing happens to be.

---

[e] I'm not inferring staying in an untenable situation. I'm referring to day-to-day interactions that are normal in every relationship.

In some cases this will involve taking action and other times it will involve changing our perspective.

The only person you are destined to become is the person you decide to be.

Ralph Waldo Emerson

For example, if someone doesn't like their age, because they think they are too old to do something they want to do, they can't reverse the clock. They can change their perspective about the capabilities of people who are their age. It turns out that our beliefs about aging affect how we age. I've been collecting examples of people who age well for two decades and my view of my potential in my older years changed significantly as a result. There are people in their 70's running marathons and even a few in their 90's. I knew a man when I lived in Idaho who was 99 and lived alone. When he died he had 60 lbs of seeds on his kitchen table that he was going to plant in his garden the year he turned 100. He did not die of natural causes. He lasted six weeks in the burn unit in Seattle before succumbing to an infection. He was born in 1897 in the Oklahoma territory and American Indians came from as far as 100 miles to see him and his two siblings because they considered triplets good luck.

Aging is not the only thing we can change our minds about. If you want a more in-depth dive on aging, Ellen Langer's *Counterclockwise* is excellent.[182] There is also research with children that demonstrates expectation affects outcome.[183]

So, if you can't change the actual thing, change the way you think about it. If you can change the actual thing, make a decision to change it. This is the process:

1. Pay attention to how you feel. Get used to doing this so that when you feel more negative emotion than normal you are aware of the feelings.
2. When the negative emotion is a response to self-criticism, say to yourself, "I don't like this about myself. What would I prefer?"
3. When you know what you'd prefer, make a decision to change whatever it is.
4. Begin doing everything you can do to change the thing you don't like.
5. You'll feel better as you move toward becoming as you want to be, even if it the process will take years.

Decisions have power. When you make a definitive decision something clicks into place that makes accomplishing whatever you've decided to accomplish easier than you thought it would be.

Two of my favorite quotes are about the power of making a decision. I've previously attributed this quote to Johann Wolfgang von Goethe but I've since learned that the correct attribution is to W. H. Murray in *The Scottish Himalaya Expedition*, 1951. That change does not make the words any less inspirational.

> *Until one is committed, there is hesitancy, the chance to draw back. Concerning all acts of initiative (and creation), there is one elementary truth that ignorance of which kills countless ideas and splendid plans: that the moment one definitely commits oneself, then Providence moves too. All sorts of things occur to help one that would never otherwise have occurred. A whole stream of events issues from the decision, raising in one's favor all manner of unforeseen incidents and meetings and material assistance, which no man could have dreamed would have come his way. Whatever you can do, or dream you can do, begin it. Boldness has genius, power, and magic in it. Begin it now.*

My second favorite quote about decisions is:

Once you make a decision, the universe conspires to make it happen.

Ralph Waldo Emerson

Self-criticism can also take the form of *shoulding* or *coulding* as in "I should have. . . " or "I could have . . . ". There are two things to consider when you realize you're *shoulding* all over yourself. One is to make a decision to become who you want to be. The other is to consider your resources.

We often beat ourselves up for not doing our best when we did do our best in that moment in time. Understanding the concept that your best potential is not the same as your best in any given moment can help you go easier on yourself and it may help you make better decisions in the future. More detail about resources to consider are discussed under the *Re-defining Your Best* chapter heading.

After adjusting my definition of my best to be "the best possible at the moment the behavior is measured" I've observed a lot of people and come to the conclusion that we all do the best we can, given our resources, in any given moment. Our "best in the moment" varies depending on the resources available to us at that point in time.

NEGATIVE RUMINATION

Negative rumination is thinking about or talking about something that brings forth negative emotions, usually repeatedly. The actual event may have lasted five minutes but our experience of it could span weeks or months depending on how many times we re-live it or talk about it.

CO-RUMINATION

Co-rumination is when you get together with others and focus on things that feel bad when you talk about them. Conversations that outline problems and then turn to solutions will be helpful. Conversations that focus on problems and simply grumble about problems without identifying solutions are not beneficial. Even worse are conversations that focus on problems and lean toward solutions that are not ethical, moral, or legal.

If your interactions typically focus on problems you are probably not aware in-the-moment that you're participating in these conversations that they feel worse than alternatives because you're used to feeling that way. Pay more attention to how you feel, both emotionally and viscerally, as you participate and you will recognize the negative impact it is having on your physiology and psychology. You can absent yourself from these conversations, attempt to steer them toward solutions, or change the subject.

LOW SELF-ESTEEM

Historically, low self-esteem has been one of the most difficult areas to change, even with the aid of a professional. That's no longer true.

Emotional Guidance does not support low self-esteem. Thoughts that reflect low self-esteem receive a negative emotional response which, given the new definition of the purpose and use of emotions, indicates the thoughts are not serving our highest good and that we should find a thought that elicits a better feeling thought.

When I am working with individuals who have low self-esteem I use two methods. The first is for them to use their emotional guidance as often as possible, but not directly on the low self-esteem issue in the beginning. The purpose of using emotional guidance frequently is to develop strong trust in its accuracy. Once this is done, the individual can begin working on adjusting their self-esteem with the guidance they now trust.

Before trust in emotional guidance is established I do not recommend using it to work on self-esteem.

The other process I find most helpful with low self-esteem is to look for counterfactual thinking and distortions that are obvious. Do you give other people the benefit of the doubt but vilify yourself? Write down your accomplishments. If you're a doctor or a nurse your accomplishments already exceed those of many people.

Self-esteem is best dealt with after you loosen it up a bit. Like an old rusted screw, it is easier if you work it loose a bit first. Giving up unhealthy habits of thought in every area you can and developing healthy habits of thought will loosen up the mental connections that have kept thoughts that support low self-esteem active.

This was an issue I dealt with myself. I will never think I am better than others so the belief I deliberately cultivated is as follows:

I am wonderful. . . and so is everyone else.

This new belief reminds me to see the potential in others rather than focusing on who they are being in the moment. That helps me inspire them to become more of their potential. It allows me to have positive self-esteem without placing myself above anyone else. It was the perfect belief for me to establish. If it resonates with you, feel free to use it. If it doesn't resonate, play with your thoughts until you find one that feels good to you. Other people don't have to be part of the equation. For me it felt better to acknowledge that my being wonderful doesn't make me any better than anyone else. It was the only way to quiet the voice in my head that wanted to dispute the "I am wonderful" belief.

People who boast about themselves and toot their own horn are often perceived as having big ego's (high self-esteem) but the truth is that these are signs of low self-esteem and insecurity. Someone who knows they have value and worth doesn't have to prove it or point it out to others. One key to healthy self-esteem is caring less about what others think of us and just being the best person we can be.

In the section on Developing Healthy Habits of Thought there is information that will help you increase your self-esteem. There is also a questionnaire in Appendix XVIII where you can learn more about your level of self-esteem. Accomplishments, even high achievements, and low self-esteem are not mutually exclusive. Many high achievers have low self-esteem. Self-esteem is about what you believe about yourself which may not reflect reality.

SUPPRESSING EMOTIONS

Suppression of emotions has long been associated with adverse health outcomes including depressive symptoms, decreased mood, and lower levels of well-being.[184] More recent research indicates that memory suffers when emotions are suppressed.[185]

Given that the purpose of emotions is to guide us toward self-actualization, suppressing emotions is the equivalent of ignoring signs like these:

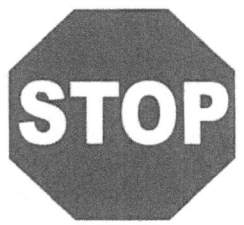   

The consequences of suppressing emotions can be as serious as ignoring these signs; it just takes longer to happen.

Many people are taught to suppress their emotions by their parents. It used to be primarily men because it was considered more acceptable, even expected, that women would express their emotions. The life expectancy gap between men and women began closing in the 1970's. Although too many factors are involved to figure out exactly what is causing it, the timing corresponds with increasing numbers of women in professional roles where they might feel they have to regulate their emotions. Individuals and society pays a cost for expectations of emotional suppression.

The expectation that we suppress emotions stems partially from the old view of emotions:

> *There are times . . . when our emotions are our worst enemies, leading us to think and behave in ways that are downright destructive. . . Consensus that emotions are functional and adaptive has reached such a level that contradictory evidence is no longer seriously considered, and the complex determinants of functionality are not fully appreciated. To remedy this complacency, the author draws attention to the nontrivial amount of dysfunctional emotion in everyday life, as well as to the many long-standing philosophical and religious traditions that counsel dispassion. This exercise is useful for tempering functionalist zeal and restoring scientific skepticism. It also demonstrates that the functionality of emotions depends critically on the appraisals that give rise to emotions, the choice and control of the behaviors motivated by emotions, and the socialization and training of emotions. These parameters, whether or not they are considered part of an emotion, must be considered part of what makes emotions functional.[186]*

The religious traditions that counsel dispassion may stem from the amount of dysfunctional emotion in everyday life. However, that dysfunctional emotion is the result of not interpreting emotions as guidance. When emotions are interpreted as guidance toward self-actualization with negative emotions being the equivalent of your global positioning system (GPS) freaking out and telling you to make a U-turn rather than telling you to punch someone or seek retribution for a wrong, they become functional. When they are interpreted correctly and a pause is applied between feeling strong negative emotion and action, during which the interpretation is adjusted, they are highly functional.

When I first began teaching people about emotional guidance many of them asked me how it coincided with their religious worldview. They seemed reluctant to use emotions as guidance unless it was supported by their religious worldview. In order to help them I researched the texts of six major religions and found support in the text of each of them. Those passages are documented in *Rescue Our Children from the War Zone*. Given the support I found in religious texts indicating that we are provided guidance and how the new interpretation of emotions as guidance fits perfectly into those passages, I lean toward accepting them as guidance which is consistent with many religious worldviews. However, they can be explained scientifically using quantum physics.

I completely agree that "the appraisals that give rise to emotions, the choice and control of the behaviors motivated by emotions, and the socialization and training of emotions" must be considered. This text provides information on skills that address these issues so that readers can be empowered with knowledge they can use to accurately interpret and regulate their emotions.

"Our emotions are often our best allies, helping us to respond energetically and effectively to the opportunities and difficulties we encounter."[187]

PESSIMISM

Most importantly, pessimism is not a fixed element of personality or an inborn trait. Pessimism arises from an individual's habits of thought which often echo those around them and especially those that were around them when they were young.

Pessimism can be changed by changing underlying beliefs and habits of thought. Pessimism is associated with worse life outcomes in health, relationships, career, and longevity. There are many aspects that affect these outcomes but the increased stress experienced by someone who has a negative mental attitude is a significant factor.

An individual may be pessimistic in every area of life or in selected areas. Pessimists often believe situations are worse than they are and may perceive solvable problems as unsolvable. In the Resilience section of this book, the habits of resilient and less resilient individuals were compared. Many of the less resilient habits of thought in that chart reflect pessimistic attitudes.

Pessimists may:

- Distrust and doubt others intentions
- Believe the worst will happen
- Not feel hope or trust that things will work out well
- Believe the world is evil
- Believe people are bad

Pessimist's lives often reflect their beliefs about life. Negative mental attitudes result in interpreting experiences in a negative light. Where an optimist sees an opportunity a pessimist sees a problem. Both optimists and pessimists live in self-fulfilling prophesies.

LOW SELF-EFFICACY

Self-efficacy is a context specific belief. Think in terms of strengths. A person can believe they are good at one thing but not good at another thing. I have many skills and talents but I need a bucket to carry a tune. My self-efficacy when it comes to singing is that I should only do it when I am alone and if I learn someone else is present I apologize for assaulting their ears.

The actions you'll take when you believe you are capable of doing a good job are different than the actions you'll take when you don't feel confident in your abilities.

". . . Meta-analyses indicate that self-efficacy is relatively strongly related to burnout components across occupational groups, countries, and professionals' age and gender."[188] Low self-efficacy is associated with lack of engagement and accounts for between 27-40% of employee engagement.[189, 190] "Exhaustion led to decline in self-efficacy beliefs over a six month period which in turn resulted in higher disengagement levels."[191]

A study that evaluated the association between exhaustion, self-efficacy, and burnout concluded enhancing self-efficacy beliefs can reduce work stress which helps prevent burnout.[192]

WILLINGNESS TO SEEK SUPPORT

Many people perceive asking for help as a sign of weakness and avoid asking for help even when it is desperately needed. Failing to ask for support is a weakness.

This is an area I've struggled with and continue to work on changing. Two things have helped me become more willing to ask for assistance when I need help.

The first is recognizing that I enjoy helping others and that by not seeking help I deprive others from the pleasure they would receive from helping me. Do you ever help someone because you want to help them? When you do, do you enjoy it? Does the level of your enjoyment increase if they are willing to accept the help you're offering? Do you find it frustrating to want to help someone but they refuse your offer?

Remember times you helped others and enjoyed it. Now turn it around and see that there are people who would gladly help you.

The other thing that helped me was when I recognized that *asking for help* is an adaptive coping strategy.

SURFACE-THINKING

Surface thinking means believing the first thought you have on a subject without questioning it. It can also involve defending beliefs with anger because you cannot articulate reasons to support your stance. The reason you cannot articulate the reason is usually because you were taught the belief and did not question it or you were influenced by others to believe the belief.

If you cannot articulate reasons you believe what you believe it doesn't mean your beliefs are wrong. It does mean you've accepted them without examination and your brain will interpret reality as if your belief is true. This may be helpful or it may be hindering you. The only way to know I to see how it feels, use your emotional guidance.

MALADAPTIVE DETACHMENT (DISENGAGEMENT)

Disengagement is associated with higher emotional exhaustion and depersonalization.[193] Disengaged employees suffer from physical health issues that are as bad as those suffered by unemployed individuals. Their actions and behaviors can create negative effects on other members of the organization and "drain the energy" of your human capital.

Being aloof and detached and/or uncommunicative are indications of detachment. This behavioral trail is not singular. One person can have a multiplier effect on many.

DEPERSONALIZATION

Depersonalization is a form of avoidance coping and is similar to disengagement.

HIGH NEUROTICISM

"Greater stress and burnout in doctors are related to the personality trait of neuroticism or 'negative affectivity.'"[194]

Scoring high in neuroticism is associated with being more likely than average to be moody and to experience anxiety, frustration, envy, jealousy, guilt, worry, fear, anger, depressed mood, and loneliness.

Although neuroticism is commonly considered one of the Big Five personality traits, after reading this book you will understand why I place it into the unhealthy habits of thought category. You cannot understand the associations between mood/emotional states and perceptions/behavior without seeing neuroticism from a viewpoint that differs from its common conception.

"I don't know why I worry so much. If ever I got 20 patients needing a house call one day, the rest of the partners would say, look come on, we will take half of them for you, stop worrying about them. Fear of the unknown to some extent, what is going to come in and see you in the afternoon" (respondent 7, phase 2).[195]

DENIAL

Denial of negative events is associated with higher emotional exhaustion and depersonalization.[196]

CAUTIOUS (OVERLY)

Overly cautious individuals are "reluctant to take risks for fear of being rejected or negatively evaluated."[197] They may perceive attending a social function as a risky activity. Over time, being overly cautious leads to lower achievement, fewer social connections, and lower levels of well-being.

CYNICISM

Cynicism is one of three symptoms of burnout on the Maslach Burnout Inventory. It is an attitude towards others characterized by distrust of their motives. The person who is feeling cynical may focus on uninspiring reasons for actions such as ambition, materialism, and greed. They may perceive someone who has an inspiring why for their actions inaccurately and attribute them with a reason they find negative for their actions.

For example, I wrote a suicide prevention book and occasionally I offer a coupon code that allows the holder to obtain an e-book copy free of charge. There is no financial benefit to me when someone obtains my book for free. I've had individuals post online that my offer was self-serving. That is something someone who is cynical would do because they would not perceive any altruistic motives.

Cynicism is not the same as skepticism. Skepticism is open to additional knowledge. Skepticism is being unwilling to accept something as fact, yet.

Emotional guidance will guide you away from cynicism when emotions are accurately interpreted.

ADDICTIONS

Addictions begin when someone who lacks skills to feel better in healthier ways wants to dull pain or feel better.

> BEATING AN ADDICTION WITHOUT BUILDING STRESS MANAGEMENT SKILLS IS A RECIPE FOR RELAPSE AS SOON AS STRESS AND NEGATIVE EMOTIONS BECOME UNBEARABLE.

If you're addicted to drugs, alcohol, sex, shopping, or other unhealthy addictions, get help but also build your resilience and advanced coping skills. If you knew that you could avoid relapse because you had better skills, you'd be more energized about beating the addiction. As long as it feels hopeless, as if you'd relapse if your level of stress got too high, there may not seem much point. When you have skills you feel more capable of resisting relapse. You are stronger with skills.

DISTRACTIONS

Although not what I would call unhealthy, distractions do not protect against burnout. "Reading outside the field of medicine, regular exercise, and taking time for family did not demonstrate a protective effect for burnout."[198] That's not to say that exercise or family time or leisure reading don't have other benefits.

HUMOR

I'm not ready to say that humor is an unhealthy coping mechanism. It depends on how humor is used. It's not universally good or bad. In one study it was associated with higher emotional exhaustion and depersonalization.[199] Humor can be healthy and help us process information. When humor is had at others' expense, it can harm both the person being targeted and the person having fun at the person's expense because it can lead to guilt.

Where humor turns to sarcasm and negative phonics, then the individual may be masking much deeper patterns of unhealthy thinking.

DON'T GIVE UP PLEASURABLE ACTIVITIES

We've been telling people to manage their stress since the strong connection between stress and undesired physical and mental health outcomes was recognized in the 1970's. One of the early recommendations was to stop doing so much but many people found that the only activities they could give up were the ones that increased their energy—pleasurable pursuits.

Don't give up activities that:
- You look forward to doing with positive anticipation, for example:
    - Vacations
    - Reading for pleasure

- Time with friends
- Sports
- Relaxation activities
• Regularly lead you to experience time in *flow*[f], for example:
  - Gardening
  - Card games
  - Learning about something you find interesting
• That leave you feeling more energized after you participate in them, for example:
  - Exercise you enjoy
  - Lively conversations
  - Comedy
• That leave you more relaxed after you participate in them, for example:
  - Massage
  - Bubble baths
  - Love making
  - Spa treatments
  - Golfing

These examples are neither exhaustive nor intended to detail right or wrong (or good and bad) activities. We all have individual interests. The examples may not apply to you at all. Use the descriptions to make a list of activities you enjoy that fit each category.

DEVELOP HEALTHY HABITS OF THOUGHT

Interventions that enhance positive implicit valuing of emotion regulation may be beneficial. Techniques that allow individuals to experience successful emotion regulation may positively influence the value they give such regulation. Training procedures that specifically enhance cognitive reappraisal would be promising as cognitive reappraisal abilities play a distinct and important role in successful psychotherapy.[200] Researchers reported:

> Although many factors associated with lower risk of burnout were also associated with achieving a high overall quality of life, notable differences were observed, indicating surgeons' need to employ a broader repertoire of wellness promotion practices if they desire to move beyond neutral and achieve high well-being.[201]

Developing healthy habits of thought are associated with better:[202]
• Moods
• Cognitive function
• Social functioning
• Social Outcomes
• Well-being
• Quality of Life
• Thriving

You can develop healthy habits of thought by using the transformational and advanced coping skills provided in this section to increase resilience and reduce stress. There are two pathways that are best used in conjunction with one another. One is deliberately cultivating healthy habits of thought that support positive emotions. The second is paying attention to

---
[f] Flow: Flow is (review)

how you feel in response to thoughts you have and reappraising those that elicit negative emotions. Your thoughts can be the result of something you do or do not do, something that is done to you, a conversation you have, or any other life experience. Recognize that it is your thoughts about the experience and not the actual experience that creates its meaning for you.

It is important to note that stress is based on perception and that different individuals will perceive differing levels of stress in the same situation. A study that involved determining the stress levels of dental students during examinations reported that the higher level of stress perceived, the greater the risk of burnout.[203] During the past two decades an extensive body of emotion-regulation literature has been produced (over 10,000 research papers). This body of work "provides evidence that cognitive reappraisal is a powerful tool to regulate emotions."[204]

Practicing cognitive or behavioral techniques and challenging self-critical thoughts can foster optimism and self-worth.[205]

Imagine that someone is piling bricks (or monkeys) on your back all day long. If you have good coping skills you can remove most of the bricks (or monkeys) almost as soon as they land on your back. If you don't have good coping skills they stay there, wearing you down, making you tired, and eventually leads to burnout.

Note about microaggressions: Instead of imaging bricks, imagine fishing weights, lots of small fishing weights.

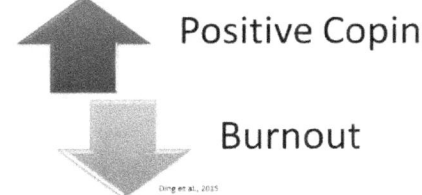

In a survey of the wellness promotion practices of primary care physicians, those who used wellness practices had greater psychological well-being. Those who developed an approach to life that minimized their stress levels had significantly higher levels of psychological well-being.[206]

The strategies shared in the following pages will assist you in developing a strategy toward life of your choosing that helps you restore and maintain psychological health. We do not attempt to tell you what to think, only to help you understand the impact of your thoughts on your well-being. The approach you choose can co-exist with any spiritual or religious practices you already practice.

Categories that have been associated with physician well-being include:

- Self-awareness
- Being positive
- Sharing of feelings
- Setting limits
- Self-acceptance
- Personal Growth
- Purpose
- Work-Life Balance
- Self-care
- Taking vacations
- Exercise
- Hobbies
- Positive self-regard
- Being in healthy relationships
- Leaving unhealthy relationships
- Pursuing and achieving goals
- Having a spiritual or religious belief system
- Developing a personal philosophy
- Reading inspirational materials
- Getting professional help when/if needed
- Avoiding drugs and alcohol
- Learning new skills
- Mindfulness
- Meditation
- Perceiving health as more than the absence of disease (wellness model)

How many of the above do you regularly do? Making small improvements many times makes a tremendous difference in the long-term results.

Shifts in one's approach to life can be very simple. I've seen many people quickly shift aspects of their approach to life after hearing an alternate view that resonates with them a single time. It is as if we become stuck in a paradigm that life is a certain way when the reality is that each of us perceives life from a unique self-created paradigm. Because we believe our paradigm is reality we don't question it. When we learn someone else uses a different paradigm and it shifts the events of our life into new patterns that make more sense, we can quickly adopt a different worldview.

The brain seems to have an amazing ability to shift the puzzle pieces when we change our viewpoint. Many significant improvements I've seen have resulted from a series of smaller changes.

Self-efficacy
Hope
Resilience
Optimism

Each characteristic (skill) is negatively related to each burnout symptom

Emotional Exhaustion
Depersonalization
Reduced Personal Accomplishment

(Ding, et al., 2015)

Approaching the information with an open mind that is willing to consider alternative viewpoints with the condition that anything that doesn't feel right can be rejected elicits the best results. In my own journey I initially rejected some ideas and came back to them later after I'd shifted in other areas and found that I was able to discard old, ingrained ideas that were factually wrong but had been strongly believed for decades.

When you consider that much of our worldview was established by age 10 it makes sense to consider alternatives from an adult perspective and make conscious decisions about what is in our best interest and what may be limiting our psychological well-being and success.

Burnout risk can be lowered using many different approaches.

RESPOND PROACTIVELY TO EMOTIONS

This is where conscious emotion regulation is applied. The first tool you need to be good at doing this is The Pause. The Pause is inserted between your initial experience of an emotion and taking action. If an emotion feels good you generally don't need a pause. However, there are short-term actions that are inconsistent with your long-term goals. In those types of situations The Pause can be applied to consider long-term goals in relationship to short-term pleasure.

The Pause can help you make good decisions about what you eat, keeping your promises, and avoiding risky behaviors. The more attention you give to your goals ahead of time the less you'll need to consider using The Pause in tempting situations.

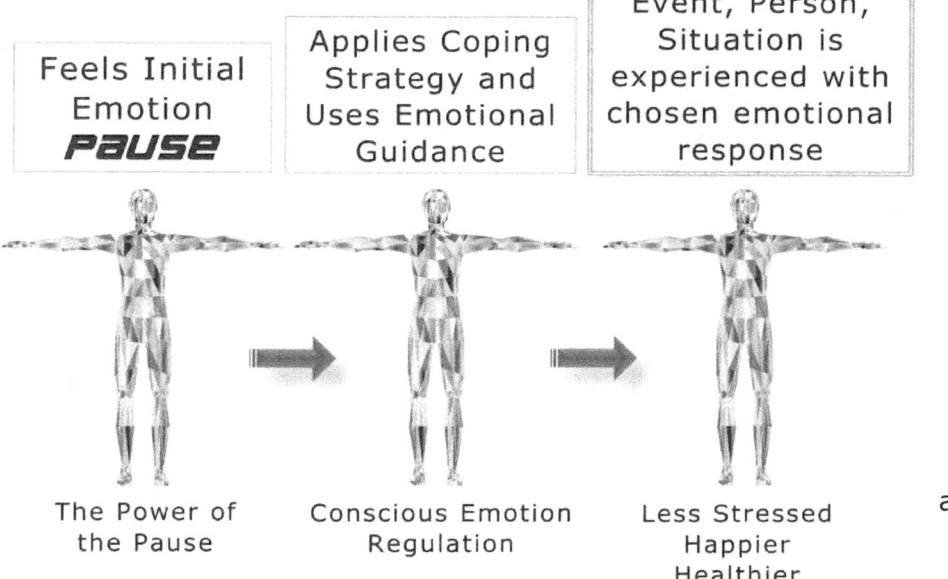

The Power of the Pause — Conscious Emotion Regulation — Less Stressed Happier Healthier

The Pause provides time between feeling negative emotion and acting on the negative emotion during which you can make better choices. You can reappraise the thoughts that led to the emotion and chose one that feels better. You can also consider the consequences of the choices available to you.

Taking a deep breath, or two or three, can help you think better during The Pause. Your pause may help you identify upstream beliefs you want to change so that your future automatic (unconscious) evaluation of situations is less stressful.

OPTIMISM

Most importantly, optimism is not a fixed element of personality. Optimistic attitudes are created and sustained by an individual's habits of thought which often echo those around them and especially those who were around them when they were young.

Optimism can be developed by changing underlying beliefs and habits of thought. Optimism is associated with better life outcomes in health, relationships, career, and longevity. There are many aspects that affect these outcomes but the decreased stress and stronger social connections experienced by someone who has a positive mental attitude is a significant factor.

An individual may be optimistic in every area of life or in selected areas. Optimists tend to focus more on solutions and what they can do than on problems. In the Resilience section of this book, the habits of resilient and less resilient individuals were compared. Many of the resilient habits of thought in that chart reflect optimistic attitudes. Optimism is a key component of resilience.

Optimists may:
- Be more likely to trust other people
- Believe that there is a way forward
- Feel hope or trust that things will work out well
- Believe the world is good
- Believe people are innately good although they sometimes do bad things

Optimist's lives often reflect their beliefs about life. Positive mental attitudes result in interpreting experiences in a positive light. Where an optimist sees an opportunity a pessimist sees a problem. Both optimists and pessimists live in self-fulfilling prophesies.

Optimists will find the silver lining in adversities. Optimists experience less stress and more positive emotions than pessimists. Optimists feel more empowered when they face difficulties which lowers the amount of stress they experience. Meta-analyses link optimism to more engagement coping.[207]

COGNITIVE RESTRUCTURING

Cognitive restructuring is the process of identifying habits of thought that increase stress or interfere with optimal functioning. Previous methods of cognitive restructuring were often labor intensive and, in many cases, required a therapist. With an understanding of the new definition of the purpose and use of emotions, the process becomes easier and immediate feedback from our emotions is understood.

We think a thought, recognize the way we feel when we think that thought is not the way we want to feel (feels bad) and know that the negative emotion means the thought is not the best thought we can think about the subject we are thinking about.

That's really a big deal. In the therapy model, the therapist doesn't know how you feel unless you explain it and even then, some of it is lost in translation. Using emotional guidance provides immediate feedback 24/7/365.

IT'S BOGUS

One of my favorite processes is what I call Bogus. When I think a thought that evokes

> *We want to make it clear that we are not advising people who need the help of a therapist not to seek the help they need. Therapy can be a life-changing process. We are pointing out that understanding emotional guidance empowers individuals with knowledge and skills that make it more likely they can make substantive progress on their own. We have seen situations where individuals who have been in and out of therapy for decades without being cured become symptom free for a decade after learning The Smart Way™.*

enough negative emotion that I pause to examine what I am thinking and why, I can often eliminate the hold the thought has on me be declaring it Bogus.

One of the reasons I can quickly and easily declare limiting thoughts as Bogus is because I deliberately collect evidence that supports empowered thoughts. I look for examples of aging that are empowering. I look for examples of women who are strong and successful. I look for examples of people who have done things I want to do. Paying attention to these examples is fun. It makes my world feel both bigger and safer. These days it is usually not my own thoughts but things others' want to convince me to believe that evoke the Bogus process. Many people have cognitive biases about subjects that I don't want to adopt as my own. I don't have to convince them that their beliefs are wrong but I do want to protect myself from adopting their beliefs and making them become self-fulfilling prophesies.

USE SCIENCE AND EXPERIENCE TO SUPPORT YOURSELF

Whether it is my belief or someone else's, I evaluate it by identifying the thought that feels better and then looking for evidence that the thought I want to believe is valid and for evidence that the thought I don't want to believe is not valid. I use emotional guidance but I also use science and experience to inform my opinion.

If you are going through a tough situation and feel isolated and alone, as if no one has ever endured what you are enduring, you can look for evidence of others who had similar, or worse, experiences to assure yourself that humans are very capable of adapting and growing during adversity.

Our world is full of inspirational individuals who have survived and thrived in spite of adversity. Unfortunately, our society tends to put them on a pedestal which makes us think they have something ordinary mortals don't have but they don't. We all have great potential within us. Believing we can makes a tremendous difference.

IF EVERYONE . . .

Another process I use to determine if thoughts make sense is carry it out in my mind as if the entire world adopted the thought. What would the world look like? Would it be good or bad? Better or worse than what we have now? This process has led to a far greater appreciation of diversity of all kinds, including diversity of thought than I had before I began using this framework to evaluate ideas.

WORDS MATTER

There are several words and types of statements that I resist using and encourage others to recognize and not use. Ought, Should, Must, Always, Can't, and Never frequently point to beliefs that may increase stress or lead to self-criticism. Definitive statements are another sign. "I'm not good at X" is an example of a statement I would challenge. The challenge is not the opposite; the challenge changes the statement to one that is recording a current event that does not necessarily reflect the future. "I'm not good at X, yet" leaves the door open to change your relationship with X.

BE FLEXIBLE

Don't accept the first thought you think about a subject as the truth. If it feels bad when you think it, it probably isn't your truth. Recognize that we all have cognitive distortions. For example, if a democrat thinks a democratic leader made a statement they will agree with it but if the same statement is reported as being said by a republican leader they object to the statement. It's not just democrats; republicans do the same in reverse.

Don't accept the first thought you think about a subject, especially if it causes negative emotion, which is an indicator that you're stressed by the thought.

When it comes to death I spent a long time coming back to my beliefs and comparing them to the emotions they evoked until I found a worldview that comforted me on the subject of death. I mention this not to convince you of any particular worldview but because people often say things like, "Well, death always feels bad so emotions that feel bad can't mean I'm looking at it in a way that doesn't serve me." Don't start with the biggest things. Use emotional guidance in areas where it is easy and work toward bigger subjects.

TRUST YOUR GUIDANCE

Cognitive dissonance is not a reason to beat yourself up. We all created worldviews as children and have added to them ever since. We don't teach children how to consciously construct worldviews that are healthy. Our society leaves it to chance. Discovering that your beliefs or worldviews could use some help is good news because changing them will make your life feel better.

ADJUST YOUR FOCUS

If you tend to look for your flaws, re-focus so that you pay attention to your strengths and successes. If you tend to look for other people's flaws, begin looking at their strengths and potential. If you're worried about what other people will think about you, focus on what you have in common with them.

Adjusting your focus can be fun. Play with it in the privacy of your mind.

GIVE YOURSELF CREDIT WHERE IT IS DUE

Many people discount their good deeds. Recognize the good in you. If you find yourself responding to a thank you with "It was nothing" you're discounting your goodness. This is an indicator that you're negatively distorting your value and worth.

LABELS

Labels take us a step further from clarity. Our society loves to label and classify but as soon as we slap a label on something we have distorted it and reduced clarity. As far as I can tell, nearly everything in our world exists along a continuum and when you use a label that does not consider the continuum, the solutions are lost. For example, burnout exists along a continuum that begins with stress and moves to chronic stress and then on to burnout. We can widen the continuum and see the distorted thinking that led to stress. The label Burnout states what is but not how it arrived or how to heal it. For the whole path to be visible one must look at the continuum.

Labels can also trap us into boxes. To many people, the label *Adult* implies that one must act mature. Playful activities that adults would enjoy are eschewed to reinforce the perception that one is a responsible adult. Yet it is possible to be a responsible adult and still play tag with your neighbors after dinner. How much more fun would that be than going to the gym and running on a treadmill?

We don't have to accept labels we don't like and we don't have to accept the limits labels would place upon us. I work with a young woman whose community bullied her because they didn't think she conformed to the racial label they put on her enough to suit them. Why would anyone willingly accept a label that tells you that you can't do things you want to do?

We will never be free to be who we are until we allow others to be who they want to be. When people aren't boxed into corners and slapped with labels that are confining they are happier and happier people treat other people better.

REFRAMING

Re-framing is one form of cognitive restructuring. I usually write about re-framing in connection with perceptions of failure. Failures can be perceived as meaning we are not good enough or failures or they can be perceived as opportunities to learn and begin again with more knowledge. Defining ourself as a failure hinders our ability to be successful in the future. Re-framing experiences as learning opportunities prepares us for greater success in the future.

Re-framing can be applied to other areas. Compare the following statements:

1. "Doctors are exposed to high levels of stress in the course of their profession and are particularly susceptible to experiencing burnout."[208]

2. Doctors are exposed to high levels of potential stressors in the course of their profession which can make them particularly susceptible to experiencing burnout.

In Statement #1, the doctor is passive and stress is something active that the physician encounters during the course of his or her work. This active agent (stress) is a threat to the physician's well-being.

In Statement #2, stress is a potential outcome. Stress is optional and may pose a threat.

Statement #2 by itself changes nothing but when physicians are taught healthy habits of thought, they are empowered to take the lower stress option by perceiving the potential stressors in low or no-stress ways which then decreases the risk of burnout.

The scientific community frequently writes about humans as if we are mechanical. If A happens, we can expect B. We know that this is not true. Not all oncologists or ER doctors experience burnout. The difference is the way they process and perceive data and professional experience. Physicians who specialize in areas where death of a patient is possible need resilience skills which are considerably different than a provider who works in a more benign specialty.

As an example, if a physician begins doubting themselves and thinks, "I'm not tough enough to handle this situation" they can use their emotional guidance to help them reframe the situation. If they've practiced with their guidance they will be reassured when they try other thoughts out and those thoughts feel better. Once an individual pays attention to their guidance for a few weeks they will be reassured when they counter this disempowering thought with, "I can find a way to handle this situation and grow in the process. I'm looking forward to seeing who I become as the result of this challenge."

POSITIVE AFFIRMATIONS

Positive affirmations are positive statements that affirm or attempt to train an individual toward a more positive mental attitude. They are useful when used correctly.

Positive self-affirmations can speed emotional recovery from slights others make toward you, including racial or gender related comments or actions. These can help employees recover from perceived stereotype threats.[209]

Positive affirmations can increase our confidence.

Positive affirmations can boost self-esteem and self-image.

A well-known affirmation that originated on Saturday Night Live is:

I'm Good Enough, I'm Smart Enough, and Doggone It, People Like Me!

Affirmations can cover any area of life, relationships, health, career, and even fun.

I love the wisdom of my body. Every cell knows what to do and does it well.

The right words come to me at the right time.

I am wise.

I am young and beautiful.

I know what to do.

I am loved.

I have the skills and knowledge I need to succeed.

My timing will be perfect today and I will make people laugh.

My emotions guide me toward my goals.

People like me because I like people.

I will do my best to see the potential in others.

I am kind.

I am love.

I am a sought after and valued employee.

I am the director of my life.

The keys to successful affirmations are to not reach too far. If you say an affirmation, in the privacy of your mind or out loud, and your mind responds by arguing with the statement you made you've attempted to reach too far. It isn't that you won't be able to get to where you want to be, you just need to take smaller steps.

For example, if the statement that you're good enough receives backlash be more specific and affirm that you're good at something specific. Once you get your mind thinking about one thing it doesn't argue about that you're good with, other thoughts will come to you.

Don't keep trying an affirmation if you get backlash. Take a smaller step. If you keep trying the arguing that happens in your mind will make your current belief (the one your mind is arguing to protect) more established and it will be more difficult to change.

The other aspect that can arise subtly is a sense of fear or lack of safety. If you're affirming, *I am safe*, but you feel unsafe as you say it the affirmation heightens your fear. Rather than your mind arguing you may simply feel the fear in sensations in your body. If you are in a safe situation, or a situation where you should be safe, use logic to increase your sense of safety. Think about the aspects of your situation that should keep you safe. If you aren't safe, it is time to take (or, at a minimum, plan) any actions you can take to get safe.

Affirmations won't keep you safe if you make unsafe choices.

REAPPRAISAL (RIGHT RESPONSE)

Reappraisal is when you apply strategies to change the thoughts you are thinking that elicit an emotion that feels bad to you. For example, you left $100 on your dresser when you left for work and when you come home it is gone. Your first thoughts may be that someone came into your room and took your money or that someone in your home took it. None of these thoughts would feel good. During reappraisal you can decide to ask the people who live in your home if they took it. You can check to see that the doors and windows are secure.

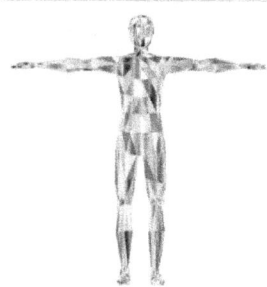

Conscious Emotion Regulation

There are many reasons the money may not be where you left it. Your partner may have put it away for safe-keeping because they didn't like it being visible. You may have forgotten to give your son money to buy the equipment he needs when soccer practice begins tomorrow and he took it to buy things he needed that you were going to buy for him. In this instance, leaving the money where he could get it when he needed it was what I refer to as a happy accident. The cat may have knocked it onto the floor and it is under the dresser.

If you don't reappraise, the attitude you bring to the conversation with others in your home may be accusatory which is not likely to turn out well. Giving people the benefit of the doubt will usually lead to a more positive emotional response.

If you're feeling intense negative emotion, you're being very specific. If you look for thoughts that are more general, you'll be able to feel better.

If you're thoughts are generally negative you may be able to find a generally positive thought that you can use. Generally positive thoughts can be very general.

I don't have to figure this out today.

I can deal with this tomorrow.

I'll figure this out, eventually.

This is not bigger than me.

Other people have dealt with things like this and found a way.

Another helpful process is to think about a camera lens. If you're feeling negative emotion

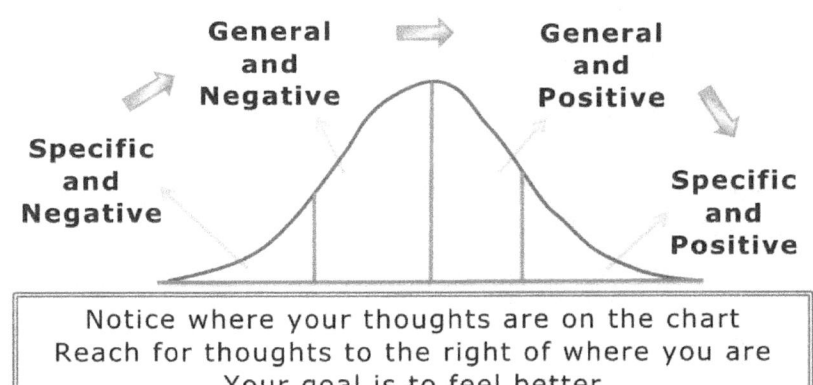

you're zoomed in on a flaw. If you zoom out to a larger perspective you'll be able to see the thing that feels bad from a different perspective.

Pivot 180^0 when you recognize what you don't want. Tell yourself that you can decide what you do want if you know what you don't want. Ask yourself:

What do I want?

Remind yourself emotions are temporary responses to thoughts and that as soon as you find different thoughts you can feel better.

PLANNING

Planning in advance is helpful. Several ways you can plan to reduce stress and increase success in advance include:

- Setting long-term goals
- Establishing mission statements for every area of your life
- Setting your intentions about what you want from your activities
- Plan to avoid temptations

For example, when someone is stressed they sometimes watch television shows for hours on end or surf the internet with the result they don't go to bed when they should. If they set a timer that will require them to get up or be continually irritated, it can serve as the nudge they need to take the action they intend.

Another example is tequila. I like the way I feel when I drink tequila but I don't like what it does to my inhibitions. I made a rule for myself that I can only drink tequila when I am with my husband. If he's not with me, I don't drink tequila.

The first time I found myself living alone as a single adult, I sat down and made a list of rules for myself. Making your own rules, ones that support your long-term goals, is very different from someone else imposing rules on you. I set curfews based on which day of the week it was that helped me fulfill my long term goal to complete my education while maintaining my reputation as a reliable employee in my full-time job.

When you're at a party and you tell people you have to get home because you have a curfew few will ask you who set the curfew.

Complying with your own rules feels completely different than adhering to rules someone else set.

Establishing our intentions is setting micro goals. Before a meeting I might set the intention that I'll have the right words at the right time. In many ways, setting intentions are situation specific affirmations made as the activity begins.

Mission statements are discussed elsewhere in this book.

Establishing clear, long-term goals helps you see the progress you're making which can contribute to your sense of accomplishment. Establishing 1, 5, 10, and 20 year plans, with as much detail as feels good and no detail that feels forced, works well. You always have the option to change your plan if your interests change.

RE-DEFINE YOUR BEST

Your best in any given moment is not your best possible. Accept this. Your best in this moment depends on many variables. You can structure your life and make commitments that will increase *your best in this moment* but you cannot always be at your best. Some of us are better in the morning. Some of us are better in the afternoon. We can't call in because we didn't get a good night's sleep—although our society should consider this acceptable in some situations. For example, if my surgeon had a hoot owl outside her window keeping her awake most of the night I would prefer she call out or come in but reschedule the surgery rather than proceed when science says she won't be at her best. I won't reiterate the negative impact of stress on performance, but it applies here as well.

Nutrition, hunger, thirst, illness, hanger,[9] emotional upset and more can make our *best in this moment* less than our best possible ever but <u>*in that moment* it is your best possible</u>.

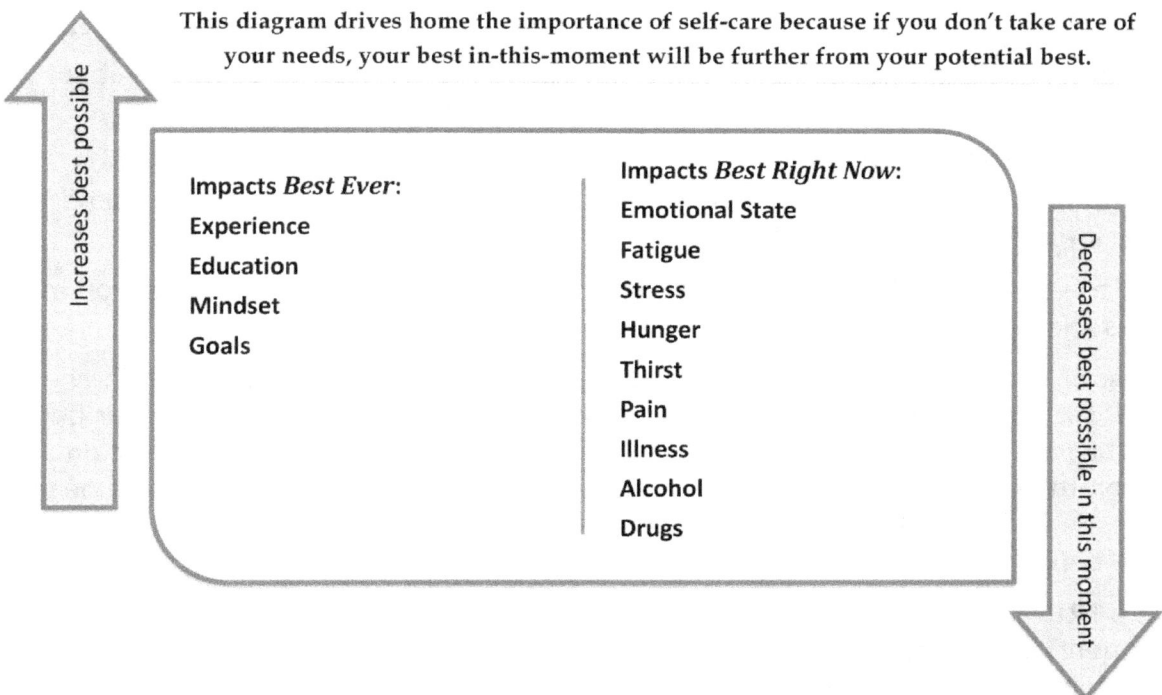

This is an important concept. It's important in deciding what to do right now because your best potential in this moment should be considered. For example, not having a discussion with someone when you're upset is a good decision, if it can wait. The outcome won't be as good as it would be if your emotional state was better if all else is equal. Also consider the other person's emotional state. If you've ever been in a disagreement with someone who became upset and you insisted on continuing the discussion you know it probably would have been better to wait.

My husband and I have a general agreement that whoever is in the better emotional state drives. However, when the person in the better emotional state is ill or tired, we shift the rule to allow the one who has fewer negative effects to drive at that point in time.

The key is to plan in advance, to the extent possible, to have as few negative hits on one's best in the moment and as many positive as we are inspired to have in the best ever category. The better our best potential is, the better we will be even if we have some hits to our best.

For example, I've been using *The Smart Way*™ for ten years. It is rare for me to be in a bad emotional state. I've developed expertise in keeping my emotional state up so that even in situations where someone who doesn't have that skill is experiencing fewer stressors, I'm usually in a better emotional state.

In most cases, a physician with decades of experience in his specialty will be a better diagnostician than a 1st year resident even if the more mature physician is experiencing

---

[9] Hanger is anger largely attributable to hunger

moderate pain, hunger, or fatigue. Increase the pain level and the 1st year resident may do a better job. It's an art, not an exact science. Understanding the relationships is more important than being precise. The understanding should be considered when deciding what your limits are in that moment.

If you blunder into your day without considering factors that may limit your best in that moment you are more likely to make mistakes and you're more likely to feel guilty about those mistakes because you will recognize that you could have done better.

Guilt doesn't help. It is an indicator of a pretty high level of stress and often leads to maladaptive (unhealthy) methods of stress relief. Commit to doing better next time and to consider your in-that-moment limitations.

Give yourself the benefit of the doubt. Realize that your best in-the-moment when you made a mistake was the best you could do in-that-moment.

Review the list of items that most frequently have a negative impact on one's best in one moment. You will probably find at least one reason you weren't capable of doing your best ever potential every time that you ever made a mistake. You did the best you could do at that time given the circumstances. You are human. Your body, mind, and spirit have needs and when those needs aren't met you can't be at your best. You are human. You aren't a machine. The benefits of your humanity far outweigh the occasional downsides.

Think about a DUI. Someone whose blood alcohol level is .03 is legal to drive but they have some impairment. The higher the blood alcohol level goes, the greater the impairment. Strong and resilient people may function okay with two or even three of the seven (low emotional state, fatigue, stress, hunger, thirst, pain, illness) but add a fourth and their performance will surely suffer. Learn your limitations and set your own rules.

I teach a class at a psycho-social rehabilitation agency where I'll often have sixty individuals with various degrees of behavioral challenges and thinking, many of whom are recovering from addictions and abuse. I cannot help them when I'm tired or a little under the weather. I make a point to eat before I go and stay hydrated. In a group like that you never know what you may encounter. One day I arrived and almost immediately put my lesson plan aside because one of the women in the class said she was in crisis (suicidal). I encouraged her to spend some one-on-one time with an available counselor but she refused stating, "I want to know what you can do for me in this situation." So I spent the next hour and a half working to bring her to a more stable emotional state in front of a fairly large audience. At first, the audience watched but in time, several of them helped by sharing their own stories. Months later she gave me a verbal testimonial that you can hear on my YouTube Channel (Jeanine Joy) with the title, *Solutions for Social Problems*. Her testimonial begins at about 16:40 into the video. I shudder to think what might have happened if I hadn't had breakfast. It was a challenging situation with not just the life of a young woman on the line, but also her child's future which would be irrevocably changed if she ended her life.

On my way to class I use the commute to get myself into as positive an emotional state as possible. I think about the people I'll be seeing and see the potential inherent within them to help me inspire them to fulfill more of their potential. I allow myself to love and care about them but not to take responsibility for their choices. They're adults and are responsible for their choices.

In the same way, a physician could think about the patients that will come for healing that day and see their potential for health, the wisdom of their bodies, and care about them without taking responsibility beyond offering his or her best possible at the moment in time when they meet one another.

The dividing line between caring and taking responsibility is very narrow but it has to be a clear line to preserve our own health and well-being.

No one decides "I could do a better job but I feel like messing up instead of doing my best." Even if it looks like someone is doing that, for example, seemingly asking to be fired, they are doing their best but their goal is not the goal others want them to have. Maybe they want to leave the job but are being pressured to stay or are staying out of guilt at what they'd give up for their family if they left so they self-sabotage.

If you've made a mistake, the takeaway should be to do better in the future which means consider factors that may keep you from doing your best and manage them to the best of your ability, which can include increasing your ability to manage them. That could be building your resilience, your ability to manage your emotional state, going to bed earlier, eating regularly, etc.

POSITIVE REFRAMING

Positive reframing is a powerful tool. It takes something undesired and finds a positive aspect to it and chooses to focus on that positive aspect. This can feel like an impossible task if you've never done it. With practice your mind will begin looking for the silver lining in the first moment that an undesired situation comes about.

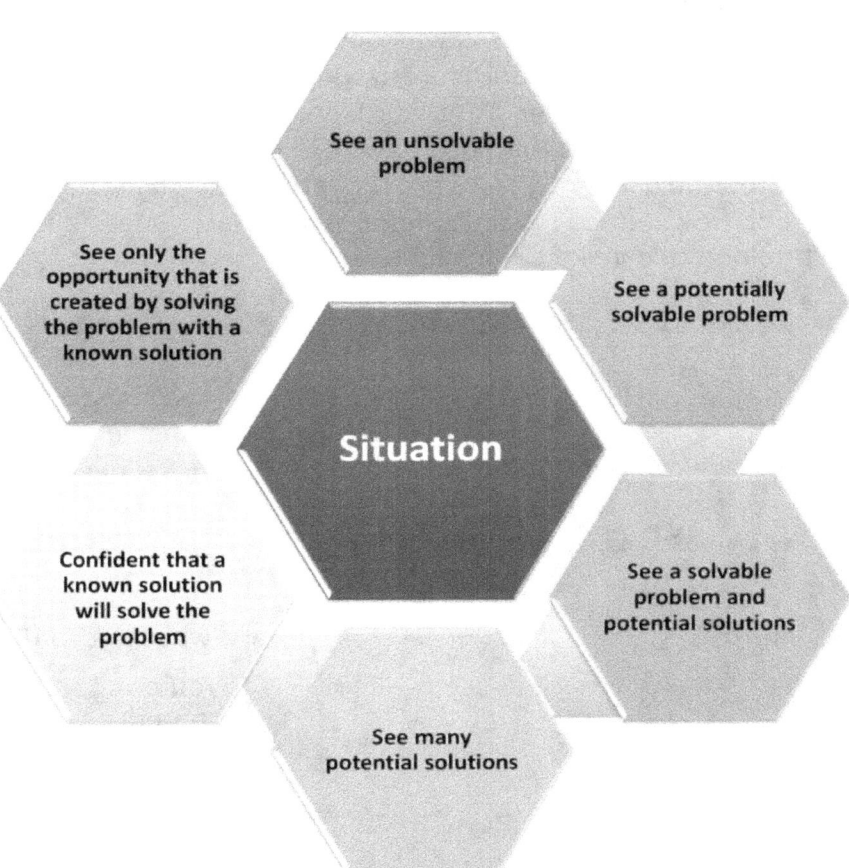

After applying *The Smart Way*™ to the way I live my life, I realized that where I would have once perceived an unsolvable problem I began seeing the potential to solve problems. The way my mind perceived situations I encountered gradually shifted until my first automatic response was focused on the opportunities the situation provided. It didn't mean I reveled in the problem but once the problem exists it is best to make the most of it. Given a choice, we would never choose the gift if it meant we would have to choose the situation that gives rise to it. But once the situation occurs we don't have a choice about whether it will happen. Our only choice is our response to it.

In reality, all the perspectives on the illustration exist. They are always there. Inspiration is being able to see the best possible perspective and helping others move to more empowered perspectives (closer to the best possible perspective).

Some people refer to the silver lining as gifts in the wound. I have come to believe that there are always gifts in the wound. When we lost Prince (The Artist) to opioid overdose the conversation changed. No longer were opioids a problem of nameless, faceless addicts. Now the problem has the face of someone the world loved and mourns.

When we lost Robin Williams to suicide I was days away from publishing my second book, *Prevent Suicide: The Smart Way*™. I held off on publishing it because I felt the world was too raw and felt some guilt that I hadn't written it sooner because then maybe I could have saved the national treasure that Robin Williams was from such a lonely and senseless demise. But his death breathed renewed life into the campaign to end stigma and to find solutions that will stop the loss of lives to suicide.

We wouldn't have chosen these situations but once they are here we must embrace the gifts they bring if we want to feel as good as we are capable of feeling.

A friend of mine lost his daughter last year, 10 years past the age he was initially told to expect her to survive. The loss was devastating to him but at the same time he can be grateful for the advances and hard work of the medical community that gave both of them those extra years together. Afterwards he realized that he had been under constant stress wondering if this trip to the hospital would be the last and that he might have enjoyed her even more if he'd worried less. It's too late to face her challenges differently but he can help others and he can face his own and his wife's later years differently than he would have if he hadn't gained this insight.

LOOK FOR SILVER LINING

In the spirit of,

If life gives you lemons, make lemonade

Situation	**Potential Silver Lining**
Make a mistake	Learn what not to do • If you don't, it is very unlikely it will be repeated • What led to it; avoid that in the future • Share what you've learned and help others avoid the same mistake • After a mistake you're better than you were before the mistake because you've learned something you didn't know
End of a relationship	Opportunity for someone better to enter your life
Disability	Opportunity to help/inspire others • Christopher Reeve • Sujit K. Reddy (empowerment speaker

	born with spina bifida)
	• Jon Morrow (can only move his eyes and mouth – inspirational writer)
Death of a child	Make it meaningful
	• Dr. Darren R. Weissman (inspirational author)
	• Candy Lightner (founded MADD)
Being fired	Find a job better suited to your skills and talents, which may mean a better job that you find more satisfying.
Being laid off	Find a job that you've grown into but wouldn't have looked for without the motivation of a lay-off.
	An opportunity to ask yourself, "What do I want to do?"
Being abused	Opportunity to realize how strong you are and to help others realize the same.

SAVORING

Wiki does a great job defining savoring in the way it is intended here:

> *Savoring is the use of thoughts and actions to increase the intensity, duration, and appreciation of positive experiences and emotions.*

Anything you enjoy can be savored. It can be the present moment. An example is mindfully savoring the fresh berries you're eating. It can be savoring a treasured memory from your past. It can be savoring a feeling, like confidence. It can be savoring anticipation of a future experience.

Savoring is deliberately choosing to think about thoughts that feel good to you and especially thoughts that do not evoke a downside. Remembering pleasurable experiences with a mate who is no longer in your life is fine if you can do it without the bitter-sweetness of the relationship being over creeping into your mind. If you can find a stance that appreciates that you had those experiences, your past becomes a treasure trove of memories to savor.

Think of savoring as something comprised of pure pleasure. There is no attention to lack when you savor. You don't wish you were elsewhere or with someone else, in a body that feels or looks better, in a different place. You appreciate what you are thinking about fully.

As long as it brings you to a feeling of pure appreciation you can savor the same thing repeatedly. If it stops feeling uplifting, savor something else. One of the things I like to savor is *Happy Places* I've created in my mind. One of my *Happy Places* is a yacht with a full crew that I use to sail around the world, always in warm locations. I do different things in this *Happy Places*. Sometimes I just enjoy the rocking of the boat as I bask in the sun. Other times I have imaginary conversations with people I love and sometimes with people

I'd like to meet. Sometimes I fish. When I go to my *Happy Places* I can do anything I want. It's an especially wonderful place to go when your body is having a root canal.

Because we now know that sustained positive emotions "predict physical heath, including lower levels of the stress hormone cortisol"[210] you can enjoy your savoring without feeling you should be doing something more productive. Savoring is good for you.

You can also plan your life so that you always have something you are looking forward to that you can savor before you do it. I love to travel and usually plan my trips well ahead of time. One time I decided to go on a cruise just six weeks before it sailed. Afterwards I noticed that I didn't get to enjoy the cruise before the cruise. Normally I spend time savoring a trip before the actual trip. After noticing a big difference I decided to plan my trips further in advance and to spend time savoring trips I intend to take but haven't booked yet.

If you make a habit of using your commute time to savor the aspects of your day that you enjoyed and connect it to your why, your work will feel more meaningful and enriched which protects against burnout.

You know savoring is working if you feel good while you're savoring. Have fun with it.

CORE SELF-EVALUATIONS (CSE)

Core self-evaluations is a high-level construct that includes self-esteem but also one's ability to perform one's job, skills, etc. Individuals with healthy core self-evaluations tend to have:
- Healthy self-esteem
- An Internal Locus of Control
- Low neuroticism
- Generally good self-efficacy beliefs

High core self-evaluations are positively associated with employee engagement. Nurses with higher self-evaluations experienced fewer symptoms of burnout.[211] Your emotional guidance will support healthy self-efficacy beliefs and the development of new skills.

STRENGTHS

Everyone has character strengths and areas where we are not so strong. Find, recognize, and embrace your strengths.

1. Wisdom and Knowledge: creativity, curiosity, judgment, love of learning, perspective
2. Courage: bravery, perseverance, honesty, zest
3. Humanity: love, kindness, social intelligence
4. Justice: teamwork, fairness, leadership
5. Temperance: forgiveness, humility, prudence, self-regulation
6. Transcendence: appreciation of beauty and excellence, gratitude, hope, humor, spirituality[212]

HEALTHY SELF-ESTEEM

Self-esteem reflects the beliefs you've developed about yourself, about your self-worth and value, about your goodness, about your lovability or desirability, about your intelligence, and you capability.

Do you like yourself?

Do you have the right to be happy?

If you're not in a relationship do you feel incomplete?

Do you deflect compliments?

Do you hold back from doing things you want to do out of fear of rejection?

Do you feel like an imposter waiting for people to figure out you don't deserve what you've achieved professionally, in relationships, or financially?

Do you struggle taking criticism?

Do you apologize frequently for things that you don't need to apologize for?

Can you accept a compliment?

Do you make decisions based on what you believe will appeal to others or get their approval instead of what pleases you?

Do you avoid arguments and disagreements by suppressing your needs and feelings?

Can you comfortably walk up to a stranger and introduce yourself?

Do you embellish the truth about yourself in an attempt to project an image you hope others will deem is good enough?

Do you act as if your opinions matter?

Can you choose where you want to eat or do you always defer to others?

Do you seem to need more sleep than others?

Do you take care of your body because you're worth it?

Do you take care of your body because others' opinions of your body matter to you?

Do you share meaningful details of your life with friends?

Do you believe people will like you if they know the real you?

Do you try to make yourself small or wish you could disappear or run away when you have a negative emotional experience with someone you care about?

Can you stand in front of a mirror, look yourself in the eyes, and tell yourself:

- *I am good*
- *I am wise*
- *I love you*

Do good things happen in your life because you prepare for opportunities so you're ready when they appear?

This section is lengthy because it is important. Every area of your life is affected by your beliefs about yourself. There is an infinite variety of undesired manifestations that occur in the lives of people who have low self-esteem that can be stopped by increasing their self-esteem. Healthy self-esteem does not seek to be better than anyone else. Healthy self-esteem is about feeling worthy and being of value for being the unique being that is you.

Self-esteem seldom reflects the reality of an individual. We are often taught to form our beliefs about ourself from the opinions of others so I'll start there. We've already talked about how our perceptions vary as the result of our emotional state when we perceive. If I meet someone when I am feeling insecure I might perceive them as someone who feels superior to others. If I meet someone when I am in a state of appreciation my mind will find and focus on aspects of them that I appreciate. We connect emotionally. That's why we love stories so much.

So if you were raised around people who were often angry or frustrated or afraid it is unlikely they focused on your strengths and helped you see them. It is likely they focused on aspects of you that matched their emotional state and that formed their opinion of you. Other people's opinions of you are, to a very large degree, a reflection of their emotional state when you interacted with them. That's one of the reasons charming, charismatic people are so well loved. They *charm* people into feeling better than they usually feel which makes the person grateful.

The thing is you can't charm someone into feeling better if you're feeling bad. Feeling good when you have low self-esteem can feel like climbing Mt. Everest and you can't stay at the peak for long.

When you really begin seeing that others' opinions reflect their emotional state you'll give them less control over how you feel about you. It isn't that others' opinions don't matter. It isn't about disrespecting them. It's about understanding where they are emotionally and the relationship between their opinion and their emotional state. It takes the sting out of harsh words. Once you understand this relationship, you can look back at things that formed your self-esteem and re-frame them as reflections that someone you interacted with didn't feel good instead of being a basis for your self-esteem.

You don't have to go back at all. You can begin where you are and move forward but if there are memories that haunt you or hurt you that you still think about often, re-framing them changes the way they feel.

When you truly get it that other people's opinions and words reflect their emotional state, your ability to hear them out grows. There is no need to defend yourself because even if they are talking about you, they are really demonstrating their emotional state and practiced habits of thought. This doesn't mean you never again listen to constructive criticism. Seeing yourself as someone who is always learning and growing makes you want to become better. What happens is someone provides you feedback and you evaluate it in a different way. Instead of criticizing yourself for not being perfect, evaluate the information using critical thinking. Is there a grain of truth in the comments? Is it something you want to change about yourself?

For example, my pubic speaking and my writing are two areas where I want to be the best I can be. If someone tells me that I could do either of those things better, I am all ears, but not as criticism of what I've done. I am all ears to pick up any nuggets of information that will make me even better. For example, several people who provided feedback on my first five books made comments along the lines of "They contain very useful information but there is so much science they are heavy reads." I now feel satisfied that I have documented much of the science that supports my work in those earlier books and am now honing my craft in writing books that are easier to read. I want this information to reach a lot of people so it's important that they are as good as they can be. I am not seeking perfection. They'd never get published and never help anyone if I waited for perfection. I don't even care about them standing the test of time in the way a classic novel can because the information shared in these pages should become common knowledge. If people still have to undo unhealthy thoughts society taught them a hundred years from now it will mean I failed to get this information to enough people to make healthy habits of thought normal.

An attitude toward your life, relationships, and work that goes along these lines, "I've always done the best I could but I will always have room to learn and become better" would serve you well.

The motivation of someone who criticizes you can run the gamut from someone who is miserable and gains a tiny bit of pleasure by making others miserable to someone who values your work but recognized that a slight change will help you accomplish your goals easier, faster, or better. If you take others opinions as information that you can accept or reject, the miserable person won't be able to make you feel bad. In fact, if there is a grain of truth that gives you an idea to improve in what is said, the person attempting to make you miserable may actually make you happy that you now have one more tool in your toolkit that makes you better.

You could even feel empathy for the miserable person because the tiny bit of pleasure someone attains by making someone else feel worse is nothing when compared to the enormous pleasure possible when we uplift others. These affirmations may be helpful to you.

I am good as I am, but I also seek opportunities to learn and grow and become even better.

I welcome opportunities to learn and grow because it is fun to learn and grow.

I do not have to learn and grow. I do it because I know moving toward self-actualization feels good and I like to feel good.

If your mind argues with these affirmations, take smaller steps toward feeling good about yourself. You can give your accomplishments more attention than you normally do. Take time to make lists of goals you set and accomplished. If you can't think of anything you've done recently, go as far back as you need to in order to find something you decided to do and then did. If you have to go all the way back to learning to walk, that's okay. As you find thoughts about setting goals and succeeding your mind will start helping you find other examples.

Accomplished goals don't have to be big. I set a goal to drink at least 80 ounces of water a day and I now do that. That represents accomplishing something that I decided I wanted to accomplish. You see, the funny thing about goals is that once we achieve anything it doesn't feel big to us even if someone else thinks it is massive. We grow into our goals. It is human nature to set new goals, often even before we've accomplished the ones we're working towards. That happens because as we move toward accomplishing our goals, we fulfill more of our potential. We become better and more capable than we were so we feel more capable of accomplishing more.

I've accomplished many things in my life but by the time I achieved them they didn't seem to be the big deals they were when the goals were set. I'm sure you have accomplished many things, too. Achieving the goal was never the point. The point was to grow into the person we had to become in order to achieve the goal.

If there is something about yourself that you truly don't like, decide to change it. There is a relatively simple and fun process I developed that can help you change aspects of yourself that aren't as you would like them to be.

Years ago I heard an interview of a famous fiction writer who was asked, "How do you write the dialogue for your characters?" His response was, "I don't. I create the character and the character writes his own lines." When I wrote my first fiction novel (not yet published, the working title is *Shades of Joy*) I discovered the truth of his comment. Somehow I leaped from fiction writing to the fact that how we define ourselves determines much of our behavior including the words we speak. Our world is filled with evidence of this playing out in lives all around us. The realization that how we define ourselves determines how we show up in the world came to me.

Two things flowed from that realization. The first was an *ah ha* moment about something I'd been saying I would write a book about if I ever figured out how I'd done it. At one point in my life, I was a 2-pack-a-day Marlboro girl who had been smoking for 14 years and after attempting to quit several times decided that it just isn't in my nature to quit. I don't quit anything.

At that point I had an inspired thought that said "I can't quit smoking but I can become a non-smoker." I then spent six weeks brain-washing myself that on a specific day I would be a non-smoker. The last two weeks of being a smoker I had to force myself to continue smoking because I was still a smoker until the day I became a non-smoker. I won't lie. The first three days were difficult but decades later I have never again smoked because I don't smoke, I am a non-smoker.

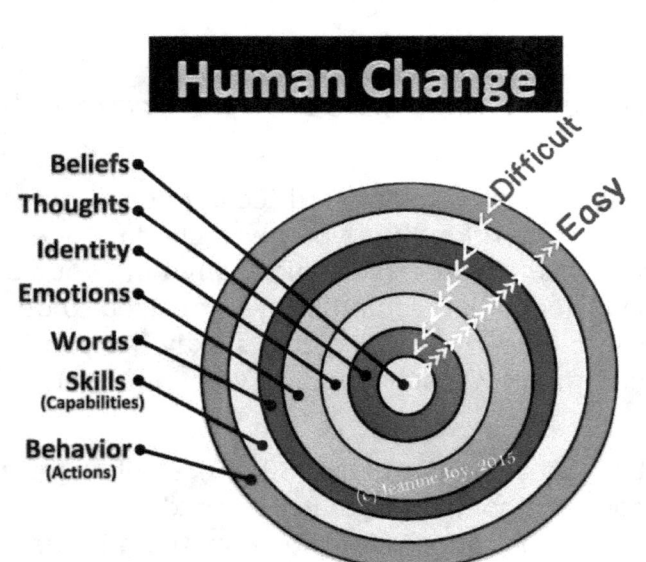

The *ah ha moment* combined with my prior experience of changing my definition of self helped me see that we can define ourselves as we want to be and we will become more of who we want to be. We usually try to change by changing our habits, but if we change from the inside out, beginning with beliefs, our thoughts, words, and actions will follow our beliefs. That's what they do naturally.

Your words reflect your beliefs. Since beliefs are just neuropathways created by repeatedly thinking thoughts, we have the ability to re-program our beliefs to support becoming who we want to be.

Evidence of the power of belief change is all around us. The Pygmalion Effect where students whose teachers believe in them and encourage them who end up exceeding expectations is because their belief in their abilities increased. Believing we can do something leads to greater success because when we believe we can the filters our unconscious mind uses to determine which data to make consciously available includes data we need to be successful.

I'd already learned how to feel good most of the time when I had this realization but sometimes I just wasn't where I wanted to be and when I wasn't I wasn't as kind or as loving as I was when I am in that really good-feeling emotional state. Once you become accustomed to feeling that way towards others it feels worse to be even a little off the mark than it did to feel miles off the mark when that was how you normally felt. So I decided to define myself in the following ways:

I am kind.

I am a loving presence.

I look for and see the best in others.

After re-defining who I am in the above ways it is easier to show up that way even if I'm not having my best day. It isn't about working (emotional labor) to show up that way. It is simply who I am. It can even help me identify when I am a little off so that I can use one of the processes to improve my emotional state. I don't pretend to be nice. I am nice. I don't pretend to feel upbeat. I feel upbeat.

Emotional labor is a work-related requirement to project emotions the worker may not feel.[213] Emotional labor drains our energy and can be discerned as inauthentic or dishonest by observers. Individuals who are required to perform emotional labor at work seem to deplete resources we use for self-control and find themselves less able to control their behaviors in desirable ways at the end of the day and especially when they leave work. This can result in unhealthy behavioral habits.

It is most obvious in the young child who behaves according to social norms at daycare but has a meltdown when in the safer company of a parent. While it is not as dramatic (usually) in adult behavior, the same underlying mechanisms are in play.

If you have a job where you are required to present a particular emotional front and it is an emotion you would like to experience (i.e. cheerfulness), you can try defining yourself as a cheerful person. It usually takes 6 – 12 weeks of daily reinforcement to change our definition of self. When I became a non-smoker I affirmed my new definition every time I lit a cigarette (40 times a day) for six weeks. I find it helpful to identify times during my day when I have a minute or two alone as well as when I wake up and before I go to sleep to affirm beliefs I want to establish and make concrete.

Comparing one's performance to others is associated to burnout. This relationship holds regardless of whether others are perceived as performing better than you or worse than you.[214]

Another way people often sabotage their self-esteem is by comparing themselves unfavorably with others. Adopting an attitude that you're not in competition with others and that you are simply becoming the best version of you that you can be will help you achieve more than unfavorable comparisons with others. If your goal is to be better than someone else it requires a worldview that puts people in hierarchies of better than and worse than one another. Your emotional guidance will support a worldview of everyone being unique and good much more than it supports one of competition.

There is nothing noble in being superior to your fellow man; true nobility is being superior to your former self.
Ernest Hemingway (or Hindu Proverb)

A final consideration about comparisons of self to others is that if your goal is to be better than someone else that is not the same as becoming the best you can be. Your self-actualized self may be far better than someone else's ability in the same area but if you stop improving when you're better than the person you're using as your basis of comparison you won't discover how much more you could have become.

If you didn't take a look at the Self-esteem questionnaire in Appendix XVIII when you read the section on low self-esteem you may want to take a look now or after you finish the book. It can be helpful in identifying areas where your attention would provide significant benefits.

SELF-COMPASSION

Self-compassion is giving yourself the benefit of the doubt. You did the best you could with the resources you had available at the time. Resources were detailed in the section on Individual Perception. Self-compassion is:[215]

- Treating oneself with kindness
- Recognizing one's shared humanity
- Being mindful when considering the negative aspects of oneself

Low levels of self-compassion are associated with higher levels of burnout,[216] psychopathology,[217] and social anxiety.[218] Self-compassion is not the opposite of self-criticism.[219] Self-compassion lowers concerns about comparisons with others, public self-consciousness, negative self-rumination, and reduces feelings of anger.[220]

Perfectionism is actually a flaw. We're human. We aren't meant to be perfect. If we were perfect we'd have nothing left to improve and we feel best when we have something we can improve. Our goal is not perfectionism. Our goal is growth, learning, and positive emotion. Attempting to be perfect diminishes positive emotion.

Another area of research that points to the benefit of using *The Smart Way*™ in conjunction with Emotional Guidance demonstrates that self-compassion is important in recovery from stressful life events and can reduce or eliminate PTSD symptoms following "severe and repeated interpersonal trauma."[221] A study of women going through divorce found that women recovered faster when they were compassionate toward themselves.[222] Give yourself permission to be self-compassionate.

Ask yourself, "How would I treat someone I love if they were in this situation?" Be as kind to yourself as you would be to a friend.

I have never met anyone who did not do the best they could in that moment when their situation is considered fully. If they failed or did not do a good job there is an underlying reason. Self-compassion accepts that we are not at the top of our game 100% of the time. We live in bodies that have needs and when those needs aren't satisfied we cannot do our potential best but we still accomplish our best possible in that moment.

Your emotional guidance will support self-compassionate thoughts. Trust it.

SELF-LOVE OR SELF-RESPECT

Self-love and self-respect go beyond self-compassion. We can feel compassion for someone for whom we don't feel respect or love. This may sound religious to some of you but the fact of the matter is that the phrase *Love Thy Neighbor* from the Bible has seeped into society's idea of what is right. The problem is that they forgot to include the "*as Thyself*" part of the instructions. In fact, in many cases, society tells us to love others more than or before we love ourself. There are a lot of self-sacrificing people who never take care of ourselves. Many healers are that way. The problem is that when you don't take care of yourself you become the one who needs help which was never your intention.

You are at your best when you take care of yourself and you have more to give to everyone else when you take care of yourself first. Loving yourself is not wrong. This is fact. We are healthier, mentally and physically, when we feel good and if you don't love yourself, you can't feel good.

Self-love and self-respect are the opposite of low self-esteem. They mean you see yourself as a human worthy of love and respect. It doesn't mean you are better than anyone else, but you're not worse either.

Two things help increase self-love and self-respect. One is your emotional guidance supports loving and respecting yourself. You can check that out for yourself by thinking self-supporting thoughts and feel how they feel.

If you need more than that, you can make a list of all the ways you'll be better for others when you feel worthy of love and respect. When you feel worthy you're not stressed and that means you can be at your best: Your best health, your best performance on the job, your best in your relationships.

META-COGNITION

The personality trait of 'Imaginative' is a positive predictor of resilience. One reason may be that it can aid in finding perspectives that feel better. A creative way to change how a situation is perceived is to make up a story. Albert Ellis found that creative perspectives didn't have to be true to provide benefits as long as the individual realized that it wasn't reality.

In a bullying prevention class I use the example of visualizing taking a space ship to another planet with the bully with you and then leaving the bully on the other planet. Students have reported that just the thought that they'd done that helps them not respond to the bully in a fearful manner, which makes them less of a target. Bullies like people who are easily frightened. I used creativity to come up with the idea because I knew I couldn't teach them to visualize doing something they could actually do because it would increase the likelihood that they'd really do it.

OPEN TO NEW EXPERIENCES

The more you open yourself up to new experiences, the bigger your world (I like to call it my playground) becomes.

Most of us have what we consider to be our comfort zones. By deliberately expanding your comfort zone repeatedly over time you can expand it so far that you can't find the end of your comfort zone.

I've done this so I know you can do it. I began my adult years as an extremely shy, socially awkward victim who didn't have a clue about much of anything. I was most comfortable lost in a fiction book. One-on-one conversations were difficult for me and led to watery eyes and a bright red face.

Being fearless and being stupid isn't the same thing. I still apply risk management strategies to my life. I don't walk down dark alleys at night. But I get on stage frequently without fear.

I think the count of countries I've visited is up to 43 and I did a lot of that travel alone or as a single mother who was also responsible for two daughters.

Between starting a business and writing a book where many of your own trials, tribulations, and struggles are laid open for any reader to see, I'm not sure which one takes more confidence, but I didn't hesitate to do either when it seemed to be the right path for me to take.

When I went on my first business trip to San Francisco as a young woman I ate room service because I was too timid to go to a restaurant alone. The week after that trip I began going out to eat alone every Thursday night until I was able to confidently walk into any restaurant and enjoy dining alone. Part of that was learning to enjoy my own company. Another aspect was deciding that I was worth a nice meal. Those first few Thursdays were tough. I would sit in my car giving myself a pep talk before going in to the restaurant. In my mind I imagined all sorts of awful things people might think about me dining alone including that I had no friends or wasn't good enough to have friends. Only by facing my fear (and learning that most waitresses are very kind to solo diners) was I able to expand my comfort zone.

Expanding your comfort zone is a lot like building up your muscles through weight and endurance training but unlike exercise, once you develop confidence it doesn't disappear if you don't use it for a while. If I could do it, so can you.

GROWTH MINDSET

A growth mindset is necessary to learn and grow. However, it is similar to PsyCap in that a growth mindset is a function of an internal locus of control

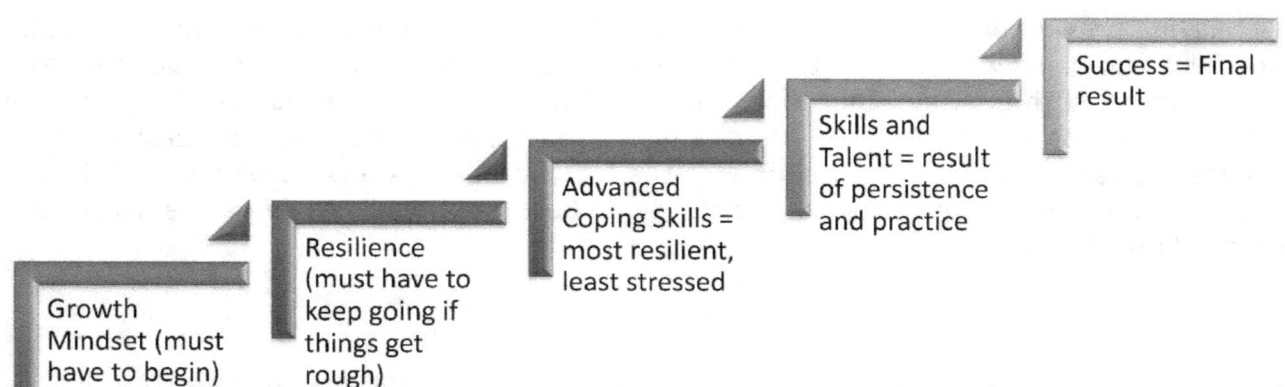

Individuals with a fixed mindset focus on protecting their self-image. They focus on not failing more often than they focus on what they can achieve.

A growth mindset is important for achieving more of one's potential and will be a natural result of meta-cognitve processes combined with emotional guidance because our guidance leads toward growth and greater achievements.

EMOTION REGULATION BELIEFS

There is an area that is related to growth and fixed mindset that may have a greater impact on well-being than a fixed or growth mindset relating to learning. Some people believe that their emotions are whatever they are and that they cannot change them. This is considered an entity belief that is very similar to a fixed mindset. Other people believe that they and others can learn to change their emotions using emotion regulation strategies, which is very similar to a growth mindset.

If you believe that emotions can't be changed, the good news is all you have to do is try using some of the techniques presented in these pages and you'll be able to show yourself that you can change your emotions because you want to change them. That will have a transformative effect on your life and decrease your risk of developing psychological disorders, which often involve some kind of emotion dysregulation.[223]

INTERNAL LOCUS OF CONTROL

Different people promote different methods of increasing human thriving. At first glance it seems that there are many paths leading to stress reduction and greater accomplishment. When you break high-level concepts down into their component parts it becomes apparent that the same lower level factors lead to success.

The names reflect different approaches but they all end up back at the core elements of resilience. Every high-level psychological factor that increases health or success includes an internal locus of control. An internal locus of control is the belief that your actions have an impact on the outcomes you experience. It is the opposite of learned helplessness[224] where a person or animal will not act in its best interest because it doesn't believe its actions will make a difference.

Using meta-cognitve strategies with emotional guidance automatically increases one's internal locus of control by demonstrating that how you perceive a situation, person, or event determines the way you experience the event. It becomes clear that you have the ability to exercise control over how your experience feels by changing your perspective about the situation.

Locus of Control

Internal — Empowered

External — Disempowered

Downward Spiral

When a situation that feels bad to you arises, remember that how you feel is determined by how you perceive the situation and begin using advanced coping skills to change the level of stress you experience. When you do this it increases your sense of empowerment.

Individuals with an external locus of control can experience downward spirals following a negative event. This is the result of using dysfunctional and maladaptive coping strategies.

High Core Self-Evaluations (CSE)	Resilience	Psychological Capital (PsyCap)	Growth Mindset	Happiness	Psychological Flexibility
Internal Locus of Control Healthy Self-esteem Self-efficacy (task & general) Emotional Stability	Internal Locus of Control Healthy Self-esteem Optimism	Hope Optimism Self-efficacy Resilience*	Internal Locus of Control	Internal Locus of Control Healthy self-esteem Optimism Metacognitive skills Hope or better Priority = happy Positive habits of thought Self-awareness	Internal Locus of Control Metacognitive skills
Outcomes:	Outcomes:	Outcomes:	Outcomes:	Outcomes:	Outcomes:
Higher motivation[1]	Greater task persistence[2]	Manager rated performance[3]	Sets higher goals[4]	Better cognitive abilities[5, 6, 7, 8, 9]	Increased Resilience[10]
Greater task persistence[11]		Job Satisfaction[12]	Open to learning[13]	Long-term success[14, 15]	
Higher work engagement[16]		Trust[17]		Manager rated performance[18]	
Higher commitment[19]		Higher work engagement[20]		Job Satisfaction[21]	
		Higher commitment[22]		Trust[23]	
		Lower absenteeism[24]		Higher work engagement[25]	
				Higher commitment[26]	
				Lower absenteeism[27]	
				Better pregnancy outcomes[28, 29]	
				Better negotiation outcomes[30]	
				Lower crime[31]	
				Better Relationships[32]	
				Better goal attainment[33]	
				Higher Emotional Intelligence	
Outcomes that are the same for all high-level constructs: Better physical health[34, 35, 36, 37, 38, 39, 40, 41, 42]; Better mental health[43, 44, 45, 46, 47, 48, 49, 50]; Better behavioral health[51, 52]; Better pro-health choices[53, 54]; Lower stress[55, 56, 57, 58]					

Individuals with an external locus of control are more likely to blame others for the undesired event. This leads to perceptions that the event is beyond their control and could happen again if they are in a similar situation. The belief that you can do something to prevent an event from happening again encourages the use of adaptive coping strategies.

Notice the common elements for the following high-level factors:

See Appendix XVI for a separate Bibliography for this chart.

POSITIVE THINKING

The way we think about the world determines our thoughts and actions. Fighting against disease is not the same mindset as testing the limits of human wellness.

Paradigms

• Prevent disease	• Wellness Promotion
• Sustain life	• Quality of life

Many people reject positive thinking out of hand because they believe it is unrealistic and Pollyannaish. These beliefs are not the result of examining the research or of reality. More people than I can remember have said they don't think positive because they are realistic. There are two responses to this.

> "If you think you can or can't, you are right."
> Henry Ford.

Although the above quote is commonly attributed to Henry Ford, the attribution stems from a 1947 *Reader's Digest* article that did not note when or where Henry Ford made the statement. A similar quote can be traced to Virgil in *Aeneid*. This 1925 Henry Ford quote can be traced to its origin:

> "**You must never, even for a second, let yourself think that you can fail**," said Mr. Ford. "**Our first principal is that failure is impossible**. You may not get what you're trying to do right the first time or the second time or the tenth time or the 100th time, but **if you shut out of your mind the possibility of being licked, then you are bound to win**."[225]

Self-fulfilling prophesies have been documented in research. Our personal expectations of self and others' expectations of us can both influence our outcome.[226, 227] Because our beliefs filter the big data that our subconscious mind sends to our conscious mind, self-defeating beliefs block our access to information that would help us if we believed we could be successful.

One study demonstrated that "beliefs about the likelihood of success in emotion regulation can shape actual emotion regulation success."[228] The field of positive organizational scholarship takes the concept forward, stating "Adopting an affirmative bias is associated with resourcefulness, or with creating, unlocking, and multiplying latent resources in individuals and organizations. Resourcefulness means that an amplifying effect occurs when individuals and organizations are exposed to positivity."[229]

The second important aspect of positive thinking vs being realistic is that the facts support positive thinking as realistic. It is only our perception, largely influenced by the media's focus on the negative aspects of our world that makes us think more is wrong in our world than right.

If your habits of thought focus on the negative aspects of our world it can be difficult to recognize the positive aspects that surround you. It isn't that our world lacks positive aspects; it is that your brain is trained to focus on the negative aspects.

The appreciation exercise is helpful in training your brain to recognize positive aspects of our world. You can also think about things that give you pleasure when you think about them and then realize how common they are.

How many healthy babies were born today?

How many people fell in love today?

How many parents told their children they love them today?

How many people were cured who would have surely died from an illness one hundred years ago?

How many people easily communicated with someone today that it would have taken months to reach just a hundred years ago?

How many people laughed today?

How many people went to bed in a safe place today?

How many people had enough to eat today?

How many people learned something today?

How many people cared for an animal today?

How many people took a breath of fresh air today?

How many people turned on a faucet and had clean water available to them at the touch of a fingertip?

How many people learned something useful today?

How many people smiled at a stranger today?

How many people appreciated someone else today?

How many people enjoyed smelling a blooming flower today?

How many flowers bloomed today?

How many pieces of fruit ripened today?

How many seeds germinated today?

I could go on like this for hours. The amount of good happening all over our planet every day is far greater than the bad happening in our world. Positive thinking does not mean we don't recognize the bad. Positive thinking means we believe we can find solutions to problems.

One trick to positive thinking is to ask yourself what you can or will do about something that you do not want in our world. For example, today we lose 2/3 of our at-risk children to prison, addiction, or death. That is definitely a negative aspect of modern society. I could lament that fact all the days of my life and not change it at all. Or, I could document evidence-based solutions that are already proven to work and to be cost effective and publish a book containing those solutions. I did the latter but I would never have done it if I thought we lived in a bad world where we can't solve our problems.

Positive thinking doesn't mean you ignore problems. It means you believe they are solvable and that you are resilient enough to deal with the problems you encounter. Maintaining a positive outlook has been shown to protect against burnout.[230, 231]

SUPPORTIVE, EMPOWERING BELIEFS

"Beliefs powerfully shape emotions via their influence on appraisal processes. . . several influential appraisal theories have posited that beliefs are one of the most important influences on appraisal process, and thereby determine when and what type of emotion will be elicited in response to environmental contingencies."[232] It is important to note that most of our beliefs were established while we were children and were not examined using critical thinking. We often share beliefs that our parents held that may come from their parents' beliefs.

Evaluating beliefs we are aware of and changing ones that do not support our highest good has the ability to change every area of our lives. Beliefs can be about the nature of our world, the nature of people, aging, our bodies, or literally anything we've encountered or heard about during our lives. Beliefs occur partially because of our experiences but it is repeated thinking about something that forms the belief, which is simply a neuropathway your thoughts can travel more easily than they travel alternate routes.

You cannot change beliefs directly because when you attempt to think about the belief and change it, your thoughts travel the same neuropathway and keep the belief reinforced.

The way to change a belief is to decide what you'd rather believe and then reinforce the new belief by repeatedly thinking about it and, if possible, talking and/or writing about it.

There are a variety of methods to use to determine what beliefs you would like to change and which beliefs you'd like to establish. The process I used is as follows:

- Identify areas where my emotional guidance indicated my beliefs were leading to emotional appraisals, including automatic appraisals, that resulted in negative emotions and/or feelings of disempowerment
- Recognize that things that were true in my life but not in others' lives were reflecting my established beliefs
- Decide what I would rather believe based on how ideas felt (using emotional guidance).
- I found it helpful to read quotes and inspirational books to help me identify empowering beliefs that resonated with me.
- Look for evidence that others could do what I was encouraging myself to believe I could do (when it came to personally empowering beliefs)
- Practice thinking the thoughts I wanted to believe through affirmations, by writing, and by speaking about them with others

I had some firmly embedded beliefs that I stopped believing but they still functioned as beliefs (impacting my words) for a while until the new beliefs were firmly established. I was easy on myself when I realized I was voicing opinions I no longer held by recognizing it was just evidence of an old neuropathway that would stop being the path my thoughts traveled once my new thoughts had created a stronger neuropathway. Eventually they stopped being active neuropathways. The process took about three months of consistent effort which consisted of affirming my new beliefs every time the old beliefs came into my mind.

As I consciously adopted a more empowered worldview my personality and emotional response to previously stressful events changed significantly. I went from being a Mom who was always worried about her children to one who allowed them age appropriate freedoms. I felt more confident and became more assertive. I stopped allowing other people's opinions of me to determine how I felt about my self-worth. I identified empowered perspectives about prior traumas that transformed them from subjects to be avoided to topics I could help others heal from their own traumas. For the first time in my life I began liking myself.

Because beliefs inform the automatic appraisal of potentially stressful events, adopting more empowered beliefs meant the initial negative emotion I felt in a variety of situations was diminished and in some cases, gone entirely. Situations I would have previously perceived as hassles or problems were immediately perceived as opportunities or useful information. I no longer had to use as much conscious reappraisal to regulate my emotions because more empowered beliefs made the initial appraisal of the situation less stressful. My experience is supported by research that indicates a single belief change can change the amount of stress experienced in a variety of situations.[233]

DIVERSITY APPRECIATION

It is not possible to dislike someone, or a group of people, and feel good while you are with them. The dislike you feel is a negative emotion which The Smart Way™ tells us is a sign post that we would serve ourselves better if we found a better-feeling perspective about the subject we are thinking about.

Remember, negative emotions are an indicator that we're experiencing stress. It is self-inflicted stress because if we liked the person or group that we're feeling stressed about we wouldn't be stressed.

Also, when we define our in-group (people like us) in narrow ways our brain sees out-groups as *other*. Our brain and physiology respond differently to *others* than it does to our in-group.

The best way I've found to get around biases we've been taught or learned is twofold.

1) Deliberately cultivate a new belief about your in-group. Expand it to be as broad as possible. The process may require an individual to gradually expand their concept of their in-group but the ultimate goals would include the human race or all sentient beings.
2) Pay attention to how you feel and when you feel negative emotion about an individual or group of people view it as a sign that the way you perceive them is not the best possible perspective you could take for your own good (best interests) and actively seek a better-feeling perspective about the individual or group(s).

There are some helpful ways to do this:

- Keep feeling good as a high priority goal that supersedes having been right in the past. This means that if you were taught not to like a group of people and now you recognize that you feel negative emotion when you think about that group but you can't feel good and hold onto your negative beliefs about the group, give feeling good a higher priority.

  For example, I was raised during the Cold War and although I had never met a Russian, I was taught to hate Russians. I dutifully did this for decades until I began understanding that my emotions were providing guidance so the emotion of hate meant there is a better feeling way to view Russians and by hating them I was depriving myself of the opportunity to feel as good as I could.

  I began seeing myself as human first instead of American first. It was about that time when I began traveling more internationally. While I was in Australia I met some

Russians that I liked quite well and they liked me. One evening at dinner our conversation strayed to the Cold War and we laughed about how we had once allowed our government to dictate how we should feel about each other when we actually liked each other. My Russian friends grew up hating Americans because they were told we were bad.

When you step outside the paradigm that allows you to decide that all members of a group are bad because they are members of the group, it immediately becomes apparent how ridiculous that perspective really is. I was happy to let go of my anti-Russian sentiments and feel good.

I could have beat myself up for all the years I spent believing that Russians were bad but that would serve no purpose other than continuing to deprive me of the potential to feel good now. I know too much to give in to the insistence that I was always right in the past because the price that extracts requires me to feel bad while learning. Learning and expanding one's awareness, especially awareness that no one should dictate to others how they should feel is knowledge worth celebrating.

2) The second technique is to see people for their potential rather than for where they are today. I've worked with quite a few people with sordid past experiences. If I wanted to feel bad I could negatively judge them for what they've done. If I want to feel good I have to see the potential for good within them. I have developed the belief (supported by research) that people are innately good and that most humans live far below their potential. I could judge people for living below their potential but that wouldn't feel good. Instead I seek to inspire them to fulfill more of their potential. That's what feels best to me.

   a. The one thing that helps me see people for their potential and not judge them negatively for who they are in this moment, or who they were in the past, is by understanding that happy people are good to others and everyone would be happy if they had the skills to achieve happiness. There is a direct link between sustained negative emotion and bad behaviors including crimes. We live in a society that does a poor job teaching people how to be happy which means we do a poor job of preventing crime.
   b. My research has led me to conclude that people would not behave badly if they knew how to feel good and since we don't teach those skills, society plays a role. It is not that people are blameless or have no moral control over themselves. This is a far different perspective from the one I had as a teenager and young adult. It is formed based on the research that shows all of us have the capacity for bad behavior when we feel disempowered and for good behaviors when we feel empowered.
   c. I understand that teaching people to feel more empowered will unleash more of their potential.

Changing your attitudes, should you chose to do so, will not happen overnight. It works best if you take small steps repeatedly to move toward a broader definition of your *in-group*. Use your emotions as the guidance they were meant to be to help you identify thoughts that will benefit you.

Even after you eliminate your biases you may find that new ones try to creep into your belief system. As long as you pay attention to how you feel it's easy to stay ahead of it. The recent election cycle with all its negativity tried to make me classify people into groups I liked and groups I didn't like. I had to consciously reject the prevalent attitudes in order to feel good. I also made my decisions about who I was going to vote for and then withdrew from as much of the negative dialogue as it was possible to avoid because engaging in the discussions felt awful.

HUMAN DIGNITY

Healthcare professionals are required to treat all patients with dignity which means with respect and as if their lives have value simply because they exist. This requirement reminds me of the Corinthians passage about love in the Bible, idealistic but impossible if the individual is not taught how to use meta-cognition to find perspectives from which the value of their life can be seen to have worth about individuals who are more difficult to respect.

What do I mean by this? It can be difficult to view a murderer, rapist, addict, racist, pedophile, or other individual who has exhibited socially undesirable behavior as worthy of respect. Just as loving someone the way love is described in Corinthians, even your spouse or child, can be difficult if you don't know how to use your mind to find loving perspectives under any and all scenarios.

Unconditional respect or love for others requires psychological flexibility and the development of beliefs that yield the benefit of the doubt to others. It is difficult to give others unconditional love or respect if we do not first give it to ourselves.

Western society holds conflicting belief structures about human dignity. There is a strong current containing the belief that respect must be earned. There is a possibly equally strong current containing the belief that respect is an inherent right of all humans regardless of their deeds. Even an individual who consciously chooses to view all humans as deserving of respect may have an internal struggle to fend off learned beliefs about earned respect.

Add the near impossible task of viewing others with unconditional love and respect when we don't do the same for ourselves combined with a society that has a strong current of protest against seeing oneself as good and there are many internal (psychological) factors that come into play.

Teaching healthcare practitioners how to find perspectives that view all others as deserving of dignity and respect would go much further in helping them find these perspectives than simply telling them it is a requirement. Your emotional guidance will help you identify these perspectives.

Why is this important? Emotional labor is pretending there are emotions that you don't feel. Treating someone you don't respect, or even despise, as if you respect them is emotional labor. Emotional labor takes energy and adds to the risk of burnout. Helping healthcare workers find perspectives where they authentically feel respect for everyone reduces the amount of emotional labor.

Treating someone with dignity and respect does not take a toll when the feelings you express match the emotions you feel. Authenticity is healthy and is received better by those with whom we interact. We can often sense when a person's words and actions differ from their true feelings. When we do, it diminishes our trust in them because we innately know they're not being honest with us.

In addition to conflicts between a physician's belief systems and the requirement to treat everyone with respect, when outside forces demand someone demonstrate emotions or attitudes that are inauthentic it reduces the individual's sense of autonomy, which is demotivating and can reduce the energy they have available even further.

I want to be clear that I'm not, in any way, suggesting that people do not deserve to be treated with dignity and respect. I am arguing that teaching people how to authentically adopt those perspectives will:

1) Allow them to authentically display those attitudes.
2) Improve the energy physicians have available for work.
3) Eliminate a potential source of diminished trust between patients and physicians.
4) Improve physician's ability to experience positive emotions.

COMPARE CBT TO THE SMART WAY

The Smart Way™ Meta-cognitive Processes used in conjunction with Emotional Guidance helps you optimize the way you use your mind and body.

Meta-cognitive simply means you think about what you're thinking. You're not thinking on auto-pilot. You think about what you're thinking and how it feels when you think what you think. It is actually natural. Some people naturally do it and thrive as a result. Like any skill, yours will get better with practice. Like any new skill, you won't be an expert the first time. But you can learn how to do it and the best part about it is that doing it feels good. Once you feel the empowerment the first time you are successful, you will want to do it again—because it feels good. The effort you exert toward self-empowerment today provides a stepping stool that provides empowerment for a higher step you'll climb tomorrow.

"One particularly adaptive type of emotion regulation is reappraisal, which refers to changing how individuals appraise the situation they are in to alter its emotional significance."[234] Individuals who engage in reappraisal tend to:[235]

- Feel a higher sense of purpose in life
- Feel less depressed
- Have strengthened social bonds
- Experience higher levels of well-being
- Demonstrate greater social adjustment

People who recently faced stressful life events had higher levels of well-being, better social adjustment, and fewer depressive symptoms if they habitually used cognitive reappraisal.[236] Several aspects of *The Smart Way*™ are designed to increase individual's motivation to use cognitive reappraisal techniques, both by overcoming common limiting beliefs and by educating participants about the benefit of maintaining better-feeling emotions. A meta-analysis of 51 independent studies with a total of 21,150 participants confirmed that cognitive reappraisal (a skill taught as part of *The Smart Way*™) significantly contributes to positive mental health and protects against indicators of poor mental health.[237] Imagine how much more powerful cognitive reappraisal is when you add Emotional Guidance to the tool kit.

When you use mindfulness and "accept thoughts and feelings without judgment and focus on the present moment,"[238] depression and anxiety decline. With *The Smart Way*™ you take the next step and change perspectives using emotional guidance to help you identify perspectives that serve your highest good.

The Smart Way™ provides a stable foundation for success throughout life. Evidence-based techniques address core skills that make the difference between choosing a path toward self-actualization and success or a less productive one.

The objectives of *The Smart Way*™ are:

- Foster skills and social competence through training that increases self-confidence.
- Increase success by providing goal setting training that reinforces inherent desires for autonomy and competence.
- Reduce susceptibility to negative external pressures and stress.
- Increase growth mindset and intrinsic desire for continuous self-development.
- Develop skills that increase happiness and resilience, which reduces stress.
- Develop a thorough understanding of how to accurately interpret emotions and respond to their signals in pro-health and pro-social ways (Emotional Intelligence Plus).
- Recognize the connection between emotional state and behaviors.
- Teach skills that lead to the development of habitual bias that allocates attention during new situations in ways that elicit positive emotions more often, essentially resulting in implicit emotion regulation.[239]

Skills that empower an individual to regulate their emotional response to the events occurring in their life (self-regulation) significantly reduce the risk of mental illnesses including burnout, depression, anxiety, panic disorders, bi-polar disorder and even psychosis. Individuals with the ability to self-induce desired emotional states "are happier in both positive and negative circumstances."[240] Regulating negative emotions to feel better reduces stress, which leads to improved physical health. "The existence of automatic, unconscious processes influencing human emotion, cognition, and behavior is widely accepted and confirmed by numerous studies."[241]

Although these processes provide regulation below our conscious awareness, the actual way they regulate emotion and whether they regulate emotion in ways that supports greater health or in ways that diminishes one's ability to achieve and maintain health varies between individuals. They are learned methods that can be adjusted to improve outcomes. When they are adjusted and begin automatically supporting healthy emotional states they are transformational. Individuals do not give themselves the dosage they need to maintain optimal emotional states when their stress levels rise when dose-dependent (Palliative) coping skills are utilized.[242] In other words, frequent use of The Smart Way™ techniques for just a few months improves automatic stress and happiness regulation. And, unlike most self-improvement techniques, The Smart Way™ feels good every step of the way so its use is intrinsically rewarded.

The Smart Way™ was designed by combining characteristics of individuals who thrive against the odds with the latest research in positive psychology, resilience, psychological flexibility, self-determination theory, emotion regulation, and other research that points to the basis of human thriving.

Happiness and stress have an inverse relationship. Research on the presence of happiness and the presence of stress reveal the following benefits of higher levels of happiness and lower levels of stress:

Increased pro-social behaviors
- Reduced anti-social behavior
- Better citizenship
- Increased kindness (even to strangers)
- Intrinsically motivated diversity appreciation (a significant step-up from tolerance)
- Reduced (or no) criminal behavior
- Increased positive goal setting

Increased pro-health behaviors
- Reduced likelihood of alcohol, drug, and cigarette use

- Increased physical activity
- Better dietary choices
- Improved sleep habits and quality of sleep

Physical and Mental Benefits
- Improved immune function
- Improved cognitive function
- Improved digestive function
- Improved Central Nervous System Functioning
- Reduced risk of mental illness (including depression/anxiety)[243] and suicide,[244] which are all are strongly correlated to stress and poor emotion regulation skills

The Smart WayTM program is designed to build strengths associated with positive outcomes including:

- Autonomous Intrinsic Motivation
- Positivity/optimism
- Growth Mindset
- Emotional Intelligence

- Authenticity
- Positive goal-setting

- Internal Locus of Control
- Healthy self-esteem
- Meta-cognitve Skills
- Physical, Mental, Emotional, and Behavioral Health
- Positive self-image
- Acceptance of responsibility for actions and results

The Smart Way™ has been compared to Cognitive Behavioral Therapy in the following way:

Cognitive Behavioral Therapy (CBT) is done one-on-one and resembles having an expert marksman stand next to an amateur who is blindfolded while attempting to hit a target by obtaining instructions from the expert, who is the only one who knows the location of the target.

The *Smart Way*™ can be delivered in large group settings where hundreds can be taught at the same time because it removes the blindfold and makes the target fully visible to each individual, who is given skills that empower them to identify the right target and continually improve their aim. Intrinsic motivation occurs naturally because each step results in positive emotional feedback. Even when the overall emotional state is still negative, the student feels the relief of feeling better and the hope that comes from knowing one has the skills to shift to increasingly better feeling emotional states.

Cognitive Behavioral Therapy is further hampered by:
- Stigma associated with mental illness
- High cost of one-on-one therapy
- Recurrent need because CBT resolves current issues without necessarily developing skills to address future issues
- Cognitive Behavioral and other types of therapies are reactive

Therapists are typically trained to move people from a minus state to zero on the following scale:

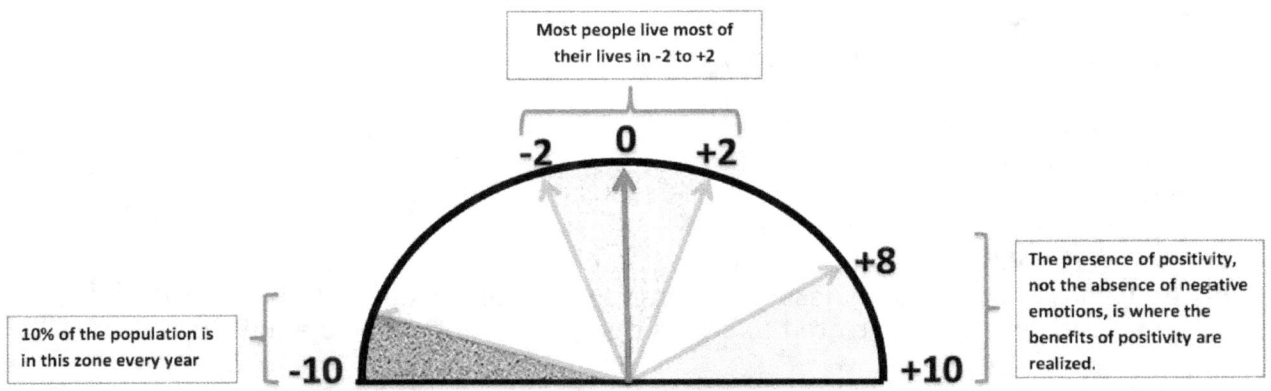

The Smart Way™ is proactive, low-cost, develops skills that improve results throughout life, and is designed to help individuals achieve and sustain emotions in the +8 range (from hope to joy). Because it is educational and structured to correct prevalent misconceptions, no stigma is attached to learning about emotional guidance or developing advanced and transformational coping skills. It is an evidence-based form of Primary Prevention. Training comes with added benefits, including improving morale, reducing burnout, enhancement of any existing wellness programs, and reduction in any existing prejudices or biases.

"Cognitive behavioral therapies can be defined as those interventions with the core assumptions that what individuals think directly impacts how they feel and what they do."[245] Despite the fact that Cognitive Behavioral Therapy is used as a curative rather than a preventative method of improving mental (and in some cases, physical), health, "it is clear that the evidence-base of CBT is enormous." Hoffman, et al. conducted a review of meta-analyses of the use of CBT to address a wide variety of issues and concluded by recommending that countries adopt it as a first-line defense against mental disorders. I go a step further in my hypothesis.

> *My Hypothesis is that anything Cognitive Behavioral Therapy is effective at treating, **The Smart Way**™ can prevent from happening in the first place.*

The Smart Way™ is not synonymous with Cognitive Behavioral Therapy provided before an individual develops a mental or physical health problem. It is **CBT Plus** because of emotional guidance. *The Smart Way*™ is delivered primarily to groups or provided as self-help using videos and books. It is significantly more cost effective than CBT because it does not require one-on-one therapy and because it prevents the problems before they happen, thus avoiding the costs associated with problems that have manifested. Also, it is more difficult to cure a condition than to prevent its occurrence in the first place and there is no relapse because the illness did not manifest in the first place. Another major difference is that Cognitive Behavioral Therapy does not include Emotional Guidance, which overturns a prevalent but inaccurate interpretation of the purpose of emotions. *The Smart Way*™ also disabuses negative beliefs about the subconscious portions of personality that often include beliefs that the subconscious is secret, dark, and frightening as well as unreliable and dangerous to explore.

The *Smart Way*™ provides information and skills that empower individuals to develop healthy habits of thought before a problem develops.

While there is a strong emphasis on prevention with The Smart Way™, case studies demonstrate that The Smart Way™ is effective in restoring mental health to individuals who were suffering from severe long-term PTSD, severe chronic depression, and that is has been effective in preventing imminent suicides. It was those successes combined with the increased experience of positive emotions in those I taught that convinced me of the power The Smart Way™ has to help people even though the techniques are delivered to groups.

After Butler, Chapman, Forman, and Beck, conducted a meta-analysis to review the existing research relating to Cognitive Behavioral Therapy in 2006, they concluded, "The meta-analyses reviewed strongly suggest that across many disorders the effects of CBT are maintained for substantial periods beyond the cessation of treatment. More specifically, significant evidence for long-term effectiveness was found for depression, generalized anxiety, panic, social phobia, OCD, sexual offending, schizophrenia, and childhood internalizing disorders. In the cases of depression and panic, there appears to be robust and convergent meta-analytic evidence that CBT produces vastly superior long-term persistence of effects, with relapse rates half those of pharmacotherapy."[246]

The robust support for persistence of Cognitive Behavioral Therapy suggests that learning meta-cognitve processes protects against the occurrence of many chronic problems our society would like to eliminate. The persistence of the results suggests (strongly, in my opinion) that prevention is possible.

Providing knowledge and skills that prevent the maladaptive cognitions Cognitive Behavioral Therapy is designed to correct will prevent the problems from manifesting in the first place, thus preventing a significant portion of the suffering that currently affects people around the world.

CBT is essentially teaching people to think in self-supporting ways, it makes sense that teaching them to do that before a problem manifests would effectively prevent many issues from ever arising. The benefits of healthy habits of health extend to both physical[247] and mental health.[248] The benefits to individuals, employers, schools, and society in general of reducing the incidences of these problems should be obvious.

If we and our children have skills and habits of thought that make us resilient, we will fare much better than those who are not resilient if we find ourselves the survivor of such an event. We will also not experience the same level of chronic stress that leads to diminished physical and mental health in those who do not have skills. Our world has changed.

Add the improvement in employee engagement and happiness that result from learning *The Smart Way*™ and it begins to look like a miracle drug, except it's not a drug. It is so effective because it corrects thinking that exists only because many common beliefs in our society are slightly off base. Meta-cognitve processes and Emotional Guidance correct those issues, helping people who learn them live up to their potential. One of the reasons so many suffer is because they know intuitively that life should be better for them, but without understanding their guidance or the false premises in their beliefs that are negatively affecting their life experience, they don't know why it isn't working out the way they feel it should. The Smart Way™ makes all the difference.

There is no need for a diagnosis before teaching *The Smart Way*™ because it is simply teaching individuals about how their brain works and how to think in ways that optimize outcomes. While learning *The Smart Way*™ may lead to recovery or better outcomes from manifested chronic illnesses, the main purpose is to prevent new manifestations of problems that can be prevented by using a skilled level of cognition that reduces stress on a daily basis.

Cognitive Behavioral Therapy teaches people how thoughts influence feelings and behaviors.[249] That is something everyone needs to know. To the average person, mental health care is shrouded in mystery, stigma, and secrecy. Just the thought of thinking about our innermost feelings can be enough to cause fear. But when one begins considering that Cognitive Behavioral Therapy is essentially about helping someone change the way they think to healthier thought patterns doesn't it make sense to teach people what healthy thought patterns are in the first place? When you see how many mental health problems can be healed, or at least improved with CBT, does it not point to the fact that information about how the mind works would be highly valuable to everyone?

How an individual uses her mind determines how much stress is felt in a given situation. Everyone who receives a lay-off notice does not feel the same degree of stress. Not even everyone with two children and a mortgage and no spouse feels the same degree of stress when a lay-off is announced. The amount of stress felt depends on the perspective the individual takes about the situation. When the individual understands *The Smart* Way™, she has control over the stress.

How our brains, emotions, and thoughts are connected should not be information reserved for the elite. "CBT is a psychotherapeutic approach that focuses on the way in which people's thoughts influence their feelings and behaviors. CBT includes a number of different approaches that share the belief that it is not the event that causes our feelings and behaviors, but rather how we perceive or think about what happened . . . Socratic reasoning is a central technique."[250]

The only aspects that really make CBT therapeutic is that it is done after-the-fact (once someone is already suffering from a diagnosis). CBT also has assessment procedures to measure progress toward healing. If done before an illness manifests there is no need for assessments to be done to determine when health is restored to a level where insurance will no longer pay and no need for a diagnosis because the point is to avoid having a diagnosable illness.

Albert Ellis developed a form of therapy in the 1940's that was much like CBT because the wisdom from philosophers such as Bertrand Russell, Marcus Aurelius, and Epictetus helped him with his own problems. His path is eerily similar to my own. I was teaching people to use early versions of *The Smart Way*™ techniques for years before my knowledge of CBT expanded and I realized that the techniques I'd developed independently were essentially a preventive form of CBT. Dr. Ellis and I even benefited from the wisdom of the same philosophers.

People are not disturbed by things, but by the view they take of them.

Epictetus

At about the same time Ellis developed his version, Aaron T. Beck was starting to lean toward a cognitive form of treatment. Both are considered founders of CBT although when Ellis's associates came to him upset that Beck was calling himself the Father of CBT, Ellis was undisturbed and simply referred to himself as the Grandfather of CBT. Now, that sounds like the way someone who has learned *The Smart Way*™ would respond to a situation many people would find highly distressing. It is a real reaction, not suppression of rage. The mind that uses skilled meta-cognition finds perspectives that feel good under almost any circumstances.

Ellis stated his use of rational referred to cognitions that "are effective and self-helping, not merely cognitions that are empirically and logically valid."[251] This is an important distinction and one I also make. In fact, I go further and under some situations, I encourage magical thinking. As long as you understand on the meta-cognitive level that you're fantasizing even when you create something that feels real on the basic cognitive level, if it feels good when you do it, it's helpful. You can't spend all your time in a fantasy world, but you can do it often enough to improve your emotional state.

"Beck's system included different classifications of thoughts. Automatic thoughts are quick, evaluative thoughts that seem to come to mind immediately, without the person being aware of them and therefore without deliberation. People tend to accept their automatic thoughts as truths . . . Individuals use their core beliefs as a lens through which they interpret life situations."[252] That is what I refer to as *surface thinking*. Beck seemed to think that people consciously accept core beliefs as true. I disagree. Many core beliefs are not consciously understood—that is one of the reasons for dysfunctional thinking—accepted but erroneous core beliefs.

The difference between Beck's "consciously accept core beliefs as true" and my hypothesis "the brain filters information using accepted core beliefs" is that Beck assumes the thinker is aware they have internalized the core beliefs and consciously and deliberately decided to view the world that way. Researchers have repeatedly found that many core beliefs are established by age 6. I don't think 6-year-olds are consciously and deliberately evaluating whether they should see the world as a good place or an evil one, or whether they should see the world as a competitive kill or be killed environment vs. one of mutual cooperation and co-existence.

My hypothesis is that the core beliefs develop based on the *back stories* our subconscious mind creates about our experiences. We could live in a mansion situated in a peaceful island paradise and have an older brother who resents us and physically harms (trips, punches, pushes, etc.) us every chance he gets and we could decide the world is a mean and violent place.
We could live in a slum where the sounds of knife and gun-fights ring out at all hours of the day and night, navigating past drug dealers and women reduced to selling their bodies to survive to get to the bus stop but have an older sibling who is protective and always there for us and feel protected and safe.

It is not our circumstances that lead to what we internalize about the world. It is what we are taught and the back stories we create about our experiences. The good thing is that our worldviews are not chiseled in marble. We can change them with a little bit of concentrated effort.

In Cognitive Behavioral Therapy: [253]	In *The Smart Way*:
Finding the client's irrational beliefs	Feeling the emotional discord and using meta-cognition to find thoughts that feel better
Automatic thoughts	When automatic thoughts don't feel good, question them and use meta-cognition to find better feeling thoughts
Assisting the client in changing them	Individual directs his or her own change. If a therapist is needed, Emotional Guidance will encourage assistance and help client overcome concerns about stigma
Verbally disputed by client and therapist	Mentally disputed by client. Individual may also verbalize (i.e. See Bogus Process)
Pragmatic: How is it working for you in your life?	Same: This question is used in *The Smart Way*™
Empirical dispute: Prove to me that this belief is accurate by just giving me the facts	Individual uses emotions to gain greater clarity about the potential perspectives of a distressing situation, leading to a less emotional and more fact-based evaluation
Elegant dispute: Generate a new more effective belief to replace the old one for client to test in homework assignments to see how the new belief works in his actual life	Individual understands beliefs are thoughts you've thought repeatedly until you've created easy to follow neuropathways. Changing neuropathways simply requires thinking new, better-feeling thoughts repeatedly until those neuropathways are easier to travel. Moment-to-moment adjustments in the new beliefs can be evaluated by how they feel—there is no need for the trial and error process to be applied in real life without knowing in advance (by how the idea feels) that it will bring improvements.
Shame-attacking	*The Smart Way*™ sees shame as an inescapable double-negative and refutes it directly. Sustained negative emotional states are inherently harmful to both body and mind, so shame is refuted as something based in unhealthy beliefs about self or others. *The Smart Way* sees beliefs that cause shame as dysfunctional.

In the above chart, CBT is compared and contrasted with *The Smart Way*™ to demonstrate how much more efficient it is to give people information they can use to effectively adjust their thoughts in-the-moment. The time they would spend recording the frequency and events that co-occur with specific beliefs and how frequently those undesired behaviors occur so they can share the information with a therapist could be spent applying the processes and making progress toward better-feeling perspectives.[254]

Often, traditional methods address symptoms of the root cause, such as assertiveness training, anger management and social skills training.[255] The problem is that these programs do not address the root cause of the problem. They help, but not as much as using the same time to improve the root cause would help.

The Smart Way™ has a decided advantage over CBT for a number of reasons:
1. It can be delivered in a cost effective manner to large groups
2. It is prevention, not mental health treatment for a manifested illness so there is no stigma. The focus is on increasing happiness and resilience, which requires healthy cognition and self-esteem.
3. Because it is not a one-on-one therapeutic relationship, cultural differences are not a significant element. The student can use Emotional Guidance to decide what is personally meaningful and best. Classes should always include the instruction to follow one's own Emotional Guidance over and above the instructor's viewpoint. Instructors will disclose that they have their own core beliefs and that having different core beliefs is acceptable, and adds to the value and worth of each individual. Diversity is recognized as a form of collective strength that is to be appreciated.
4. It empowers the individual with skills and knowledge that leads to more functional thinking capabilities.

CBT focuses on client empowerment, positing that the client is capable of change by controlling her/his thoughts and emotions, conveying respect for the client's abilities and understanding.[256] *The Smart Way*™ does the same but reinforces it by putting the knowledge and power in the client's hands, helping to develop and reinforce a healthy internal locus of control. Despite its limitations, Cognitive Behavioral Therapy is highly effective, but *The Smart Way*™ has greater potential because it can be delivered as a preventative measure and it overcomes some of the objections that our most vulnerable populations have about mental health services.

The *Smart Way*™ is **Cognitive Behavioral Therapy Plus** because it adds Emotional Guidance and a direct understanding of how the mind works, not just insights garnered by a guided tour led by a therapist.

I'm not suggesting mind-control—at least not by anyone other than the individual controlling his or her own mind. In fact, when individuals do not understand how the mind works or how what they expose themselves to affects their outcomes and the very thoughts they think, they make decisions that harm themselves without any awareness of what they are doing. We're careful about exposing ourselves to toxic chemicals, but most people do not realize that over a period of time, negative habits of thought are just as toxic as the chemicals they try so hard to avoid. Not understanding how the mind works is no different than giving someone the keys to a car without a map when some paths take them through hostile and even deadly territories.

We encourage providing *The Smart Way*™ training classes and materials to both employees and their families because it increases consistent reinforcement and the techniques help families manage their own stressors, contributing to a more supportive and harmonious home environment. Improving the emotional state of any member of the family benefits every family member and the evidence suggests it can reduce family problems that eventually affect the quality of work and absenteeism.

The *Smart Way*™ can be taught to large groups, which reduces the cost of implementation.

EXPECTANT QUESTIONS

Expectant questions are more powerful than positive affirmations.

Positive Affirmation:

I can do this.

Expectant Question:

How can I do this?

I was excited as soon as I read this research. It makes sense given the way our brains work. Asking a question prompts the brain to look for answers.

Affirmations can backfire if the person stretches further than they believe is possible and the mind will affirm the existing beliefs.

Questions that stretch too far might do the same thing but I'm not sure and in playing with my brain I asked it "How could I get to the moon?" The first thoughts I had in response were trains of thought that could lead to actionable answers. I didn't follow those trains of thought because I don't really want to go to the moon.

When I ask other questions, such as "How can I get this book to best seller status?" a lot of actionable answers immediately come to my mind.

When I ask "How can I best help clients with a specific issue?" actionable thoughts come to mind immediately.

I read this new research during the past month but I've pulled 500 studies for this book and right now I can't find the specific study I read. If I find it before this goes to print I'll add the citation.

It won't hurt you to try this process the next time you need a solution. Just turn it into a question and see how your mind responds. Although I'm new to using this process I like the results I am getting so far.

Here are some lead in's to questions that seem to get my brain working productively:

How can I . . .

What should I do in order to . . .

Who should I contact to help me . . .

What do I need to accomplish . . .

How can I best . . .

Where is the best place to . . .

When should I . . .

Which method would be best in this situation . . .

Which breakout session should I choose?

Why should I use this?

Is there something that would be better than what I am considering?

How can I illustrate this simply?

What analogy will provide a clear example?

How can I heal. . . ?

How can I help this patient decide to adhere to instructions. . . ?

I like using expectant questions. To me, it ties in with Appreciative Inquiry which has proven to be an effective form of organizational change. It also ties in with the origins of my own work.

A professional asked me why I was so resilient in 1995. I didn't even know I was resilient when he asked me that question. I recognized that if I was more resilient than many others and I could figure out why, I would be able to help other people. I began asking "What makes people thrive in spite of adversity?"

Over the years many people told me it was not possible to answer a broad question like mine but my intuitive guidance contradicted their perspective. Today I feel I know the answer fully and it began with asking a question and continuing to ask the same question until I was satisfied.

Today my guiding question is "How can I best communicate what I've learned about human thriving to as many people as possible?" As I began asking this question analogies and diagrams began coming to me even though I never considered myself to be good at creating either of these.

I would love to hear from you about how you use expectant questions and the results you notice.

APPRECIATION

Simple appreciation is one of the most powerful tools. It hasn't been researched nearly as much as gratitude but for 2/3 of the people appreciation is more powerful than gratitude and for the remaining 1/3 there is no difference between gratitude and appreciation.[257] I prefer appreciation but if gratitude makes someone else feel better I encourage them to use what feels best to them.

There are two appreciation practices I encourage.

Appreciation Process I

Every morning tell yourself (set an intention) that you will find at least three things to appreciate during the day. If you want to use an expectant question you can ask, "What will I find to appreciate today?"

Then plan a time at the end of the day (both dinner and bedtime work well) to remember what you found to appreciate during the day. Don't just remember what it was. Pause and actually allow yourself to feel the emotion of appreciation and any visceral feelings in your body that correspond with the things you found to appreciate. If you have dinner with someone sharing what you found with them is another good practice. Writing, as is journaling, is another good way to practice appreciation. Some studies show that journaling can become routine so make sure you are present when you journal. If you choose to journal then you have actually chosen to spend time feeling appreciation.

Appreciation Process II

The second appreciation process involves stream of consciousness writing. It does not replace the 1st process but supplements it. In this process you decide to focus on one thing you appreciate and begin writing about what you appreciate/love about it until you run out of thoughts of appreciation on the subject. I do three of these each day and am often high from the release of good feeling bio-chemicals in my body by the time I am finished with the process.

If you want to keep falling in love with your partner over and over again do this process about your partner at least once a week. It doesn't have to be about your whole partner. You could focus on one aspect of your partner one time and another aspect another time. If you find yourself feeling irritated by your partner you can use this technique to help you remember what you love about your spouse. Being irritated is a reflection of your emotional state more than anything else.

What to appreciate? The world is full of things to appreciate. It does not have to be a big thing. You can appreciate that you have running water, that your body knows how to transport oxygen to cells that need it, that your heart pumps without you having to think about it, that you have food to eat, that the sun came up, that you have a comfortable pillow, that you can smell a flower. The list is endless. The key is to focus on things that make you feel good. I love sitting on my deck in the morning feeling the sunshine and looking out over the golf course in my backyard, listening to the birds chirp and catching sight of cardinals and finches.

Appreciation Process I works to focus your brain to look for the good in the world. There are lots of people that want us to focus on the negative and we can easily become unbalanced in our perspective. Many people think a negative bias is realistic but the truth is that there is far more good going on everyday than bad.

Appreciation Process II reinforces positive emotions and as I mentioned, it's a great way to get a natural high. There is something very powerful about knowing you can feel great just because you want to.

There is no more powerful foreplay than to express appreciation for your partner, in writing or verbally. I'll leave that there. You can apply the same process to enjoy your job more.

SOCIAL SUPPORT

Social support is a protective factor against burnout and many physical and mental health issues. It is important to note that, in general, people who feel good emotionally have better relationships with others in every area of their lives. Rather than attempting to develop relationships in order to improve your health and lower your risk of burnout, work on improving your emotional state and then do what flows naturally from your better feeling emotional state. Individuals who use reappraisal as a coping skill have better interpersonal relationships and those who use suppression have worse interpersonal relationships.[258]

It is also important to understand that the perception of emotional support is the source of its benefits. In studies that looked at how individuals perceived social support by comparing their perceptions with the actual support the people they perceived as supportive were willing or able to provide, it was the perception of the presence of support that mattered.

Use the benefits of social support to give yourself permission to take the time to develop relationships if you need a reason. Also, be mindful of whether you have close relationships.

Just knowing that help is available and you don't have to jump over hurdles to get it or feel like a failure can go a long way to reducing stress.

As a busy professional raising two children on my own, who had relocated across the country from life-long friends and family, I realized that I had not developed any real friendships (outside of work hours) when I had been in North Carolina for about three years. I had met a number of women at work with whom I would have enjoyed spending more time because I enjoyed our time together at work.

I arranged a Ladies Slumber Party at a lake house about three hours away and invited several of the women I wanted to know better to join me for a weekend. We had a blast. We planned to go into Charleston (about an hour away) early on Saturday but we stayed up half the night talking so we didn't head out until later in the day. The weekend was a wild success. I made some good friends who were no longer just work acquaintances. One of my guests got such good advice from others on her love life that she changed her mind about which of the two men she was dating to see again and they're celebrating their 10th wedding anniversary this year.

I'd never heard of a Ladies Slumber Party before I planned one. It was so much fun. We did it several more times.

Be open about the goal if you decide to plan an event. I was very upfront. "I like you and I'd like to get to know you better because I think we could be real friends; not just work friends." I was also very clear about who I wanted in my circle of friends. My priorities were that the person be nice and intelligent. The group was diverse with respect to age, religion, race, and background. The nice requirement ensured that we were able to get along. The intelligent requirement ensured that we could learn from one another.

Use criteria that are important to you. It amazes me how many people go out of their way to socialize with people they don't really enjoy. Be neighborly with your neighbors but if you don't enjoy their company or share interests in things you love, don't plan to spend your evenings with them. It's possible to get along with nearly anyone. It's also possible to survive on cheap fast food but so much more enjoyable to sit down to a meal with a server who provides top notch service and a memorable meal. If you make plans with people and find yourself forcing yourself to go it's probably because you didn't choose your friends wisely. It doesn't make them bad people. They just aren't what you want or need now.

When it comes to family, do your best and be satisfied with it. The strategies in this book can smooth out acidic family relationships. Remember, you have to change your perspective. Attempting to change someone else is a lesson in frustration.

People who have good social support tend to be optimistic, have healthy self-esteem, an internal locus of control and are more resilient.

MAKE HAPPINESS A PRIORITY

Our society doesn't support making our personal happiness a priority. There are many reasons and ways this message is conveyed to us so that it becomes part of our belief system.

One way is to project personal happiness as selfish. This common belief is blatantly wrong for a variety of reasons. Our happiness is good for others for the following reasons:

- When we are happy we are naturally nicer to others.

- When we are happy our immune function is better which improves our physical health which makes us less likely to become a burden to others.
- When we are happy we naturally make better choices about food which also improves our health.
- When we are happy we naturally make better choices about exercise which also improves our health.
- When we are happy we naturally make better choices about sleep which also improves our health.
- Positive emotions are associated with greater resilience so when bad things happen we rebound faster making it less likely we will become a burden to others.
- Positive emotions protect against mental illness which helps us be a better citizen, spouse, parent, etc.
- When we are happy our cognitive function is better so we make better decisions which make us of greater benefit to our families, employer, and community.
- When we are happy our digestive function is better which reduces the likelihood we will develop chronic illnesses associated with digestion.
- When we are happy our central nervous system functions better which reduces the risk we will be involved in or cause an accident.
- When we are happy we have a greater capacity to have good relationships with others which is good for us and them.

Our unhappiness leads to the opposite—detriments to our families, employers, and society. Everything mentioned above that is improved by happiness declines when we are unhappy. In addition, we are more likely to commit a crime or be violent when we are unhappy. Productivity and customer satisfaction decline when we are unhappy.

Think about arguments you've participated in with a spouse or co-worker. How often were the arguments because you wanted to prove your rightness about something that, in the greater scheme of things, was inconsequential? How would you have perceived the situation if your first priority was to be happy instead of be right? Could you have let it go? Do you argue with someone about their opinion? Do you have heated discussions when you're really talking about different perspectives, both of which are right from the perspective from which they are being viewed?

When arguments become heated, how often do hurt feelings and decrements to relationships occur? How often are perceived social connections damaged by arguments or other disagreements?

Now take those arguments to a larger arena. How much is society harmed by people demanding that others think like them or behave like them? Is it possible to get everyone to think the same or behave the same? Is it a desirable outcome to whittle everyone down until all people have only one opinion amongst them? Are any problems solvable when only a single perspective about the situation is available?

SET LIMITS: SAY NO

Saying no can be one of the most difficult things for someone who has been taught to be selfless or someone with low self-esteem to do.

There are a variety of methods I've used to increase my ability to say no to extraneous activities that don't support what is most important to me.

The first step is being very conscious about your own priorities. When I was creating the mission statement for Happiness 1st Institute the idea to create mission statements for all the important areas of my life came to me.

I created mission statements for:

- My life (an overriding statement of purpose)
- My business
- My primary relationship
- My relationship with my body
- My relationship with me
- My relationship with my health
- My relationship with my children
- My relationship with my parents
- My relationship with my friends
- My relationship with my home
- My relationship with strangers

Mission statements aren't long, drawn out missives. They are concise statements of intention.

Once I had my mission statements I could compare requests to my mission statements and ask if the request fit into any of my missions or if it was outside my core missions. I am interested in many things so filling time is never something I want to do with things that don't fit my core missions. I do ask if a new request is something that calls to me (using my emotional guidance as a guide).

There are volunteer activities I used to participate in for causes I care about that I no longer do because they didn't support my core missions. When you're a caring person there is a never ending list of causes you'd like to support. One way I make the decisions about which volunteer activities I participate in is whether it is the highest and best use of my skills, knowledge, and talents. For example, I joined my husband volunteering for a USGA golf tournament. I enjoyed the four days I worked and had fun but I kept thinking about the greater contributions I could be making elsewhere and decided I wouldn't do that again.

For years, I volunteered for a conservation organization but the contributions I made could have been done by anyone with basic skills so it wasn't the highest and best use of my skills.

If I'm going to be thinking about other things I would rather be doing while I do something I will say no. This was a difficult skill for me to learn.

It is helpful to have kind answers when you decide to say no.

"I would love to but my other commitments don't allow me enough time to give you the commitment you're asking for. I hope your event is very successful."

"I'm sorry but I'm already stretched thin. I am honored that you thought of me."

Sometimes somebody wants to do something for me that would take time I don't have and I use "I'll take the thought for the deed. I so appreciate your kindness."

When my children were younger I would use, "I am spending as much time with them now while they still want to be with me."

You don't have to give a reason but I found that doing so stopped repeated requests. Just be authentic.

It's easier to say no if you have established your priorities in advance. In a study that interviewed physicians who were known in the community for their resilience, one of the findings that supported their resilience was the ability to set limits.[259] Learning to set limits increases job satisfaction which decreases burnout.[260]

MINDFULNESS

I live the techniques I teach. Numerous people, including clinical psychologists, have remarked that I am very mindful. I want to differentiate between mindfulness and *The Smart Way*™.

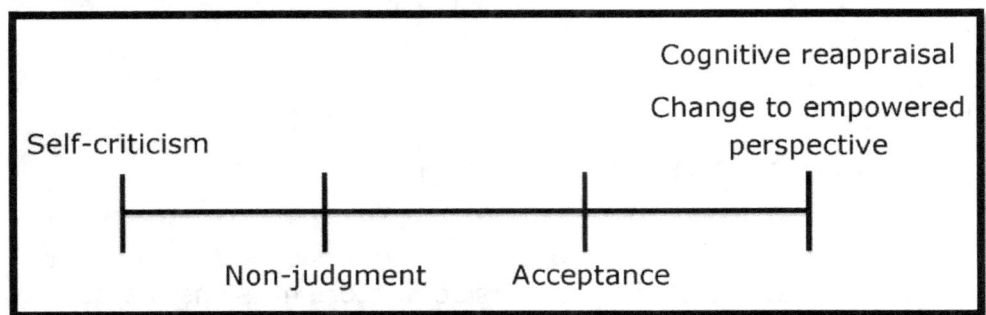

Mindfulness strives to focus on the present experience without judgment or evaluation.

The Smart Way™ doesn't care if you're focused on past, present, or future. It encourages you to focus on things that feel good and to find the best feeling thought you can find about what you're focused upon. There is an absence of negative judgment. Negative emotions simply mean that you're looking at a situation or individual in a way that is not the best way you could perceive the situation or person. In that regard it is not judgmental and emotions are seen as guidance so they can be appreciated for providing guidance even when they don't feel good. Emotions are not indicating that someone else is bad when our gaze upon them feels bad to us. It is the thoughts we think about the person/situation that cause our negative emotion.

The Smart Way™ encourages savoring future events that you are looking forward to so that you can enjoy them now and when they actually occur. The trick is not to become attached to the outcome. For example, I enjoyed the things I had planned for my wedding day enormously but when things didn't go exactly as planned I immediately felt for thoughts that felt better which ensured our day wasn't ruined because of a few things that weren't exactly as I wanted them. Reaching for the better-feeling thought ensures that savoring in advance doesn't lead to disappointment when the anticipated situation doesn't manifest exactly the way you'd hoped.

The Smart Way™ does not discourage recalling the past. It discourages negative rumination. But there is nothing disadvantageous about savoring memories of good times in the past as long as it is done while feeling good. If it is done while feeling melancholy or missing the good old days, think about something that feels better. It is also okay to pick up memories from the past in order to reframe them but only do this if it is a subject you still think about. For example, if you never think about the classmate that was mean to you in sixth grade don't dredge that old memory back up. If you were abused as a child and you still feel like a victim, finding more empowered ways to view the past would help you. I've previously written about how to do that in *Rescue Our Children from the War Zone* and those instructions are beyond the scope of this book.

Mindfulness has been heavily researched and implemented in a wide variety of situations. It is a helpful practice but I believe time will show that the practice of using Emotional Guidance and Meta-cognitve Strategies provides better short and long-term results. In 2016, *The American Journal of Occupational Therapy* reported that abbreviated practices of mindfulness are not supported in the literature[261] (as being effective at reducing stress).

A Medscape report shared that Primary Care Physicians learned mindfulness by attending a weekend immersion and two follow-up evening sessions. They could learn *The Smart Way*™ with the same time commitment. A Huffington Post article reported that a conference attendee shared "how the hospital where she works had introduced a MBSR program to help minimize job stress. The program appeared to make a difference in the mental states of the staff. But instead of bringing about higher productivity in the workplace, greater mindfulness about what they were doing led a surprising number of the employees to conclude that their pathway to stress reduction was to leave their jobs."[262]

The time commitment for mindfulness is not less than that of learning *The Smart Way*™. A 2016 study on mindfulness for occupational therapists suggested "reading mindfulness books and websites, watching or listening to mindfulness prompts and tutorials, attending local mindfulness groups (e.g. meet-up groups, spiritual groups), and enrolling in a mindfulness course (e.g. college or continuing education offerings, MBSR program).[263]

I've worked with clients who used mindfulness before learning *The Smart Way*™ who have reported that their lives improved with the addition of *The Smart Way*™ and I've never had a client with a mindfulness practice who reported that learning *The Smart Way*™ did not provide stress relief beyond what they were already experiencing. This is as good of a place as any to remind the reader that extensive research on a specific practice does not mean it is the best practice, just the most researched practice.

MEDITATION

There are many different meditation techniques. Like Mindfulness, meditation can be a compliment to *The Smart Way*™ but unless one's practice is very rigorous (daily), it isn't likely to reprogram your brain.

Meditation is a wonderful practice. I use a couple of types of meditation in my own practice including one that simply allows my mind to rest and a loving heart meditation that helps me find peace and love for all of humanity in my own heart. Loving-Kindness meditation has been shown to improve compassion and resilience in healthcare workers.[264]

Instruction in meditation is beyond the scope of this book.

RELIGION/SPIRITUALITY

Many studies indicate benefits of spiritual or religious beliefs. A survey of interns at Yale indicated that belief in the utility of prayer and meditation and a belief that their life has a purpose during times of hardship (indicating flexibility and purpose in the belief system) were protective against burnout.[265]

What I encourage is that you use your emotional guidance to determine if your worldview uplifts you or makes you feel worse. If it makes you feel better, it is beneficial to you.

VOLUNTEERISM

Volunteer activities are associated with lower burnout rates. This may be via a higher sense of purpose from volunteer activities. Thirty-seven percent of physicians who were not burned out volunteer compared to twenty-eight percent of physicians who are burned out. It could also be that being burned out robs them of the energy to devote to volunteer work.

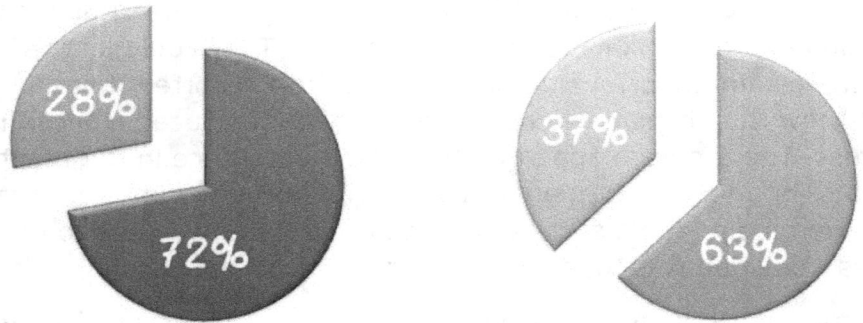

If a specific volunteer activity appeals to you, participating should be beneficial. The worst thing you can do to yourself is feel guilty if you don't volunteer. If your beliefs are that you should and you'll feel guilty if you do not, volunteer. If you enjoy volunteering, volunteer. If it feels as if doing so adds to your burdens, don't volunteer. There isn't a one size fits all answer. The answer may be different at different times of your life. You'll find more information about volunteering in the *Set Limits: Say No* section.

PRACTICE IS IMPORTANT

People apply the strategies they know provide relief that carry the least risk. Generally, someone who knows how to improve their emotional state in a healthier way won't use dysfunctional or maladaptive coping styles. When new, healthier styles are initially learned it is important to practice them. Strategies, such as keeping visible reminders where they will be seen, can help the healthier styles become the new default response. It is possible to forget about new methods if they aren't used enough to form habits.

The good news is that even if someone forgets for a while, as soon as they remember they have better options they can apply those methods. They don't have to begin at the beginning all over again. When a new bad event occurs it can take me a little while to remember to apply the healthier methods if I haven't encountered that sort of situation previously. When it is something I've dealt with previously it is easier to remember.

I'll share two examples. My 26 year-old daughter is currently on a solo 65-day journey through England, Wales, Scotland, and Ireland. Last night it was well past midnight in her location and I hadn't heard that she was in for the night and I felt a little anxiety about not hearing from her. As soon as I felt the negative emotion I began soothing myself. I went more general. I reminded myself that negative emotion meant my guidance was telling me to have better expectations. She had posted new pictures to Facebook the day before and I hadn't yet viewed them so I went to Facebook to see if she'd posted there and started viewing her new pictures. She looked so happy in the pictures and that was very soothing to me. Within a few minutes my concern had dissipated. A little while later she texted to let me know she was back in her Airbnb room.

Contrast that with last week when I found out my mother's cancer has returned and the physician told her to expect it to be aggressive which threw me for an emotional loop. The first time they caught the cancer very early and there was little concern that it could be eradicated. I forgot an important meeting that day and spent much of it trying to work but realized later that I had been in what I would call a "fog."

It wasn't until the next day that I began soothing myself. I *forgot* that I had skills. Sometimes you're just not ready to be soothed immediately and that's okay. I've had to go very general in my thoughts about her condition. She is a fighter and that soothes me. I can also be soothed by her long life and marriage. I also seek solace in my faith. I won't detail my personal faith here but will encourage you to have beliefs that you find soothing when it comes to death. In an occupation that deals with death frequently that seems essential for self-care.

In both situations, my prior practice finding better-feeling thoughts helped me self-soothe and find perspectives that were less stressful quickly.

Remember, most of our thoughts are habitual not thoughtful. In order to make your habitual thoughts feel better you have to consciously practice the techniques that will develop the habits of thought you find to be less stressful.

Keep the book handy and if you find yourself feeling stressed look through this chapter and find strategies to apply. If the first one doesn't work, try another one.

ADAPTIVE COPING

Adaptive coping strategies are complimentary to advanced coping skills. Applying advanced coping skills first makes implementing and following through on adaptive coping strategies easier. For example, using advanced coping skills to reduce stress without requiring a situation to change before your level of stress can be decreased makes the cognitive capacity you have available for problem-solving higher. You will literally be able to identify better solutions when after you use advanced coping skills than you would have if you went straight to problem solving.

Anger management is an adaptive coping style that can become unnecessary when you frequently use advanced coping skills. When you practice your emotional state into good feeling emotions frequently, anger is not near the surface. Things that would have once made you angry (because they seemed like big problems) no longer make you angry because they seem like minor inconveniences that you are fully capable of handling.

In my own journey, my level of assertiveness increased naturally as my confidence increased. I notice this primarily in my personal relationships but it is has also changed in my professional relationships. For example, when a comment is made that I would have previously ruminated about and worried it meant that my spouse's eyes were wandering, I'll address directly but not in an accusatory manner. I'll inquire directly and be open to the answer and won't be stressed about what it is.

When I teach a class or give a speech I ask for feedback including the good, bad, and ugly because if I don't have the bad or ugly I can't improve what I don't know isn't up to the standards I want to meet. When there is negative feedback, I take it as useful knowledge, not a vilification of me or my value or worth. The feedback is incorporated into my goal setting. I don't feel I have to defend what I did or didn't do; my job is to learn from it and become more of my potential.

Conflict resolution needs disappear because when you're no longer viewing one person as right and the other as wrong because you realize that in most cases we just perceive the same situation from different perspectives there is no conflict. There is simply more work required to understand one another's perspectives but that work is not about determining who is right; it is about identifying a way forward that is mutually beneficial. The goal of the conversation is communication.

When it is a factual, right or wrong, the ego isn't involved in the answer. If I learn I've been wrong about something I focus on the fact that I now know something I didn't know in the past which I always perceive as a good outcome. The amount of information that exists today is far beyond the ability of any one person to know. If we continue to cling to the insistence that we are always right we diminish our capacity to be happy. Also, new research has made many "facts" we were taught in school inaccurate. Examples include Darwinism which won over Lamarck's view of soft inheritance and is now being reconsidered due to advances in epigenetics. The determination to be "right" is further complicated by the continued teaching of concepts that were never validated as "facts" and the continued teaching of concepts that have been invalidated. A common one is Maslow's Hierarchy which was never validated and has been partially invalidated but is still frequently taught. In Rescue Our Children from the War Zone I proposed a modified version of Maslow's Hierarchy of Needs that fits modern knowledge.

Giving up the need to be "right" isn't about discarding facts. It is about not forming opinions that are so strongly held you will defend them even when new evidence suggests prior information was flawed. Our brains naturally protect our beliefs, regardless of whether doing so is beneficial to us. By adopting an attitude of curiosity toward new information the brain's automatic rejection of new information that conflicts with existing beliefs can be bypassed.

Your emotional guidance will support the curious approach and it will let you know when you're arguing for beliefs when it is not in your best interest to do so.

Some skills, such as time management, community living skills, meditation, mindfulness, Yoga, Tai Chi, asking for help, and goal setting are very beneficial when added to advanced coping skills. There are many excellent sources of knowledge for these skills.

ANTICIPATED CHANGES

Educating physicians and other staff on healthy habits of thought and emotional guidance should result in numerous changes in the culture, burnout, and outcomes experienced in your organization.

Employees will feel more empowered so instead of resenting things they don't like they will feel empowered to speak up about them. But they won't just complain, they will offer solutions that will contribute to the success of your organization and better patient outcomes.

If you are aware of the benefits of an Appreciative Inquiry approach,[266] *The Smart Way*™ results in the same sort of outcomes on an individual basis but at a greater degree than those observed when the goal of Appreciative Inquiry is focused on the organization. The empowered individuals then extend the benefits to the organization and to patients.

Physicians can train themselves to focus on the areas of their work that they find personally satisfying. That is often the use of their expertise, their relationships with patients, and making a difference.

> *Stress reduction programs focusing on cognitive behavioral techniques were found to be of utmost significance when it comes to preventing and treating burnout in healthcare professionals.*[267]

Given the correlations between The Smart Way™ and CBT as well as salutogenesis, it is likely to be a more cost effective method. When emotional guidance is added to correct the misunderstanding about the purpose and use of emotions that permeates society, it should exceed the results of one-on-one CBT therapy in many cases. The case histories of success alleviating long-term chronic depression and PTSD that remained resistant with traditional therapy suggest the combination is a more powerful remedy.

When under stress people who have a greater sense of control over what occurred in their lives remain healthier than those who feel powerless. We never really have control over what is going to happen but we can have control over how we respond.

A word of caution is in order. When someone is new at learning these techniques they can often feel enormous excitement at how easy it is to feel better than they have in a long while and in some cases, ever. It is natural to want to share their delight and what is working with friends and family but as newbies they often don't understand it well enough to explain it and when they try to get their friends and family to come along questions they can't answer come up and their friends and family begin building a wall against the information.

This is unfortunate but I've seen it happen hundreds of times. There are two recommendations to counteract this. When I provide a program for an organization, I offer to include significant others and mature teenagers in the training at near cost. The employer benefits because work-family conflict that already exists declines more when the whole family learns The Smart Way™ together and new conflicts aren't created by attempting to teach something they don't understand well enough to teach.

For family and friends who aren't in the class the solution depends on their level of interest. If they want to learn and are good at learning from a book, any of my books will provide sufficient information that they will be able to begin using The Smart Way™. They will then be able to compare notes on what works and how they solve various issues and both will progress faster.

If the friend or family member is not interested don't talk about it at all. They will soon notice that the rough edges in your life have somehow smoothed out. Depending on how long they've been watching you they may continue observing you for quite a while but eventually they will ask what changed because they will notice that it seems you are enjoying life more and that in many ways your life looks easier. When they ask is the time to share the information. Also, by then, you'll have enough practice using the techniques that you'll be able to answer questions that would have stumped you at the beginning of your journey.

PHYSICIAN'S POWER

As we visited with physicians it became clear that the boiled frog theory has led to *subject-specific* learned helplessness among physicians and possibly, healthcare administrators when it comes to the myriad demands placed on physicians.

> *Imagine a pot filled with cold water. A frog is quietly swimming in it. The fire is lit under that pot. Water starts warming up. Soon it becomes lukewarm. The*

frog finds this rather pleasant and keeps swimming. The temperature keeps rising. Water is now warm. It's a little more than what the frog enjoys; it becomes a bit tired, but it doesn't panic. Water is now really warm. The frog finds that unpleasant, but it has also become weak, by now, so the frog stands the heat as it can and does nothing.

The temperature will thus keep rising up to the moment the frog will simply end up being cooked and die, without ever extracting itself from the pot. Plunged in a pot half-way through boiling temperature, the frog would immediately give a powerful and salutary push with its legs and find itself out of it.[268]

Whether a frog would stay in the water is not the point. The point is that psychologically, if things are introduced gradually that are close enough to our existing comfort zone we will adapt if we feel adapting is the right course of action or the least problematic choice.

Physicians want to please and they want to serve. They want to be respected. Fighting against demands that they adhere to new requirements counters these desires. A physician who won't subject him or herself to scrutiny from payers, well, what is he or she attempting to hide? That's the society we live in. We don't give people the benefit of the doubt even when we should. We view real reasons, such as not wanting to spend the time away from actually practicing medicine, as excuses rather than valid reasons.

As more layers were added to the increasing demands, the boiling frog analogy became the perfect example of what had happened. As a result of long exposure to unhealthy conditions, a form of learned helplessness has developed—a sense that there is nothing that can be done. Learned helplessness is associated with an external locus of control and learning about and using emotional guidance will develop an internal locus of control. Also, not all physicians are burned out and those who aren't can be of great assistance in leading an organizing effort. I've seen some calls for unionization but that is not the answer. Why? Because physicians don't want to go on strike and deprive people of health care anymore than they want to be perceived as untrustworthy. A physician strike would be portrayed by the media as being about money and would further damage physician's reputations in the community.

Not unionizing does not mean that organizing is the wrong solution. But the purpose of the organization is not to represent an underpowered group of individuals. The purpose is to represent a group of learned, service-oriented individuals who have been taken advantage of by organizations that didn't concern themselves with the welfare of the people their organization's demands impacted. Organization could lead to drafting and passage of legislation that requires insurers, the government, and employers to use the same source of information so that it does not have to be input multiple times. Clinically sound requirements could be sought instead of the current ill-informed requirements that aren't healthy for some patients. Could reviews be scaled back to best practice scenarios instead of attempting to micro manage every step? Physicians themselves are better able to identify what should be done and guide us toward a better future. Collectively, you have the power.

CORE CONCEPTS

Healthy habits of thought will help you develop some core concepts. Don't worry if you can't believe the core concepts at first. The core concepts will feel natural once you develop skill at using your emotional guidance together with advanced and transformative coping skills.

I am strong.

Problems are opportunities in disguise.

Everyone is good at the core of who they are.

I am wise.

I am capable.

I can find a win-win-win-win in this situation.

There is more good in the world than bad.

I can thrive even if most people are currently choosing to struggle.

Other people's opinions reflect their emotional state; not my value.

These are both actionable steps and areas where attention could bear fruit.

PART IV - RETENTION STRATEGIES

> THIS SECTION FOCUSES ON ACTIONS HEALTHCARE
> ORGANIZATIONS CAN TAKE, INDIVIDUALLY AND COLLECTIVELY,
> TO REDUCE BURNOUT.

Although individuals can learn skills that have a significant impact on the stress, burnout, depression, and anxiety they experience as the result of workplace stress, organizations have a responsibility to understand how their decisions, culture, and support help or hinder individual efforts. Organizations that want to thrive will incorporate that knowledge into their processes and culture. Healthcare worker well-being affects both patient outcomes and the health of the organization that employs them.

The goal should not be to develop resilient employees to see how far they can be pushed; it should be to develop resilient employees and organizations so we can see how good life can be. A unified model should "increase worker's ability to deal with complex problems and constantly changing demands resulting in increased job satisfaction, improved patient safety and care, and reduced staff sick-leave and turnover."[269] Using emotional guidance will help employees find better-feeling perspectives about their work environment and they will be intrinsically motivated to do so in order to feel as good as they can under the circumstances.

An employee who doesn't understand how to interpret their emotions accurately may feel negative emotion is validating their distress at changes in their workplace. An employee who understands how to interpret their emotional guidance will see the same emotion as an indicator that it is possible to find a different perspective about the situation that will feel more empowering and elicit better-feeling emotions.

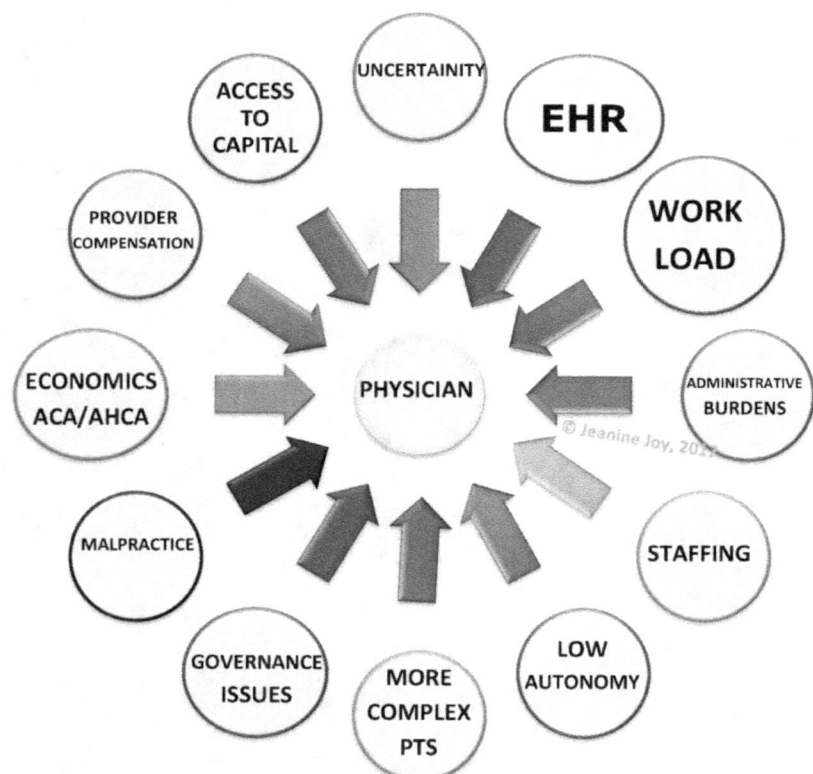

In 2012, the Achieves of Internal medicine reported:[270]

The fact that almost one (1) in two (2) US Physicians has symptoms of burnout implies that the origins of this problem are rooted in the environment and care delivery system rather than in the personal characteristics of a few susceptible individuals.

The solution will not be found solely in the care delivery system. If it were only the care delivery system, all physicians would be burned out, not half of them. A 2-pronged approach makes more sense than just attempting to change the work environment. Also, the importance of an internal locus of control was highlighted in the section describing the development of individual resilience. Since the 1970's, the number of college students with an internal locus of control has been trending downwards. That is relevant to this discussion and relevant to patient health and well-being.

The high prevalence of burnout amongst physicians is opposite that observed in other occupations with high education levels where advanced education is associated with lower levels of burnout.[271]

As payment for services is increasingly tied to things like electronic medical records (EMR) physicians can experience a loss of control and in terms of intrinsic motivation, a decrease in autonomy. When a society begins imposing what some have termed draconian requirements on some of the most highly educated citizens it is time to push back. The negative impact on physician health and wellbeing and therefore, their ability to provide quality care justifies alternatives and giving physicians' greater autonomy.

Physicians also feel squeezed on both fronts. Physicians report that the requirements of EMR result in less face time with patients. At the same time compensation is being affected by patient outcomes. Physicians cannot improve patient outcomes by typing data into a computer. Face time with physicians is valuable to both patients and physicians. My doctor reported that time on the computer and less time with patients has decreased his satisfaction with his professional life—an opinion and reality which research confirms is common.

Higher stress results in higher intention to leave. Since *The Smart Way*™ strategies lower stress, they will increase retention and improve physical and mental health.

There are several factors to consider that directly target retention.

MEASUREMENT

Many companies spend a lot of money measuring employee engagement but they are measuring a high-level factor that they already measure the low-level factors. When you understand the relationships between engagement, burnout, turnover, absenteeism, co-worker incivility, patient satisfaction, productivity, errors, disability, accidents, and more you can recognize the role burnout and engagement play in these areas. The level of control over workload, time pressures and the amount of chaos that is normally present in the work environment are additional factors that should be measured.[272]

We want you to be aware of these relationships so you're making an informed decision about where you spend your money. Engagement surveys can lower engagement if there is a perception that you ask the question but don't change anything. Employees want changes that help them maintain a positive outlook about their work. Physicians who have a more positive outlook and/or find their work meaningful experience lower levels of burnout.[273]

One question you can ask employees that provides significant insight into how they feel about your organization is: "How likely it is that you would recommend our company to a friend or colleague?"

A suggestion box that lets employees know that you want feedback and then a post of suggestions made, the decision (actions to be taken) about the suggestion and considerations that were taken into account in making the decision would go a long way toward giving employees the sense that they are being heard. The reasons are probably more important than the decision in many instances. When providing reasons it is important to remember that not all employees, even highly educated employees, have an understanding of business decision-making processes.

In my decades working in corporate America there were many instances where co-workers complained about a change where it was obvious they didn't understand the background and why the decision was the best one the company could make given the circumstances.

One easy way to develop this feedback would be to gather a group of employees and have them interview someone who knows the reasons for the decision and record responses to their questions. Use the interview to create a FAQ (frequently asked questions) document will increase the level of understanding by employees with different backgrounds.

When people know why something is decided it makes it easier for them to accept the decision. We accept decisions when we can see how we might make the same decision given the same circumstances.

A suggestion box without feedback can reduce engagement because employees who don't see their suggestions being acted upon feel ignored.

THOUGHTS ON THE BUSINESS OF MEDICINE

Finances are one of many factors that contribute to physician burnout. Other factors include:

1) Lack of adequate coping skills (could/should be trained in school).
2) Low levels of resilience (could/should be trained in school).
3) Increased mandates from government, employers, insurance companies, regulating bodies (i.e. Medical boards).
4) Malpractice stress (fear of making an error which actually increases the likelihood since stress reduces cognitive function).
5) Increased paperwork (22 - 40+% of physician time).
6) Income uncertainty due to government mandates, increased arduous medical board certification requirements, insurance company mandates, PQRS related reductions, medical necessity reviews, hospitals penalized for re-admissions, clinical decisions being made by insurance companies, MIPS, HIPAA updates and increased policing, ICD-10, EMR and the cost of establishing EMR, not knowing how to effectively negotiate contracts with insurers, marketplace contracts accepted without understanding reimbursements, Medicaid managed care, straight Medicaid, etc.
7) Clinical decision making conflicts between Hospitalists and the patient's primary (admitting or referring) physician.
8) Reduced autonomy.
9) Long work hours, lack of control of your schedule.
10) Health insurance interferes with developing long-term relationships with pts (insurance may require a change of provider); Out of network financial impacts
11) Inconsistent shifts.[274]
12) Culture that discourages use of earned vacation time.
13) Stigma surrounding obtaining mental health support and/or counseling.

14) Secondary trauma and compassion fatigue.
15) Lack of training about the business requirements of medicine (labor laws, contract law, etc.).
16) Co-worker incivility.
17) Lack of understanding of how to negotiate their own employment contract, contract clauses to have and avoid, etc.

Finances have a role in burnout but they are only one leg on a centipede.

PSYCHOLOGICAL CONTRACTS

Relationships include:
1. Written agreements
2. Verbal agreements
3. Psychological contracts

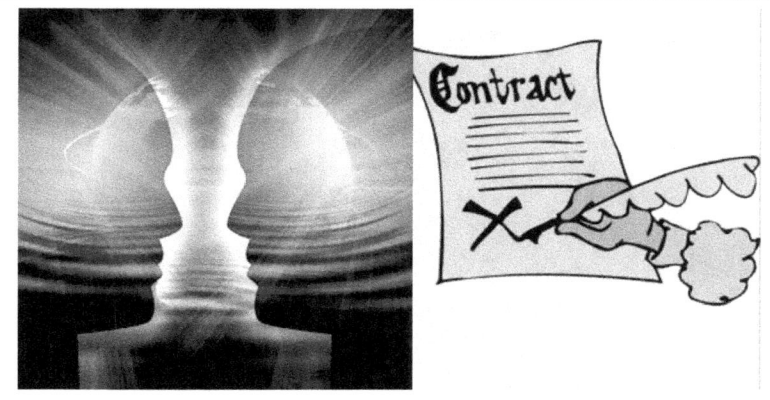

Violations of psychological contracts between an employer and employee decrease the energy an employee has to fulfill the written and psychological contract with the employer.[275] Violations of a psychological contract can feel as if one has been violated. "Over two decades of research has firmly established that a Psychological Contract (PC) breach—or the awareness that the employer fails to fulfill one or more obligations included in the PC—has negative consequences such as reduced job satisfaction, organizational commitment, performance, and increased turnover intentions."[276]

For example, a physician is highly trained and feels 100% responsible for accurately diagnosing and treating patients to the best of his or her skills and ability. This responsibility is supported by the Hippocratic Oath and, to many physicians, feels like a sacred duty. When insurance companies or employers begin interfering with this duty, by limiting what a physician can or cannot do for a patient, it violates the psychological contract. This can psychologically and physiologically feel as if the physician is being abused and destroy trust in any other psychological, written, or verbal agreements between the physician and employer. Even if it is an insurance company interfering with treatment, the physician may perceive the healthcare organization as more powerful and have a psychological contract that requires the employer/healthcare organization to protect the right to practice medicine in the way the physician perceives is best for the patient.

Healthcare organizations need to be cognizant of these psychological contracts, do their best to uphold them and when they are unable to do so, communicate, communicate, and then communicate some more. Realize that this can be (emotionally) as much or more of a violation of the psychological contract as learning one's spouse has been unfaithful.

Healthcare workers can learn to adjust their perspectives about implied psychological contracts in order to feel better and to ask explicit questions that satisfy their sense of right and just behaviors.

Another common psychological contract is an agreement that a healthcare worker will do their best to heal and cure patients but that the healthcare employer will provide adequate resources that support providing that level of care. When the healthcare employer fails to provide adequate resources in terms of staffing or life-saving equipment, the worker may feel that the psychological contract has been violated. This can contribute to burnout and turnover. It feels unjust to require the worker to do their job with insufficient resources to do the job well.

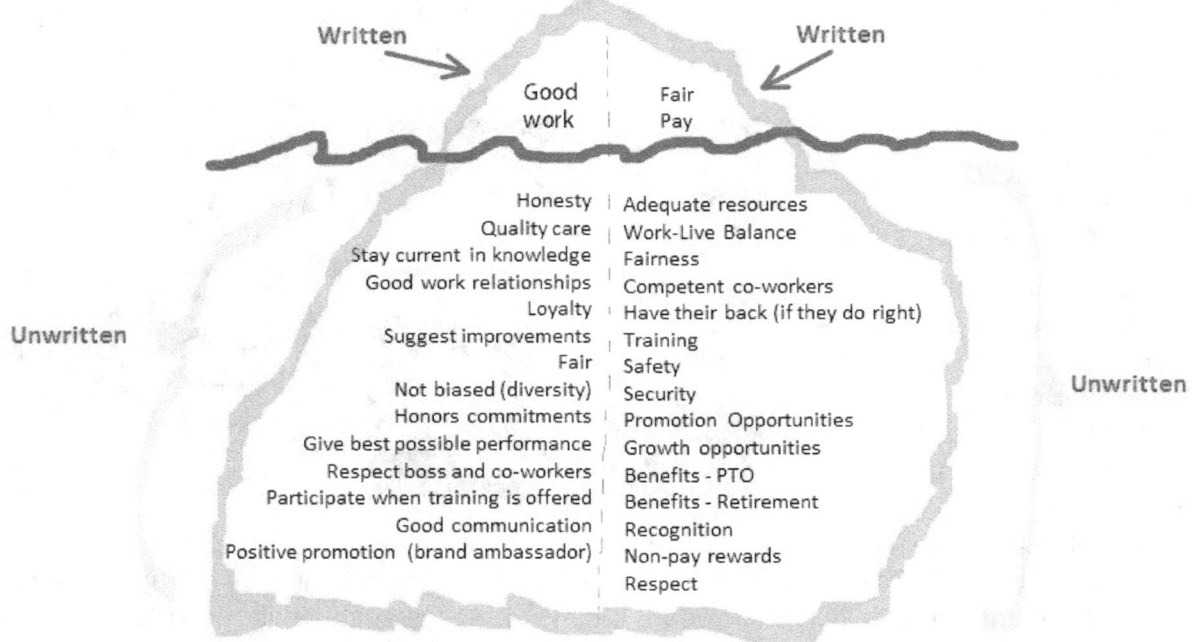

Psychological Contracts between Employees and Employers in Healthcare

Every change initiative should include the questions:

Does this change have the potential to affect psychological contracts with employees?

How will this change affect psychological contracts with employees?

Ideally, employees should be given the opportunity to provide feedback BEFORE changes are announced as a done deal.

Employees should be taught about the concept of psychological contracts. When you make the implicit explicit they are better able to identify and articulate violations and in many cases, better able to adjust their viewpoint to reduce the sense of violation. Understanding the "why" behind decisions helps employees accept violations of their psychological contract.

For example, employees expect that they will have job security if they do a good job and maintain, increase their skills. When this can't happen they are better able to accept it and maintain a positive view of the employer if they understand the reasoning that went into the decision.

It's outside healthcare but BB & T, a large regional bank recently announced that they are closing 100 branches of their bank. The employees in those branches probably feel as if their psychological contracts with BB&T have been violated. If BB&T explains that customers aren't coming to branches the way they once did and that if BB&T can't remain competitive in the emerging online banking space that they will eventually fail. The loss of some jobs to prevent the loss of all jobs in the organization is something employees can understand because if they were the decision-maker they would have made the same decision. If the employee doesn't understand the reason behind the decision they cannot determine that the actions are fair or just.

Your employees will judge your decisions based on what they believe they would have done under the same circumstances. The more information they have, the better they are able to understand why you arrived at the decision you made. It also makes them more able to provide suggestions that might allow you to avoid an undesirable outcome.

Here is an example of a physician whose psychological contract with his employer was broken:

> *The answers to these questions do not convey my very real sense of despair and exhaustion. I believe that most physicians unconsciously contracted with society to pursue their profession to the utmost of their ability and energy, to keep up their skills and do whatever was needed to promote patient care. In return, we expected respect, the equipment to do the job and freedom from financial anxieties. All 3 of these expectations have been abrogated, yet we continue to fulfill our side of the contract in confusion, disbelief and a sense of betrayal.*[277]

STOP THE SILENCE

Given the tendency of surgeons to underestimate the severity of their own stress and burnout levels,[278] their employers would benefit from educating them by providing assessments and tools like *The Smart Way*™ to equip them with skills that reduce the psychological stress they experience on a daily basis.

Bring the conversation into the open. Physicians tend to believe they are doing as well as or better than their colleagues even when they are doing the worst. Silence keeps them in the dark about methods that can improve their lives and prolong their careers.

WORKLOAD

Tasks that require a physician's direct involvement could use a re-evaluation and new best practices should be developed across the board. Administrative and bureaucratic tasks have been incrementally added to physician workloads from a variety of sources and the weight is approaching the final straw.

In one physician's words, "I still like seeing patients in the exam room but as soon as I walk out the door to the piles of paperwork I could just keep walking."[279]

"81% of physicians describe themselves as either overextended or at full capacity, up from 75%in 2012 and 76% in 2008.[280]

44% of physicians plan to take one or more steps that would reduce patient access to their services, such as cutting back on patients seen, retiring, working part-time, closing their practice to new patients, or seeking a non-clinical job, leading to the potential loss of tens of thousands of full-time-equivalents (FTEs).[281]

WORK/LIFE BALANCE

Work/Life Balance has permeated discussions of stress for decades. Two articles I reviewed while writing this book resonated with me. Both of the articles approached work/life balance from an unexpected direction that immediately makes sense. The first was from an intensivist who described her three maternity leaves. During the first she worked frequently while her baby slept and returned to work feeling energized and rested but colleagues judged and criticized her for working while on leave. She also felt grief and remorse for working despite being motivated to work. During her second maternity leave she "followed the rules" and disconnected. She once again returned to work energized and rested but was again overwhelmed with guilt, this time over the mountain of work that had piled up during her absence. They say the third time is the charm and for her it was. During her third leave she "wrote when she was motivated to write, slept when tired, and parented when it seemed fitting." She wrote, "My days were fluid, unencumbered, productive, and loving. When I returned to work, I was energized and rested and guilt-free."[282]

She explains:

> *As intensivists, we make hundreds of decisions daily and I would venture to guess that most decisions are good ones. Finding the key to work—life balance for me was having trust in my skills as an intensivist; acknowledging that these decision-making skills guide me in all my life decisions. I mostly make good decisions when deciding how best to spend my time. The most efficient and meaningful way to spend my time is to combine all aspects of my life and let them ebb and flow as naturally indicated.*[283]

I recognized how I live my own life in her comments. The next article I read echoed her thoughts on work-life balance as an illusion:

> *Since entering medical school over two decades ago, I reached the conclusion that the concept of work-life balance acts as quicksand in our professional and personal lives resulting in slow drowning in frustration, depression, and exhaustion. . . As we follow our peers' instructions trying to balance work and life, the question arises: when should we achieve this balance and How do we know we achieved it? . . . I concluded that the never-ending chase after work-life balance actually accumulates much more frustration than satisfaction. . . the absence of an objective outcome measure makes the chances of ever achieving this goal rather elusive.*[284]

If work-life balance feels elusive to you, let go of the goal. Replace it with taking a few minutes each day to savor the wonderful life that you have. Savor your loved ones; savor the food you eat and the air you breathe. Savor a sunrise and a flower. Appreciate your skills and the lives you touch. Listen to your emotional guidance and if something isn't working for you, believe you can change it and then work toward the goal of making things better. Let me know how it goes.

TIME MANAGEMENT

Organizations can provide:
- Time management training to physicians and staff,
- Opportunities to learn time management strategies from other physicians who have found successful methods of utilizing their work hours

The training should include:
- Goal setting, both short and long-term,
- How to minimize and deal with time wasters
- Managing conflicting priorities

- Planning and organizing
- Reassessment strategies

Being specific about long-term goals enhances the value of your emotional guidance. The feedback it provides changes when you are conscious about your goals. It can also help you navigate conflicting priorities. I've even found that it will help me plan. If I wait until I feel an inspiring nudge to make a call the person I connect with is fun and knowledgeable whereas if I push ahead and make myself call when I don't feel the urge things don't always go as well.

COMPLEX TASKS

In an automated world, some occupations or specialties within occupations can be designed to be routine and in ways that lack complex tasks. Complex tasks are somewhat protective against burnout.[285] This should be considered in job design such that care is taken not to create roles that lack variety or complexity.

STRESSFUL TASKS

Because some work is inherently stressful, employees should be given skills that help them deal with the stress encountered on the job. Whether it is law enforcement officers, fire fighters, or military personnel facing danger, surgeons who operate on humans, or teachers working in inner city schools, advanced and transformative coping skills will help them do their jobs well and pay a lower price for the work they do. A situation doesn't have to be unusual to create emotions that should be skillfully managed. "Surgeons' emotions (including anxiety, fear, distress, guilt, and accountability) occur even in the absence of an adverse event and pervade surgeons' relation with patients, families or colleagues."[286] *The Smart Way*™ reduces stress which should improve outcomes for patients and surgeons.

Physicians must have the right to "fire" patients. If a patient makes the physician's heart sink or if the physician feels uncomfortable with the patient, the right to end the doctor-patient relationship should exist and be supported.

EMPLOYEE ROLE FIT

When an employee does not perceive their role as aligned with his or her purpose the likelihood of burnout increases. This can be remedied in two ways. One is by using cognitive reappraisal to align with the work the employee is doing. The other is to change roles or change some of the responsibilities associated with the employee's role.[287]

TIME TO SLEEP

Sleep is critical to our well-being.

> *Individuals who are well rested have better quality work because they have a better mood, are more focused, have better mental performance, and feel less fatigued and stressed at work. Sleep also reduces memory decline, workplace injury, cyber-loafing, and unethical behavior, while lack of sleep increases the likelihood of obesity, heart disease, diabetes, and depression.*[288]

"Sleep loss is cumulative and by the end of the workweek, the sleep debt (sleep loss) may be significant enough to impair decision making, initiative, integration of information, planning and plan execution, and vigilance."[289]

At a minimum, in the short-term, shifts should be planned so that employee's have adequate time to eat, sleep, bathe, and commute between shifts. In the long-term view, time for family and building/maintaining social connections and leisure time should be considered in scheduling. Employees should not be expected to respond to electronic communications during their normal sleep times.

In 2008, the Institute of Medicine made recommendations to improve sleep quality and quantity for residents including restricting duty hours to no more than 80 hours per week, restrictions on continuous work hours to 16 without an uninterrupted sleep break of at least 5 hours that will count toward maximum duty hours for the week. Requirements for minimum duration of time off following a completed duty period ranged between 10 – 14 hours depending on the type of shift (night, day, or continuous).[290]

The ACGME Board of Directors Approved New Requirements for Residency Programs effective July 1, 2011 but did not adopt the recommendations in their entirety. Organizations that want to improve this area for the well-being of their staff and patients will find the original recommendations informative.[291]

One option that has helped with fatigue is brief naps, especially for individuals on evening shifts.

AUTONOMY

> *69% of physicians believe that their clinical autonomy is sometimes or often limited and their decisions compromised.*
>
> – The Physicians Foundation

Nomos is Greek for *law*. When a person has autonomy the person makes its own rules to live by. An individual feels a sense of freedom when they have autonomy. Autonomy is more important in some areas of life than others and some areas are more important to one person than they are to another. For example, my husband will happily consume whatever meal I prepare. My youngest daughter wants a say in what she eats and on specific holidays will balk if we decide to have a meal that differs from our family traditions.

Likewise, in the workplace, some people want full autonomy over their work while others simply want to be told what to do and some even want to be told how to do it.

The feeling of autonomy is a combination of two main factors:

1. How much decision-making latitude an individual has in the situation, and
2. How the individual perceives the situation.

Both are important but personal perception has the final say in how much autonomy the individual feels. For example, in a prior life I supervised people who sold stocks and bonds. It is a highly regulated industry and supervisors have many requirements imposed by regulations and are at risk of criminal charges if they fail to perform their duties. Despite being in a role with very little control over what I had to do on a day to day basis, I was able to maintain enough sense of freedom to feel comfortable. I have always been a freedom loving person. Ask my mom if you want verification of this as it made me the bane of her existence during my teenage years.

How was I able to have a rigidly regulated role and feel free? By viewing the job from a broader perspective, instead of seeing it as something others were forcing me to do, I saw having the job as a choice I was free to change at any time. By reminding myself that I was free to do something else, I continued to feel free while performing a job that had low autonomy.

Anyone can shift their perspective. Physicians often struggle with the concept of being able to change careers because they have invested so much time, money, and energy in becoming a physician. The thing is, they don't have to leave the practice of medicine to give themselves permission to do so when and if they make that choice. It is the attitude that one is not stuck, not actually moving to a different role, that changes the level of autonomy experienced.

Healthcare organizations can change practices to give physicians a say in:

- How they organize their work
- The equipment they use
- Office design and décor
- Work hours and schedule
- How they complete their continuing education credits
- The pace of their work
- Establishing their work related goals
- Organization goals
- What they wear
- Music in their office

In a study of over 3,000 physicians, "work control was correlated with job stress and satisfaction."[292] In a study of 1,461 nurses, increased job control increased retention.[293]

"Pressure on us to reduce our ability to make clinical decisions. We are bombarded constantly with guidelines on everything. Restrictions on our prescribing choices. Doing tasks we see as useless, like, one we all wish we could be rid of is the over 75 annual health checks, which we see as totally useless and a waste of time . . . What else? Constant change. Higher patient expectations. Pressure to audit absolutely everything, which I agree is a good idea, but it is actually quite difficult to do it with no extra resources in terms of money to spend on staff to help" (respondent 4, phase 2)."[294]

Clinical decision-making should be made by the physician who has been with the patient, not by someone at an insurance company or an administrator. To factor in how disheartening it is to have someone who didn't endure the rigor of medical school and the sacrifices medical school typically entails, you have to consider those sacrifices.

> *Physicians who perceive greater control over the practice environment, who perceive that their work demands are reasonable, and who have more support from colleagues have higher levels of satisfaction, commitment to the HMO, and psychological well-being. Interventions and administrative changes that give physicians more control over how they do their professional work and that enhance social supports are likely to improve both physician morale and performance. Factors that predict psychological wellbeing, satisfaction, and professional commitment, all measured using validated scales. The single most important predictor for all three outcomes was a sense of control over the practice environment. This included the opportunity to participate in decision making, to work autonomously, and to dictate the work schedule.*[295]

INTRINSIC MOTIVATION

Intrinsic motivation leads to self-directed effort toward achievement of one's goals. When others impose the methodology or proscribe the goals, intrinsic motivation diminishes and can be lost all together. Autonomy is essential to maintain intrinsic motivation.[296] Many aspects of the practice of medicine reduce intrinsic motivation. If organizations considered what is known about motivation in making decisions that affect the practice of medicine the burnout rate might be lower.

EMOTIONAL LABOR

Emotional labor is the requirement that a person exhibit an emotional face that differs from their current authentic emotional state. It is essentially a requirement that one not be authentic when the emotions being felt differ from mandated emotions. Lack of authenticity is associated with higher stress and worse health outcomes. Positive emotions are associated with better psychological functioning but only when the expression of positive emotions is an accurate reflection of internal emotional experiences.[297]

Emotional labor is a common requirement in healthcare when a cheerful countenance is required while doing tasks that may invoke disgust or when assisting patients whose prognosis is not good. At its essence, emotional labor is an employer mandated requirement to regulation one's emotions in a proscribed fashion. Given that some regulation strategies are known to be harmful to physical and mental health, employers who mandate employees present specific outward emotions should provide training to protect employees from potential harmful effects of unskilled emotion regulation.

Suppressing emotions is associated with a decreased memory.[298] This creates a conflict for employers who want their employees to have their full cognitive capabilities available and project proscribed emotions. Increased PsyCap reduces the negative impact of emotional labor requirements, decreasing the risk of burnout and increasing job satisfaction.[299]

ADMINISTRATIVE BURDENS

The Physicians Foundation survey of over 13,000 physicians revealed they spend 22% of their time on non-clinical paperwork.[300] We caution against only addressing administrative burdens. The physician burnout crisis was looming before the regulatory and other administration burden increases of the past decade. They may be the straw that broke its back, but reversing those won't heal the wounds or prevent new ones.

The Annals of Internal Medicine provides insight via *Putting Patients First by Reducing Administrative Tasks in Health Care: A Position Paper of the American College of Physicians*, which includes an overview of the administrative burden and suggestions for reducing that burden.[301]

The burden of paperwork is heavy with pre-certs, pre-auths, and scheduling other procedures and visits for the patient, let alone the demands and requirements of documenting the work each provider does with/for their patients and populating their respective EMR systems with clinical data. Staff hired to handle paperwork require more training which means they are more expensive.

Physicians are often required to document the same condition or services in multiple ways. In an era of electronic records, this should be automated.

The administrative burdens in healthcare are too numerous to enumerate here.

Our recommendation is that a team that includes all interested parties that understands the basis of motivation and stress as well as many myriad regulations from the government, medical boards, insurers, CMS, and other parties that impose administrative burdens on physicians and healthcare organizations as well as a number of physicians, practice administrators, nurses, allied health personnel, and IT experts form a task force with the driving force being to create a streamlined way to handle healthcare documentation efficiently, to identify redundancies, to question requirements that don't serve useful purposes or that could be managed in less burdensome ways. The task force could make specific recommendations to legislators and regulators to modify burdensome requirements that don't improve patient care.

The task force could solicit comment from the industry. It would be a monumental task but in an industry that loses the equivalent of 1.6% of new entrants to suicide each year and countless more to burnout, it is a task worth doing. The process should be done in an apolitical manner with the goal being to establish best practices and where appropriate, recommending law and regulation changes to support best practices.

Where it exists, peer reviewed research should also be considered.

This should not be about dictating clinical decisions, but about the administrative burden placed on the healthcare system and demoralizes providers while adding unnecessary time and financial burdens.

ELECTRONIC MEDICAL RECORDS (EMR) (PAPERWORK)

Forty-six percent of physicians indicate Electronic Medical Record (EMR) requirements have detracted from their efficiency.[302]

Paperwork is part of the physician's role. As a child, long before insurance company mandates and the ACA, I remember my physician writing in my chart each time I saw him. There are certain aspects of paperwork that it makes sense for physicians to do because it would take as long to tell someone else what to write as it would to write it and clarity could be lost in the translation. Additionally, the provider is responsible and liable for the content of the record, thus, each provider must have a process of review and "sign-off" on each record. It is the redundancy of paperwork and unnecessary paperwork that can feel as if you're wasting your time and erode intrinsic motivation.

There are options that can be incorporated in the practice that shift responsibility for many paperwork tasks to others.

My dermatologist has an assistant that is in the room with us when she sees me. The dermatologist and her assistant have developed a system that does not interfere with communication with the patient. During natural pauses my dermatologist would say a few words, no more than a sentence or two, and the assistant would enter data into an EMR. The paperwork was completed during our visit, although later review by the doctor may have occurred to verify the materials.

She also had a multi-tasking way of reviewing patient charts with a treadmill desk. Multi-tasking walking with paperwork could make the time feel more meaningful and productive.

Physicians surveyed about implementation of Electronic Medical Records (EMR) reveal conflicting opinions. The number of physicians who think EMR improved the quality of care is about 40% higher than those who think EMR decreased the quality of care. Nearly half think EMR improved patient interactions and a nearly equal number think EMR detracts from patient interactions.[303] This seems to indicate that sharing of best practices by organizations that are seeing success with EMR would benefit those who are experiencing decrements in patient interactions.

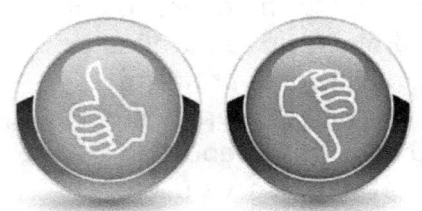

A Medscape article quoted Dr. Dean Sittig, "Electronic health records have brought new types of problems, when you have a drop-down list of medications, it's easy to select the one right above or right below." The article went on to mention that a patient died after receiving a paralytic instead of an anti-nausea medication.[304]

The worry that an innocent mistake could be so easily made would be trying on most people. It makes sense that the system could ask follow-up questions to greatly reduce the possibility of another life threatening or deadly error. If the system followed with a question from a drop down box asking why the drug was being prescribed it would alert the doctor if the reasons that could be selected did not match the patients' condition. It could also follow-up with a verification screen.

GOVERNMENT MANDATES

Beyond paperwork requirements is the distrust the government displays towards physicians. Failing to trust physicians to uphold the Hippocratic Oath is de-motivating. In the healthcare reform process, the impact on physicians' emotional well-being seems to have been missed.[305]

Medicaid regulations are ten times larger than the USA tax code. ICD10 is cited as a factor that contributes to physician burnout in comments on the 2016 Medscape survey. The frequent and extensive government mandated changes to health insurance is another factor that is leading to increased physician burnout.

Too many Federal and State regulators have oversight of physicians, for example:

Office of Civil Rights

- Prosecutes HIPAA violations (Federal crime)
  (e.g.. accidentally send protected health information)

Office of the Inspector General of Health and Human Services:

- Billing errors can be considered fraud or abuse depending upon the nature of the violation and "intent."

Federal Trade Commission:

- Doctors can't talk about fees with other doctors.
- Doctors can't refuse patients who are self-pay and only take insured patients.

Are you single and the only doctor in a small town? Forget about dating anyone because dating a patient is an ethics violation.

The Sunshine Act means you have to think about who picks up the tab or you may be in violation of another Federal law.

If you've been sued for malpractice, the Federal Malpractice data bank lists you as a criminal.

Medicare requires audits with auditors who are expected to have findings. They also mandate that you provide them with data and penalize you if you make a mistake.

Prescribe the wrong drug or too many of a narcotic to a patient and the Drug Enforcement Agency will Monday morning quarterback your decisions with possible criminal charges.

MEDICAL BOARD MANDATES

Medical Board recertification requirements are time consuming and expensive, both in out of pocket costs, travel costs, the cost of closing the practice for a day or several, and study time.

Kaiser Health News reported, "Supporters contend the new process will ensure doctors incorporate the latest medical advances into their practices, but many critics dismiss it as meaningless, expensive and a waste of time."[306]

I doubt the testing means physicians are keeping up because I'm not meeting physicians who are aware of 10-year old research about the new definition and purpose of emotions or about the 5-year old research about the benefits of positivity. That research isn't in the medical silo so it's not on the medical board's radar even though it is important to prevention of both physical and mental illnesses.

It would seem a different system might make more sense. Perhaps a data base that researchers could contribute to that provides searchable information to physicians. Physicians could then be trusted to review and document their review of new information. They could share their practice of keeping up to date in brochures with patients or on their website. With so many physicians now hospital based the healthcare institutions themselves could mandate internal updates.

The concept of keeping up with all the new information is impossible. When I first started Happiness 1st Institute I decided I wanted to read all the research published on happiness. The first year wasn't too difficult but by the second year the happiness industry had exploded and there weren't enough hours in the day to read all the new research and books being published about happiness even if that was all I did. I'm pretty sure you'd find the same scenario in many medical specialty areas.

People like me, who love to read research and pull all the pieces together into a cohesive whole could sift through the massive amount of information that is being created and provide it to physicians in condensed formats.

> *We create as much information in two days now as we did from the dawn of man through 2003. – Eric Schmidt*

I looked at the number of papers on Medline that are "in process." The number is currently 1,081,595. It is not humanly possible to read that many journal articles.

In 2016, physicians were asked to rate the causes of burnout in a widespread Medscape survey. "Maintenance of certification requirements" tied for fifth place with "feeling like a cog in a wheel" as a cause of burnout.[307]

Given the sheer quantity of new data available we may need to consider a coalition to determine best practices for maintaining and increasing physician knowledge without imposing requirements that physicians attempt the impossible. Consultative teams come to mind as do accessible and searchable data bases.

INSURANCE COMPANY MANDATES

Without standardization of processes and "paperwork" (forms, submissions, pre-authorization requests, etc.) the commercial insurance companies place a broad range of demands and restrictions on providers. If the provider wants to be paid for services delivered to a subscriber, then they must accept the nuances of these processes and comply with a multitude of documentation and clinical data. A prime example is the process of credentialing the provider. Most insurers have their specific processes and materials to complete, although NCQA has helped some in standardizing information, the provider may be subject to weeks if not months of delay before you are "recognized" as a provider who can bill for services and be paid.

In the 2016 Medscape survey, the most frequently noted free-form comments related to insurance issues and their contribution to burnout.

Insurance companies need to recognize that their role in healthcare is optional. The more onerous they are the more they push us towards socialized medicine and concierge medicine. Medical malpractice insurers should recognize the role of burnout on errors and become strong advocates for streamlined processes and other burnout reducing changes.

EMPLOYED PHYSICIANS

More than half of physicians are now hospital or medical group employees. That's an almost 25% increase since 2012 and nearly a 50% increase since 2008. The number of physicians in solo practice has declined to 17% of all physicians.[308] This change requires psychological flexibility because the mindset of an employee is different from that of a physician who owns the practice.

LEGAL ISSUES & MALPRACTICE

Legal intrusions into healthcare have many adverse results.

- Negative impact on physician income from high malpractice liability premiums
- The stress and time involved in defending malpractice suits
- Unjustifiable demands
- Impact of "defensive medicine" actions generating high volumes of testing which may not be warranted.

Malpractice worries are constant for many physicians. 60.3% of physicians see defensive medicine as a factor that is most likely to contribute to the rising healthcare costs. Only 37.4% cited the aging population as a likely factor.[309] Tort laws and public opinion both contribute to defensive medicine.

When a physician is sued for malpractice the risk that suicide ideation will occur increases. Organizations may wish to consider mandatory counseling sessions to assess the mental health of physicians being sued and provide them with training that can help them with the stress of the situation. Even if the physician is likely to be found innocent, in an untrained mind negative ruminations can lead to adverse psychological and somatic physical illness outcomes.

In January, Medical Economics published an article I wrote about a Florida physician who was being held liable for a patient suicide.[310] The physician was a family practice physician treating the patient for depression. A large percentage of depression patients are treated by family practice physicians. In the United States, 3,000 counties have inadequate resources to meet the demand for mental health services. About 30% of all depression treatment is provided by medical doctors. This Florida case has a chilling effect on physician willingness to provide this much needed care.

The need for Tort Reform is beyond the scope of this book, however, we do note that the behavioral influence of these legal parameters have a direct effect on providers and customers (patients).

Fear of malpractice suits and the cost of malpractice insurance increases burnout. Malpractice insurers have a vested interest in reducing burnout.

FLEXIBILITY

Flexibility is an aspect of autonomy but it deserves separate mention. Employees at different stages of life and with different goals will be more likely to stay if work does not create undue conflicts between work and other important goals.

An employee with young children might want to have a shift that allows her and her partner to share child care responsibilities without relying on paid care. One parent might work the day shift while the other one works a night or evening shift. With the cost and stress of finding child care this flexibility will make some employees more loyal as long as this benefit is important to them.

An employee who has parent care-taking responsibilities may want an evening shift so they can take their aging parent to frequent doctor visits without having to constantly worry about time away from work and arranging coverage in their absence.

The flexibility of roles that are conducive to work at home strategies may appeal to the parent with middle or high school children who they do not want unsupervised after school. Shift flexibility can include part-time work and schedules such as 4 – 10's or 3 – 12's work schedules.

Predictable schedules also allow employees to feel more in charge of their own life. Schedules that change from week-to-week make both work and home feel more out of control.

Finally, there is autonomy in how one accomplishes the tasks included in their role. Autonomy is a significant human need and the more flexibility an employee can be afforded in their role, the better seasoned workers usually like their job. Clear goals are important. For newer employees who are learning, incorporate flexibility into the training provided. Show the employee multiple methods of accomplishing goals and allow the employee to adopt the one(s) that feel best.

WORK HOURS

32.4% of physicians work over 60 hours per week.[311] Less than 20% of physicians work 40 or fewer hours per week.[312]

The greater control an individual feels they have over their schedule the lower the levels of stress they experience related to their schedule which improves career satisfaction which decreases burnout.[313] Burnout is a complex issue. Understanding the connections between scheduling, job satisfaction, and burnout helps organizations make the best decisions.

One practice reported a strong commitment to developing a flexible work schedule that supported physicians ability to adjust their schedules to suit their needs including "nonmedical endeavors, spend more time with their family or for health reasons."[314] They used a combination of a flexible compensation system, great communication, and the opportunity to adjust their work schedule.

Twice a year they meet to discuss and adjust work schedules and reassign their work loads. Despite the work involved in this process and the initial need for facilitators to help them communicate they continue the practice because it adds more to their satisfaction than it costs in terms of time and effort to manage. They focus on consensus building to attain group commitment each time schedules are adjusted.

While this sort of flexibility would require time and effort, given the level of physician burnout, the cost of burnout to physicians, their patients and employers, and the growing shortage of physicians, the effort appears worth accomplishing.

CONSISTENT SHIFTS

Shift work that varied between daytime and nighttime shifts had a greater negative impact on sleep quality and burnout. Consistency in the time of day of shifts (all daytime or all nighttime) reduced the negative impact on both sleep quality and burnout. Sleep deprivation and burnout are correlated and may feed into one another.[315]

Changing work schedules (from continuous to having weekend breaks) reduced stress.[316]

Planning schedules in advance so employees can plan activities with family and friends is helpful but leave room for flexibility so that they events that are not planned that far out can be accommodated when possible. This is especially true if shifts change from day-to-day. Be sure there is adequate time for commute, sleep, and food between shifts.

Ask staff for their suggestions about how to meet scheduling requirements that satisfy the organization's and staff needs. Even difficult schedules obtain more buy-in if employees feel heard.

VACATION CULTURE

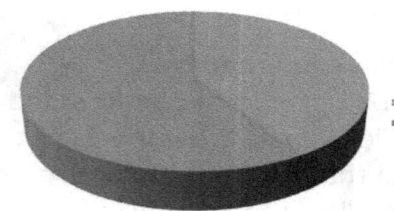

70% of non-burned out physicians take at least two weeks of vacation a year (Medscape, 2015)

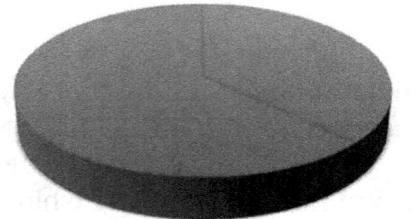

59% of burned out physicians don't take at least two weeks of vacation a year (Medscape, 2015)

Vacations can provide an opportunity to recover from consistent stressors. A workplace culture that encourages workers to take vacations would be helpful. Also, policies that combine sick leave and vacation time into one construct, Paid Time Off (PTO) can have a dampening effect on taking vacations if the person feels uncertain about future needs for sick leave. This can be especially true of physicians with young families that may need time off to care for sick children. Using creative ways to address concerns could lead to increased usage of PTO for vacation.

It also doesn't make sense to lower employee's vacation if they've been ill. The restoration of vacation can help them recover. Some organizations are beginning to increase physician vacation time and mandate taking vacations.

LONG HOURS

Being on call is not the same as being off work. The psychological difference between the two has a discernible effect on whether "time-off" is restorative.

"There is a very large, strong body of evidence showing that insufficient sleep has adverse effects on cognition, performance, and mood."[317]

"The evidence is overwhelming that nurses who work longer than 12 consecutive hours or work when they have not obtained sufficient sleep are putting their patients' health at risk; risk damaging their own health; and if they drive home when they are drowsy, also put the health of the general public at risk."[318]

A 2-year study of 186 physicians revealed that patient adherence with prescribed medication for diabetes, hypertension, and heart disease was affected by the number of patients the physician saw per day.[319]

ON-SITE PSYCHOLOGIST

One CEO at a teaching hospital that I spoke with hired an on-site psychologist to address physician burnout. She was booked solid within two weeks. For physicians who are experiencing a stressful life event or have been diagnosed with a mental illness this solution may not be ideal. The organization has over 500 physicians and a psychologist can see roughly 27 clients per week so although the on-site therapist may be sufficient to handle the physicians experiencing negative life events, it is unlikely she has the capacity to assist the (statistically) 250+ doctors who are experiencing symptoms of burnout, the 100 who (statistically) are experiencing anxiety, the 100 (statistically) who are experiencing anger issues, or the 50 (statistically) who are experiencing depression.

An on-site psychologist is a good step but there are more affordable ways to effectively help large numbers of physicians and other employees.

COACHING ENVIRONMENT

Creating an inspiring environment where staff performs their best because of intrinsic motivation is the ideal work environment. Understanding the nature of inspiration helps create this environment.

For example, if an employee is at Noon on the following diagram, attempting to inspire her/him by talking about accomplishments that someone who is at 8 o'clock on the diagram can achieve will just make her/him feel overwhelmed. Even if you can see the employee's potential to achieve at 8 or 10 o'clock, inspiration works better when you help them see the next step. Think of it in terms of a road. They can see a mile ahead but not 100 miles away. Unless there are big mountains in the distance and that will just look intimidating.

You'll probably recognize this diagram from the earlier one on finding silver linings that inspired this interpretation.

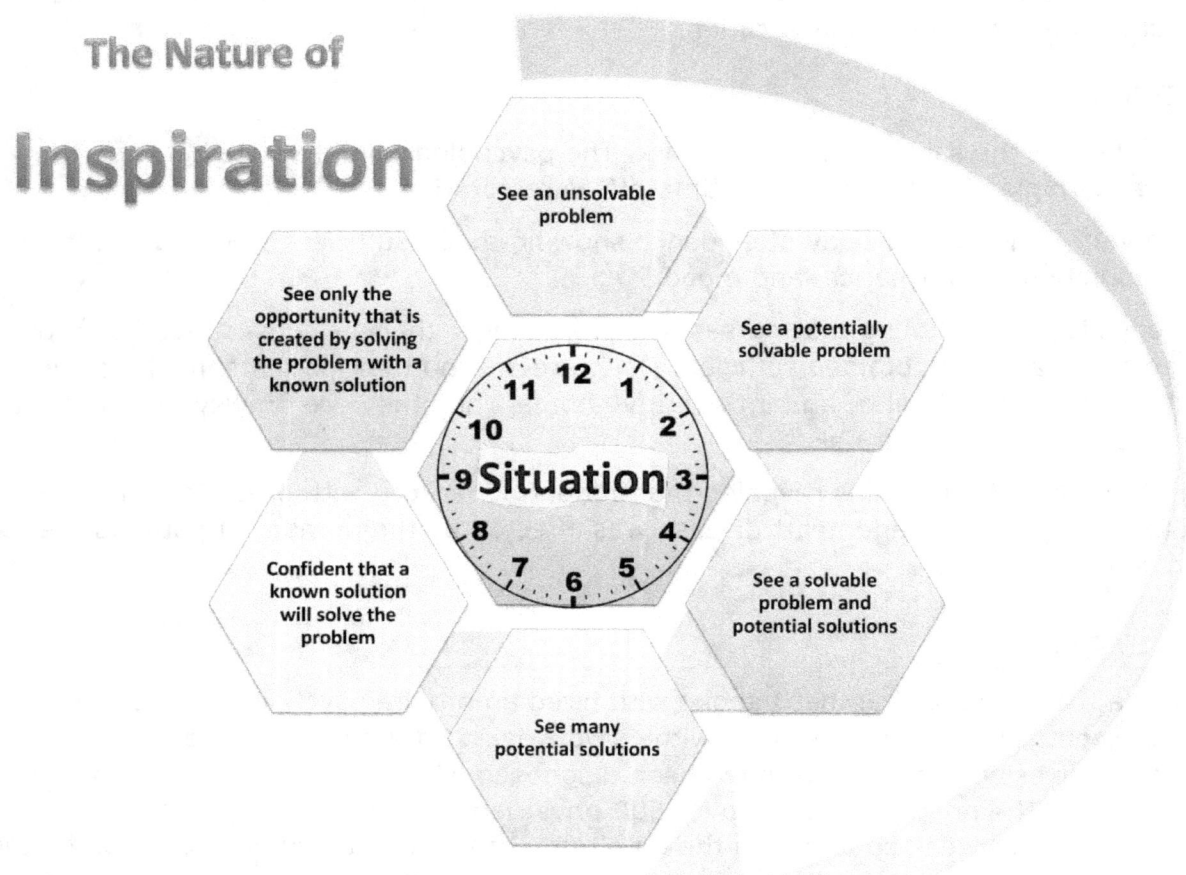

Here are some examples of how emotional guidance and advanced and transformational coping skills can be applied to a variety of situations. These responses can be done in the individual's own mind (self-coaching) or with the assistance of a peer (peer-coaching):

Feeling/Perspective	**Questions, alternatives**
I'm tired. The demands on my time are more than I can handle. I'm exhausted and don't have anything to show for my efforts.	*What does your emotional guidance say about that?* *Does that thought feel good?* *Can you find a perspective that feels better?* *Are you being too specific?* *Who did you help today?*

How will you or your family benefit from what you've done this week?

What are your resources? How are they affecting your perception? How are they affecting your accomplishments? What can you do to improve your in-the-moment resources tomorrow?

What can you appreciate about this week?

I'm not as smart as I should be. I don't have what it takes to be successful.	*What does your emotional guidance think about that? If it feels good when you say it, your emotional guidance agrees. If it feels bad try to find your truth by rephrasing it in a more positive frame.* *Are you being specific?* *How could you be kinder to yourself in this situation?* *Are you learning something new? We all make mistakes when we are learning new things; no matter how old we are.* *Is this an old belief that you were taught that isn't serving you?*
I'm so upset. I was rude and mean to some of my staff. That's not how I should or want to treat them. Why do I do that?	*Remember your resources? You wouldn't behave this way if you were at your peak performance, your best possible today is not your best possible.* *Apologize. Explain that the way you behaved is not how you want to behave and you're going to work on being more aware of situations when your resources are low so you can take time for self-care before you behave in ways you regret.* *Don't beat yourself up with guilt. Make the decision to change and then take steps to change. Make a list of the resources that affect your ability to do your best and check in with them.* *You may want to establish a few barometers that let you know if you're off-kilter. When I leave my neighborhood I pay attention to whether I'm paying attention to my neighbors' flowers or seeing their weeds. If I am seeing weeds I need to work on my*

	emotional state.
I feel like a cog in a wheel. I don't think I really matter.	*Why did you become a physician? If you refocus on your why you'll probably feel better.*
	Check in with your emotional guidance. Turn the question around. How do you feel when you tell yourself that you matter?
	Are you violating your own ethical standards in some way? If so, what can you do differently?
	What energizes you?
	When was the last time you felt energized?
	Can you do more of that?
	Give yourself permission to do what you need to do to feel better even if it is unconventional, like taking a sabbatical.
	Are you holding back from sharing what is bothering you about your work environment because you don't think anyone will care? What does your emotional guidance say about that? Think about how it would feel to speak assertively?
	How would it feel to point out the problem and offer a viable solution when you point it out?
	If you don't know the solution, does the idea of doing some research to see if anyone knows the solution make you feel more interested?
I haven't been to the gym in months. I never seem to have time to go.	*Make a decision. Ask yourself what you want to do. Then decide that you will do it. Take every action you need to take to support the decision right now. If you are going to go to the gym three times a week during your lunch break put it on your calendar as a recurring meeting. Pack your gym bag and put it in the car. Plan how you'll eat and exercise during your lunch break. Will you pack your lunch? Drink a nutritious meal replacement? Have a protein juice drink at the gym? Tell others you expect them to respect your time and not double book you for your gym time. Think about how you'll feel energized for the rest of the day after your time at the gym. Check*

to see how your emotional guidance feels and feel the validation (positive reinforcement) for your efforts.

TEAMWORK

Constant Communication:

The expectation that one is constantly available via electronic communication has an adverse impact on employee engagement. Teams should collectively decide non-work time expectations of availability. This approach has been successful in "enhancing teamwork, work-life balance, and client satisfaction."[320]

Entering Data is not communication, but it does require time and effort to complete, thus, "you are still on the clock" until the tasks are done.

Individuals who perceive a sense of community with their co-workers have lower incidence of burnout.[321]

An active, task-oriented approach has been shown to increase resilience.[322] Make the scheduling and completion of patient visits a joint endeavor such that the organization, the providers and the staff feel part of the process, "not just a pawn in the results".

POSITIVE COACHING TEAMS

In an organization where *The Smart Way*™ has been introduced it is possible to establish an agreement where employees are able to coach one another. There should be an opt-out for individuals who do not want to participate as coaches at all, or on specific days. Individuals trained in *The Smart Way*™ prioritize reducing stress more than having been right or knowing all the answers (they're more open to learning and coaching). Those who do want to participate could have an indication on their name badges that means, "If you catch me in a coachable moment, feel free to ask me if I'd like to be coached. I'm open to making the most of myself."

If someone didn't want to participate on any given day they could opt not to wear the identifying participant pin on that day. It requires training to make employees comfortable with the idea that everyone is a coach and coachable. It works because the coach doesn't attempt to solve the person's problem. Coaching is more about reminding one another that everyone has guidance and to check in with the guidance and use it to assist them in lowering the stress they're experiencing. If the person chooses to share details with a coach the coach then uses their knowledge of advanced coping skills to suggest techniques that might help the person being coached find less stressful perspectives.

Preliminary work on the connection between burnout and loneliness shows they are correlated.[323] Developing positively focused teams with a shared understanding of the effect emotions have on behavior and a shared language on advanced and transformational coping could also help combat loneliness. Since we can feel lonely when surrounded by other people, I have a theory that we feel lonely when we are surrounded by people are not in an emotional Zone close to the one we are experiencing.

Coaching is not about telling anyone what they should do. It may involve sharing what worked for the coach in a similar situation. It is also helpful to have an internal (electronic) board where people can share their success stories and ask questions.

Using the term Coaching in relationship to burnout prevention and recovery efforts has added advantages:

1. It avoids any stigma associated with counseling,
2. It avoids having to answer "yes" to questions concerning counseling on medical board applications or insurance applications.

ENVIRONMENT

It is important to recognize that one's perception of environment is not factual. It is perceptual which means different individuals will have different thoughts and feelings about the same environment. Since most researchers are not yet considering the impact of emotional state on perception, it is not possible to determine whether workers who find an environment objectionable are negatively or positively focused in general. This is important because a negatively focused person will find something objectionable in an improved environment.

For example, you survey your workers and the majority of them cite one aspect of their work environment as the one that causes the most stress. In this case, let's assume that having to keep potentially violent patients in E.D. while waiting for a room is cited as the biggest stressor by most E.D. employees. You spend the money to build a special holding area with safe, secure, locked rooms visible through windows from a main station.

A negatively focused employee would turn their attention to the things they find stressful that you have not changed and give little time or attention to appreciating the elimination of a significant stressor. A positively focused employee would feel appreciation for the change every time they think about it, which means every time they are at work.

I'm not saying there aren't environmental factors you can change to improve working conditions and lower stress but unless and until the employee begins using his or her mind to reduce stress, the improvements will not have a significant effect on negatively focused employees.

The medical environment does what it is paid to do. Individually physicians cannot do much to change a system that incentivizes activities that aren't always the best solution. Individually they can recognize issues where their actions would be different if the way they are compensated were different. For example, if ordering an MRI results in income but reviewing an existing MRI is not compensated, many physicians will opt to have their time compensated. Being compensated is fair.

Also, the vast majority of the increase in life expectancy during the past century is the result of primary prevention efforts. Given the contribution of stress to mental and physical illnesses including multi-generational illnesses, perhaps it is time to consider adopting practices that are mandated in England.

In England, employers have a duty of care for work-related stress in both statutory and common law.[324]

Identifying a problem   **Protecting individuals**

- Monitor working conditions to spot signs of stress
- Being aware of working conditions that could cause ill-health
- Consulting with employees to get their views on the workplace
- Giving consideration to employees with specific health needs or disabilities

Preventing Harm

- Assessing the potential impact of workplace stressors
- Identifying measures that could prevent ill-health
- Ensuring employees are aware of preventative measures
- Taking action where harm to individuals is foreseeable
- Considering the needs of individuals
- Making reasonable adjustments to meet specific health needs or disabilities

Managing the workplace

- Monitoring the ongoing impact of work on vulnerable individuals
- Avoiding discriminating against individuals because of their health needs or disability
- Preventing workplace bullying and harassment

SUPPORTIVE MANAGEMENT

Supportive leadership includes authentic leadership. Authentic leadership was correlated to lower burnout in 1009 nurses.[325] A "low level of manager support was a significant predictor of higher levels of burnout" in a 2015 study published in the *Journal of Nursing Scholarship*.

Many healthcare institutions are focused on transactions and push physicians to see more patients and provide the type of care that generates the most revenue. I interviewed a young psychiatrist who tried working for a healthcare system where she was pushed to prescribe medications but not provide therapy because they could make more off her work with that approach. She is now happily running her own practice.

Healthcare systems would do better to focus on the long-term and employ transformational leaders who inspire, influence with ideals, provide intellectual stimulation and consider the needs of individuals. There is a misalignment between an organization focused on making money and most physicians who have broader reasons for practicing medicine. Leadership must balance the business requirements and aspects of their organization with the delivery of high quality, compassionate care. They need to focus on the people delivering that care, include them in the business of medicine decision making processes, and, listen. On the other hand the providers need to appreciate the myriad complexities of "running" a medical organization and be part of the solutions, not the problems.

Pushing physicians to focus on transactions is about as steady as pushing a ball with two times your mass up a steep hill. You won't get any momentum and you'll always have to work hard for every step you take.

A transformational leader can tap into the physician's heart and mind in order to lead the physician and the organization to become more than it will ever be if its focus is primarily transactional. When you tap into your employees' passion they become intrinsically motivated. Ideas flow. Work becomes less stressful because it is what you want to do. It doesn't mean transactions won't happen, but the driving purpose will be broader, deeper, and inspiring.

Traditional employee engagement strategies attempt to make employees feel more valued but there is one caution. Research indicates that 27-40% of employee engagement depends on the employee's own core self-evaluations. Low core self-evaluation can predict academic burnout.[326] Core self-evaluations are a combination of the employee's level of self-esteem and sense of self-efficacy (how competent the employee feels).

The way an employee processes a compliment or positive feedback about their work will vary significantly depending on their core self-evaluations because the *back story* their mind creates to explain why the compliment was given, whether the employee believes it (even when it is truthful and authentic) depends on the employee's core self-evaluations. Managers who follow traditional employee engagement strategies will not understand why they don't get the results they want from employees with low core self-evaluations.

This diagram illustrates the process the subconscious mind uses to arrive at the *back story* received by the conscious mind:

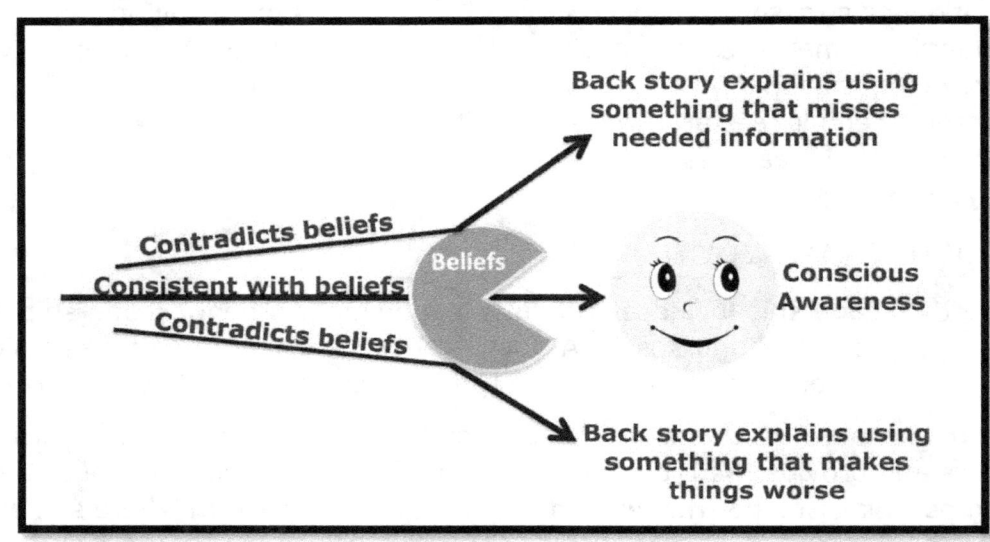

A manager has no power to change an employee's core self-evaluations. Only by teaching the employee how their brain works, about emotional guidance, *back stories*, and techniques that help the employee find more positive perspectives can low core self-evaluations be improved. Considering this accounts for between 27 – 40% of engagement it represents low hanging fruit for improving engagement and decreasing burnout.

Tapping into employee's passions inspires their best.

MORBIDITY AND MORTALITY MEETINGS

Surgeons report that mortality and morbidity meetings have an undercurrent that is looking for blame rather than understanding and lessons learned. The sense of being judged when they did the best they could in the situation they were in weighs on them.[327] Changing the tone of such meetings to be one of learning rather than judging would leave room for surgeons to be human.

Positive growth occurs when negative events are viewed as opportunities to grow that can make the individual and organization better in the future. This stance supports resilience and would be a better framework for these meetings.

INVESTING IN YOUR PEOPLE

"To a large degree, the choice about which investment opportunities to pursue remain contingent on how financial outcomes are assessed and reported."[328] If businesses are going to make the best possible financial decisions, they must begin understanding the effect of stressed employees on critical areas including patient and customer satisfaction, productivity, turnover, absenteeism, errors, and risk of being held liable for workplace stress.

Organizations that invest in their people become the world class organizations.[329]

EMOTION MANAGEMENT

See the sections on developing healthy habits of thought for advice on managing emotions.

PERFORMANCE FEEDBACK

The importance of frequent performance feedback has been recognized. Millennials in particular want more frequent feedback. However, the best feedback comes in the form of a response to every thought you think. Your emotional guidance lets you know whether your thought is leading toward self-actualization and self-determined goals. As long as your role is aligned with your personal goals, your emotional guidance will consistently provide reliable feedback about your work performance.

NEW TECHNOLOGY

When new technology is considered, employee well-being should be one of the considerations taken into account in the decision-making process.[330] Adverse impacts on the employee's well-being do not happen in isolation. Adverse impacts spread to patients, co-workers, the organization's success at long-term goals, and to the employee's family.

Technology can take time away from patients that could be used to discuss treatments, listen to the needs of patients, and determine the best plan of care.

PHYSICIAN WELL-BEING COMMITTEES

In light of the significance of burnout and its impact on the health and well-being of both employees and patients, healthcare organizations should form well-being committees that go far beyond what corporate wellness plans ordinarily consider. The level of autonomy, intrinsic motivation, alignment of goals and values[331] should be considered when organizational decisions are made. Physicians and other high-risk employees should be trained in advanced and transformative coping strategies.

In addition to their role as a confidential access point for persons who voluntarily seek their counsel and assistance, The Well-Being Committee should provide "educational resources for medical and other organization staff in matters related to maintenance of health."[332]

The industry should make physician self-care a priority for a variety of reasons:
- Preserve the health and well-being of physicians
- Ensure patients receive the best possible care
- Set a good example for patients
- Reduce medical costs

Given that the pathway from chronic stress to substance abuse is the same as the path from chronic stress to burnout it is logical for them to proactively provide physicians and other healthcare workers with training that empowers them with knowledge and skills that prevent both rather than wait for them to develop problems that are more difficult to address. Given

the available data on burnout amongst medical and nursing school students, the long-term best practice would be to provide this training at the beginning of their education.
It is important that physicians know:
1. They can regulate their emotions, and
2. Techniques to employ for successful emotion regulation.

Both treatment seeking and the success of treatment are affected by beliefs about the ability to regulate emotions.[333]

Although exercise increases well-being and reduces psychological distress,[334] we caution against using it in isolation without skilled stress reduction instruction. The American Psychological Association found that 43% of people who regularly exercise and know it reduces their level of stress don't exercise when they become too stressed.[335]

PRIMARY PREVENTION

Today we are harvesting the fruits of our ancestors focus on primary prevention while we ignore significant evidence that we could do as much good as they did by increasing our attention to primary prevention.

Misperceptions about Medical Care and Life Expectancy

"Life expectancy has doubled over the past 150 years. How is that possible? A recent study showed that most Americans would credit 80% of the improvement to advances in medical science. Historians would disagree.

The greatest increase in life expectancy occurred between 1880 and 1920, before the advent of antibiotics, chemotherapy, drugs to reduce blood pressure and advanced surgical techniques. In fact, most of the credit mathematically goes to improved supplies of clean (or chlorinated) drinking water in urban areas. In 1854, a cholera epidemic in London was linked to a water pump next to a leaky sewer. By the early 1900s, big public works projects had the immediate result that more children survived infancy and childhood. In addition, better nutrition, better (less crowded) housing, better understanding of germ science and food contamination and better standards of living were also big contributors.

In 1999, the Centers for Disease Control (CDC) estimated that of the 30 years in life expectancy gained since 1900, only five of those years might be attributed to medical advances. The rest could be attributed to: vaccination, motor-vehicle safety, safer workplaces, control of infectious diseases, decline in deaths from coronary heart disease and stroke, safer and healthier foods, healthier mothers and babies, family planning, fluoridation of drinking water and recognition of tobacco use as a health hazard. Based upon this analysis, more than 80% of the increase in life expectancy can be attributed to public health initiatives and improvements in other social determinants of health, rather than to advances in medical science. In other words, Primary Prevention led to significant increases in life expectancy.

The danger, of course, is that the lack of public understanding could "predispose a society to overfund the healthcare sector of the economy, which focuses on treating rather than preventing public health problems. Conversely, such misperceptions may reduce public support for contemporary public health programs and efforts to address social determinants of health."[336]

The *Smart Way*™ is psychological primary prevention. In studies of police officers, an occupation exemplified by high stress and similar secondary trauma to that experienced by healthcare professions, primary prevention was found to provide a significant difference in depression compared to a control group.[337] In that study, the positive effects were no longer present at 18 months. This is a consistent finding that is often seen in studies but when you factor in the understanding and active use of emotional guidance it is the same as receiving a booster lesson many times each day. I am actively seeking an organization that is interested in participating in research of the long-term benefits of *The Smart Way*™.[338]

ACCOMMODATIONS FOR ILLNESS

The number of physicians and APPs who go to work while they are sick and even contagious is over 80%.[339] One of the many reasons cited was that being out puts their workload on their colleagues. They feel they are expected to be there unless they are on their death bed. They may be required to find the person to take over their duties. The last thing I want to do when I'm ill is call and have to talk to people. I understand how it would be easier to go to work.

There have to be ways that could be established to reduce the occurrence of sick and contagious physicians going to work and treating patients. Perhaps the system schools use for substitute teachers would work for physicians.

PERCEPTION OF PHYSICIANS

During recent decades, the perception of physicians has been under attack on many fronts and is now a far cry from what it used to be:

> *There are men and classes of men that stand above the common herd: the soldier, the sailor, and the shepherd not infrequently; the artist rarely; rarer still, the clergyman; the physician almost as a rule. He is the flower (such as it is) of our civilization; and when that stage of man is done with, and only to be marveled at in history, he will be thought to have shared as little as any in the defects of the period, and most notably exhibited the virtues of the race. Generosity he has, such as is possible to those who practice an art, never to those who drive a trade; discretion, tested by a hundred secrets; tact, tried in a thousand embarrassments; and what are more important, Herculean cheerfulness and courage. So that he brings air and cheer into the sick room, and often enough, though not so often as he wishes, brings healing.*
>
> Robert Louis Stevenson, Preface to *Underwoods*.

Physicians have become more knowledgeable, more able to save and prolong lives, yet the respect with which they are held had declined. There are myriad causes, few of them attributable to physicians.

1) The mistaken belief that someone else's success can deprive you of success has become a predominant belief in society is one reason many people resent physicians relative high social and financial standing.
2) There is a tendency to believe that physicians should be willing to sacrifice anything to heal others with almost no recognition of the effort they had to put into becoming physicians.
3) High profile malpractice cases being reported in the media.
4) Physicians get caught up in research changes. (i.e., for a long while physicians encouraged some patients to restrict their consumption of eggs based on research that was later overturned.) People receive more news than ever before so they are more

likely to learn that something their physician told them to do is no longer considered the right answer.
5) Television shows that offer medical advice to millions of viewers they've never examined whose advice researchers determine is wrong[h] half the time.[340]
6) Failure of celebrity physicians to disclose conflicts of interest.[341]
7) The way the media portrays physicians, from *Marcus Welby, M.D.* and Bones (*Star Trek*) to *Grey's Anatomy, House*, and *Code Black*, have informed the public's perception of physicians. The influence of television on the portrayal of physicians is so strong that the University of Chicago created a class for first-year medical students to help them unlearn unacceptable behaviors they may have picked up by watching medical drama shows.[342]
8) The media sensationalizing medical errors and unethical physician conduct.[343]

If Tylenol could recover and survive following its PR nightmare, physician associations and healthcare systems could develop a PR campaign to reverse the downward trend of physicians as highly respected professionals. Care should be taken not to encourage the White Coat Syndrome's return but the middle ground is vast.

The lack of respect and esteem adds to the wear and tear on physicians that leads to burnout. While many people deride physicians, physicians still love their patients. In a 2014 survey, the relationship with their patients was cited as the number one factor that added to physicians' job satisfaction by 78.6%. Intellectual stimulation came in second at 65.3% 69.7%. Financial rewards were a distant 4th with only 15.2% of physicians citing it as one of the top two factors in job satisfaction.[344]

Every day there are success stories that could become PR success stories.

WORKPLACE JUSTICE

The concept of justice at work has gained significance. Our world and its institutions are increasingly judged by how the public perceives them and justice has become a common theme. There is not, however, a standard that measures justice. It is a matter of how a situation is perceived and public outcry often occurs without waiting for the facts to surface.

If the concept of justice becomes well-defined it will improve outcomes. Justice is often misread due to misunderstanding the purpose and meaning of emotional guidance. In many instances, it is the perception that should change. Jonathan Haidt's book, *The Righteous Mind*, is an excellent source of insight about the concept of justice.[345]

When policies are developed and changes made it is best to obtain input from diverse groups of people before a final decision is made to ascertain how it might be perceived. Workplace injustice has been proven to increase the incidence of psychiatric morbidity among workers.[346]

Perceived injustices relating to performance evaluations increase nursing turnover.[347]

INCOME NOT HIGH ENOUGH

The government and insurance companies are playing with physician incomes. In some cases, physician practices are losing money despite serving patients in busy practices.

---

[h] Wrong could mean that it was not indicated by the symptoms described, that the recommendation was not supported by research, or that the recommendation was inferior to an alternative.

Medicaid and Medicare recipients are some of society's most vulnerable citizens and they need medical care. The way the Affordable Care Act was written bumped primary care visit payments related to Medicaid enrollees up by 40% in 2013, 2014, and 2015 but in 2016 they returned to the old fee schedule rates.

On the surface, the increased rates may look like a windfall for physicians but the fact is that Medicare and Medicaid reimbursements were so low many physicians could no longer afford to take new patients. An individual's perception of the reward received for the work performed is one of six key domains that influence the development of burnout.[348]

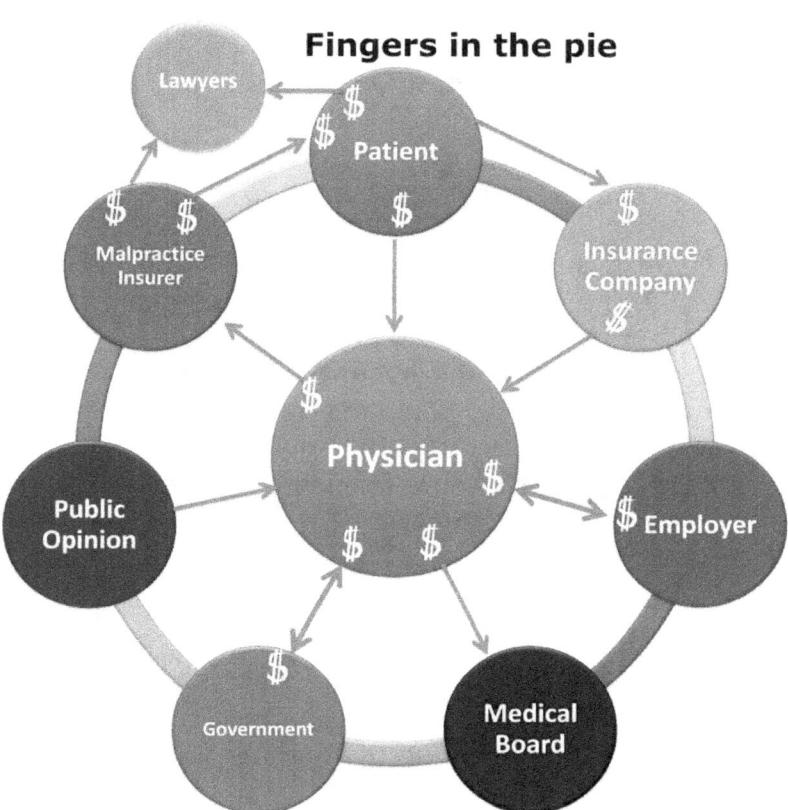

In a physician's own words, "We are on the brink of a provider revolt, doctors will quit before they take a 10% pay cut. I can happily drive a bus and live in a trailer in Florida."[349]

A public perception that physicians are wealthy and make great incomes still exists but it is a flawed perception. Few physicians are making enough to be considered wealthy and many are struggling to make ends meet. Many report that they can't afford to send their children to college. This diagram is simplified because there are many other providers in healthcare, but the number of non-clinical organizations and employees who are supported by healthcare is enormous.

Is there a better way?

I don't know the answer. I don't think it is socialist medicine like Canada or the UK. Their physicians are just as burned out as ours and they report higher staffing shortages than we are experiencing. There are reports that during economic downturns the government pulls back funding for socialized healthcare. During economic downturns more people are ill because increased stress reduces immune function. In England where employers are mandated to control workplace stress, one of the first citations issued for work-related stress was to West Dorset General National Health Service Hospitals.[350]

Malpractice insurance premiums will not decline unless and until physician stress is lower because stress increases medical errors. Do we need tort reform? Well done tort reform would help but how is that defined?

What about helping poor families become more prosperous? If fewer people were on Medicaid, the low reimbursement rates and hoops the government makes physicians jump through would be less of a burden.

There are many approaches. Physicians need advocates that look deeply at these issues and begin changing things that can be changed.

> "The Medicaid cuts are going to have an important impact on family physicians, particularly those who have increased the number of Medicaid beneficiaries in response to the parity with Medicare payment," Robert Wergin, MD, president of the American Academy of Family Physicians, told Forbes January 1. Medicaid is not the only area in which physicians will see reimbursement shrink. Several Medicare cost and quality measurements and mandates, courtesy of the Centers for Medicare & Medicaid Services (CMS), that will likely reduce payments will kick in this year.
> It's something that worries the American Medical Association (AMA). In a statement issued back in October, the AMA warned the CMS about the "regulatory tsunami" facing US physicians that could cut Medicare payments by more than 13% by the end of the decade."[351]

One physician commented, "In 1979, liability insurance for a surgeon was $13,000, equivalent to 6 or 7 hernia operations. In 2007, the same insurance is $80,000 and must be paid by performing 120 hernia operations."[352] Imagine you are that surgeon and the first 120 hernia operations you do each year provide zero income to you, they just pay for insurance against the possibility that someone will sue you. You don't have to be in medicine for the money to find that disheartening. Sometime in February, if you perform surgeries full-time, you'll be able to begin working to pay for your income taxes because your malpractice insurance premiums for the year have been earned, if all your patients pay their bills.

Physicians are creating new care delivery methods. Seven percent of physicians now have a form of direct pay or concierge medicine and thirteen percent indicate they are planning to transition, at least partially, to this type of practice. The percentage increases to 17% when physicians younger than age 45 are surveyed.[353] Physicians are also limiting access for Medicaid patients by not taking any Medicaid patients or limiting the number of them they will take.[354]

We have to recognize the many sacrifices it takes to become a physician. If they look forward to financial stress, other occupations will be more appealing.

PATIENT CENTERED CARE

Patient centered care is probably a good trend but there are some disconcerting trends that physicians find frustrating. Patients often show up for the appointment having researched their symptoms and decided the course of treatment desired based on information provided on the internet. Many patients don't know how to determine whether the information is reliable or even if it is appropriate for them. Physicians have to spend time explaining why the plan the patient arrived with may not be the best plan.

Patient compliance with treatment plans is often not good enough to prevent further deterioration of their condition and/or hospitalizations. This may be a good place to put psychological contracts in writing. A contract between the physician and the patient that spells out what the responsibilities of each person are could help patients recognize that they have accountability for the care and maintenance of their bodies. The physician is already on the hook legally for anything that would be put on the physician's side of the contract. The process could be explained by advising the patient that patients sometimes think their doctor is responsible for their health and the contract is to provide clarity.

HOME-WORK INTERFERENCE AKA WORK-FAMILY CONFLICT (WFC)

Both work interference in home life and home life interference with work increase the risk of burnout.[355, 356, 357] Developing healthy habits of thought improves relationships so it should smooth some of the rough edges in these relationships. We now know how "positive work–family interconnections enhance well-being in both contexts and how positivity spills over, enriches, and facilitates resourcefulness in work and family life."[358, 359]

Other strategies include:

- Flexible work hours
- Part-time options
- Child care provision or assistance
- Control after hours requirements to respond to patient portal inquiries
- Telehealth can add flexibility where physicians see patients via the internet during scheduled times or when a patient doesn't show for an appointment. This can also provide a work from home option in some situations.

Psychological Capital reduces burnout associated with work-family conflict.[360]

In the Netherlands, "75% of women physicians work part-time."[361] Research shows that part-time physicians are satisfied with their careers and have lower rates of burnout.

Recent research reports that Parental Burnout is a separate construct from professional burnout.[362] For a burned out parent, work may be a refuge. For the burned out professional, home may be a refuge. Individuals who are experiencing both professional and parental burnout don't have a refuge.

Recent incidents of home-work conflict are associated with higher reports of burnout.[363] "Reducing nurses' work-family conflict will increase nurse retention."[364]

DEATH AND DYING

In any occupation that deals with death and dying on a frequent basis it is critical to identify a worldview that allows you to experience those situations without the situations causing frequent emotional trauma and stress. Whether that perspective is religious, spiritual or Atheist is up to you. Your Emotional Guidance will help you find a perspective that you can live with and I mean that literally. You must have a way to handle secondary trauma that keeps you from suffering. You must also make sure the way you choose allows you to remain empathetic.

Organizations should recognize and address specific situations known to increase secondary trauma. Health care professionals generally experience a greater negative impact from patient suicides than other forms of sudden death.[365] Palliative medicine specialists who focused on meaning-making and emphasized the rewards of their work were able to resist burnout better than those without this focus.[366]

A discussion of how to create a worldview would add fifty pages to this book. It is a great workshop. See Compassion Fatigue for more related to this subject.

SECONDARY TRAUMA AND COMPASSION FATIGUE

Patient safety, risk managers, and clinical staff are beginning to recognize the adverse impact of the "emotional distress workers can experience as 'second victims' of the same incidents that harm patients."[367] A survey of 135 frontline staff at Johns Hopkins revealed nearly 90% would prefer to receive support within the first 24 hours after an event and their preferred source was:[368]

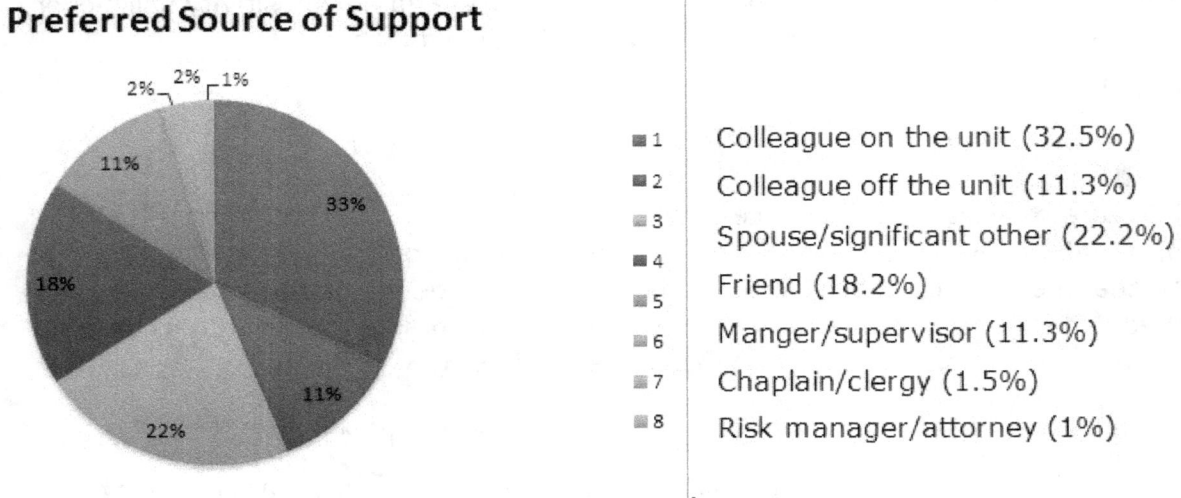

Preferred Source of Support

- 1 Colleague on the unit (32.5%)
- 2 Colleague off the unit (11.3%)
- 3 Spouse/significant other (22.2%)
- 4 Friend (18.2%)
- 5 Manger/supervisor (11.3%)
- 6 Chaplain/clergy (1.5%)
- 7 Risk manager/attorney (1%)

In a pilot program, the events that led to staff reaching out to a secondary support program included the following:[369]

- Death of a patient
- Adverse event
- Difficult decisions
- Burnout
- Staff assault
- Intrastaff conflicts
- Medical error

An individual who understands how to use his or her emotional guidance will be more capable of self-soothing but an ideal situation, given the dominant preference for reaching out to colleagues, would be to reach out to colleagues who also understand emotional guidance and advanced coping skills because they'd have a common, effective framework from which to work. A Positive Team Coaching climate would provide this type of foundation.

If the spouse also understood emotional guidance and advanced coping skills the individual would have skilled support at home. The way the event is interpreted (given meaning) or re-interpreted (given an alternate, reappraised meaning) can lead to post traumatic growth. Individuals exposed to trauma should be trained to find meanings that support their ability to thrive in the future, not meanings that bury them in guilt.

A silver lining can often be found, or created, from a tragic event. MADD is an example of someone who created a meaning for her daughter's senseless death as the result of a drunk driver. There are gifts in many wounds, even horrendous wounds have gifts but they can only be opened when they are assigned the meaning the gift provides. When an individual who lived through tragedy, trials, tribulations, or trauma helps others believe they can move forward it is an opened gift that was in the wound.

Rates of reported secondary traumatic stress in ICU range from 0% to 38.5%.[370] Whether a healthcare organization implements a program like John Hopkins RISE program or *The Smart Way*™, it is clear that secondary trauma contributes to burnout and other undesirable outcomes. All employees should be educated on the unhealthy consequences of negative rumination and negative co-rumination. Compassion fatigue can be prevented.[371]

There is another issue when it comes to support and that is when the healthcare system or their attorneys demand that the provider not speak about an incident out of fear of increasing the potential legal repercussions. The mental health (and subsequently, the physical well-being of the healthcare worker) is important and should be protected. If healthcare organizations banded together they might be able to obtain federal legislation that provides the same sort of confidential information privilege as that which exists between attorneys and clients. Healthcare workers are doing their best to help patients. They should not have to pay with their mental and physical health when something goes wrong.

Finally, despite the low inclination to seek professional counseling, there should be programs that encourage healthcare workers to access counseling or coaching when they feel a trained ear would be beneficial. We think no one knows about our mental suffering but anyone who understands *The Smart Way*™ sees right through us. When I first began understanding the strong connection between behavior (the words we speak and the actions we take and even the perspectives we assume about events) and our internal emotional state I felt like a voyeur. Awareness of that connection makes human behavior make a lot more sense and gives you access to insights that aren't available when behavior is viewed as merely a function of personality. When personality is viewed as a result of one's habits of thought and not who the person is, the ability to read people expands.

Seeing so much more was very uncomfortable until I realized there had always been some people who could see more than others. Recently I gave a speech to a State Chapter of the Medical Group Management Association about building resilience and afterwards a woman approached me and during our conversation she mentioned that she could tell I'd experienced trauma. I asked her how she knew and she said, "You can tell the difference between someone who has learned the facts and someone who has lived the journey." While I wouldn't wish my experiences on anyone, I appreciate that they allow me to help people I couldn't otherwise help.

Learning healthy habits of thought and Emotion Regulation Skills provided in this text can help you deal with secondary trauma (and 1st person traumas). The more skills you have the more flexibility you have available in your response. "Emotion regulation that is context-sensitive, effective, and flexible will facilitate positive outcomes (resilience, recovery, post-traumatic growth) following trauma and loss, whereas emotion regulation that is context-insensitive, ineffective, and inflexible will hinder positive outcomes, and promote negative outcomes (posttraumatic stress/depressive symptoms and related dysfunction)."[372]

WORKPLACE BULLYING

Someone who is authentically happy will never bully someone because it would make them feel worse and all human behavior is in pursuit of what we believe will make us feel better.

That's why kindness, better corporate citizenship, less crime and higher ethics are associated with positive emotional states.

Teaching employees skills that improves their emotional state will reduce the incidents of bullying. It will also help minimize the impact of any verbal abuse that does occur. When an employee understands at more than an intellectual level how closely emotional state and behavior are tied, it is easy to not take negative comments personally.

What we think, say, and do reflects our current emotional state. If we find fault with a co-worker it means our emotional state is one that is finding faults (i.e. frustration, blame, and anger). If we were in a state of appreciation we would find something about our co-worker to appreciate. It is easy to feel empathy for someone, even someone who is attempting to lower our emotional state by being rude, when we are in control of how we feel and understand that their words and actions are simply indicators of their emotional state in the same way that our emotions are indicators of our emotional state.

Workplace bullying prevention laws have been introduced in many states but none passed so far. We are one vivid incident away from an onslaught of workplace anti-bullying legislation. If a workplace incident catches the attention of the media or social media, much like the recent incident with the physician on United Airlines did, lawmakers will bow to public sentiment and pass legislation making employers responsible for workplace bullying.

I don't think anyone should be bullied but when you consider that it is the employee's emotional state more than anything that makes him or her behave in a bullying fashion and that an employee's self-concept that determines what is perceived as bullying, it puts the employer in an unmanageable situation. I've always been highly resilient. I've had experiences (more than one) when a workplace friend mentioned something that happened a few days previously that they were angry about <u>on my behalf</u> that I hadn't given a second thought because I didn't feel slighted or angry about the words that were spoken. If those same words had been directed at my workplace friend they would have felt bullied.

Paradoxically, there have been times when I was angry about words spoken to a workplace associate that angered me on their behalf that I wouldn't have been upset about if they were spoken to me because I knew I could handle it but they were hurt by the words. I tend to be a bit of a mama bear when it comes to anyone I perceive as being picked on by someone who they perceive as stronger (physically, in authority, in mental strength). In my 20's I'd defend them. Today I will teach them how to feel stronger and stand up for themselves which is more effective and gives them more confidence. Bullies don't pick on the strong. Increasing someone's confidence makes them less of a target.

ROI: BURNOUT PREVENTION AND RETENTION

The cost of burnout extends from the individual to co-workers, family, community, and employer. This makes preventing and recovering from burnout an imperative. The good news is that preventing burnout prevents a lot of other problems. Organizations that choose to spend training resources on reducing burnout also improve patient outcomes, co-worker relationships, overall productivity, employee wellness, and performance. When the true cost of burnout is understood, preventing burnout becomes an easy decision.

An article in the *Canadian Journal of Psychiatry* concluded, "Everyone could benefit from investment in improved mental health in the workplace. However, because the benefits associated with improved worker mental health are often distributed among several stakeholders, the incentives for any single stakeholder to pay for additional services for workers may be diluted. As a consequence, no one invests. Nevertheless, there is a role for all stakeholders, just as there are potential benefits for all. Along with government, employers, employees, and the health care system must invest in promoting good workplace health."[373]

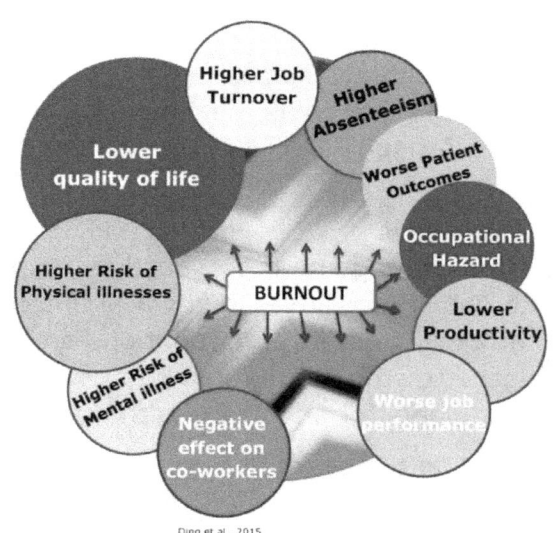

Burnout can lead to the ultimate personal sacrifice but organizations also experience numerous problems as the result of burnout. Addressing burnout is a necessary aspect of any healthcare organization's strategic planning process. An organization that ignores employee burnout is unlikely to achieve other goals because burnout has negative impacts in every area:

- Workplace relationships[374]
    - Between boss and employees
    - Between co-workers and teams
    - Between workers and customers/patients[375]
- Reduced productivity[376]
- Lower quality[377]
- Higher absenteeism[378]
- Higher turnover[379], [380]
- Increased accidents and errors[381]
- Lower customer/patient satisfaction[382]
- Higher customer/patient complaints[383]
- Burned out physicians are more likely to order tests and procedures[384]
- Hindered performance on difficult tasks (think diagnosis/surgery)[385]
- Physician disability insurance premiums increased 20 – 30% in 2001 in the Netherlands because of increasing burnout and stress-related claims.[386] Evidence suggests that stress and burnout have increased since then.
- Decreased productivity[387]
- Decreased practice revenue[388]

A research study that was a combined effort from respected universities in the United States estimated the cost of replacing one physician at "at least $250,000 per primary care physician."[389] You don't have to look much further than lowering turnover to see that it would not be difficult to achieve a positive ROI. Increasing engagement reduces burnout.

HEALTH CONSEQUENCES

Physicians who are burned out are more likely to have adverse health outcomes including:

- Increases in stress hormones[390]

- Coronary heart disease[391, 392]
- Circulatory issues[393]
- Mental health problems[394, 395]
- Susceptibility to colds, headaches, and fevers[396] (see stress symptom chart)
- Chronic fatigue[397]

RISK MANAGEMENT

From a risk management perspective, employers must recognize the potential exposure they have for liability for adverse physical and mental health outcomes. The health outcomes from chronically stressful occupations are as bad as, if not worse, than the health outcomes from cigarette smoking. We all know what happened to the tobacco industry as the result of being held liable for adverse health outcomes from smoking.

When we didn't know the affect it was different. Now we know, or should know, for example, the findings from a systematic literature review published in the *International Journal of Environmental Research and Public Health* in 2013 provide "strong support for the relationship between work-related stress, burnout and general health."[398]

> *The most chronic stressors were associated with the most global immunosuppression, as they were associated with reliable decreases in almost all functional immune measures examined. Increasing stressor duration, therefore, resulted in a shift from potentially adaptive changes to potentially detrimental changes, initially in cellular immunity and then in immune function more broadly.*[399]

If you want support to fund training, show the above to risk managers in your organization.

Now that we know the risks, it is only a matter of time before class action suits for chronic workplace stress, especially avoidable chronic stress, are brought against high-stress employers. Avoidable will be defined by the courts and juries in two ways, one will be avoidable by changing processes so that they are less stressful and the other will be providing stress reduction skills building. Best practices will be viewed more favorably than dose-dependent strategies.

> *Exposure to chronic stress markedly increases vulnerability to adverse medical outcomes. This holds true across a wide variety of mental and physical conditions. For example, persons facing chronic stress are more likely to develop an episode of clinical depression, experience symptoms of an upper respiratory infection following viral exposure, suffer from a flare up of an existing allergic or autoimmune condition, and show accelerated progression of chronic diseases such as acquired immunodeficiency syndrome and coronary heart disease.*[400]

From my perspective, the focus on technological advances and (in the USA) the myriad new payment/billing requirements are distracting physicians and health care systems from the low-hanging fruit that research in other areas has produced.

Since as early as the 1970's we've known that stress is at the root of 65-98% of all illnesses and diseases. We know more today because we understand that stress has an adverse impact on immune, digestive, CNS, and cognitive functions. We know that stress can make a healthy meal unhealthy via the body's biochemistry. We are also far more adept in reducing stress now than the early, off the cuff, recommendations that were put forth when the connection between stress and health was first recognized.

Psychological resilience is a valuable tool in high strain work environments providing protection against stress, burnout, sleep problems, likelihood of depression, intent to quit, and absences.[401] Psychological resilience also increases productivity and job satisfaction.[402]

Human relationships and caring interactions reduce stress. The machines distract the physician from the caring/healing touch.

We're plunging ahead at a rapid pace, doing things because we can without evaluating whether we should. It's time to pause and put some thought into where we are going and why.

EPIGENETICS

Our genes are not a predetermined map of our destiny. "Epigenetics is the contemporary study of how the environment influences gene expression both within and, through heritable changes in DNA, beyond the lifetime of an organism."[403] Stressful environments can lead to adverse genetic changes that last for generations. Stress during pregnancy and early life can have significant effects on lifelong health and well-being.

Unlike the tobacco class action suits, workplace stress suits have more potential targets because of the multi-generational impact of stress on physical and mental health and the ability to develop and maintain healthy relationships. If I was a betting person I'd bet that I'll see suits against employers for workplace stress from children whose genetics were affected by their parents' work stress levels. In the United States that more than doubles the potential claimants. Will they win? I don't know. The more employers know about the effects and the less employers do to mitigate known workplace stressors, the higher the assumed risk.

You should document the ways you attempt to mitigate the risk of adverse epigenetic changes as the result of new research in this area. If you prepare your defense now, by improving the work environment as much as possible and documenting what you do, it will reduce the risk of an adverse court decision

HUMAN THRIVING

Thriving employees:[404]
- Tend to be healthier
- Report fewer physical or somatic complaints
- Have far fewer doctor visits
- Experience less burnout or strain
- Facilitate reduced health care costs.
- Missed 74 percent less days of work
- Sustain their performance over time
- Are more beneficial than employee's experiencing job satisfaction or organizational commitment

WIN-WIN-WIN-WIN

When you understand your Emotional Guidance and develop advanced and transformational coping skills, you create a scenario where everyone can win.

You win because you feel better and can reap the benefits of better health and wellbeing.

Your family wins because a happy you, or, a you who doesn't demand that they change to make you happy, makes them happier and that improves their health and wellbeing.

The greater community also benefits. People who have better health and relationships contribute more and take less. They are less likely to become a burden to others and more likely to be kind, ethical, and law-abiding.

Your employer wins because you become a better employee with improved customer feedback, productivity, more intelligent decisions, better relationships with your co-workers, better corporate citizenship, and lower turnover, absenteeism, and burnout.

There are no losers. I like that.

FINAL THOUGHTS FOR HEALTHCARE PROVIDERS

As you read and begin applying the strategies in this book you probably recognized that many of your stressed, depressed, burned out, victim-mindset, and anxious patients would benefit from applying the same knowledge. We recognize that suggesting a patient read a book about physician burnout could be uncomfortable so we wanted to let you know that we are simultaneously working on another book that contains much of the information provided herein written with a lay audience in mind. That book will be available by July, 2017 and is titled: *Mental Health Made Easy*. It includes sections on Emotional Guidance, unhealthy habits of thought and healthy habits of thought that are very similar, and in some cases, identical, to the ones included here.

REVIEWS

If this book has helped you we ask that you pay it forward by writing a review on Amazon, Good Reads (goodreads.com) or another online bookseller's website. In the competitive publishing world, books without reviews seldom make it into the hands of the people they are designed to help. Your review helps us help others. You never know whose life will be positively impacted because you chose to share your thoughts about this book. Thank you ever so much if you choose to write a review.

DR. JOY'S BOOKS

Mental Health Made Easy: The New Science of the Mind: Develop Healthy Habits of Thought

Empowered Employees become Engaged Employees

Harness the Power of Resilience: Be Ready for Life

Prevent Suicide: The Smart Way

True Prevention—Optimum Health: Remember Galileo

Is Punishment Ethical? The Fallacy of Good and Evil

Rescue our Children from the War Zone, Teach them Social and Emotional Skills, Applied Positive Psychology 2.1

Psychology from the Pulpit

"Trusting One's Emotional Guidance Builds Resilience", Perspectives on Coping and Resilience. Ed. Venkat Pulla, Shane Warren, and Andrew Shatté. Laxmi Nagar: Authors Press, 2013. 254-279

ABOUT THE AUTHORS

JEANINE JOY, PHD

Dr. Joy followed a non-traditional path to mastering the knowledge she shares by pursuing a passionate interest with determination for more than two decades. After an expert told her she was more resilient than most and asked her how she managed it she concluded that if she was more resilient and she could figure out how or why, she could help a lot of people.

As a citizen scientist, she was not bound by the silo's that constrain most researchers. If information helped her thrive or communicate how to thrive more to others, she looked for ways to incorporate it into her repertoire. Adding evidence-based support to the experience-informed processes and techniques she'd accumulated was the last step in her journey. When she turned to reading peer reviewed research she was delighted to find support for all the major strategies she was teaching.

She's been teaching classes to diverse audiences, from bank presidents to homeless recovering addicts, for more than a decade. Many fields of science have made great progress in emotion regulation, motivation, organizational behavior, positive psychology, organizations, and teams, resilience, self-determination and self-control but none have put together as many pieces of the puzzle to form a cohesive picture of human thriving as Dr. Joy.

It wasn't until the last step in her journey that she learned about existing bodies of work that closely parallel her own work. Cognitive Behavioral Therapy is a one-on-one version of what she effectively teaches to groups as educational content. From a broad perspective, we can and should teach people how to develop healthy habits of thought rather than waiting until they experience physical or mental illnesses from the stress they incur as the result of unhealthy habits of thought.

Her doctorate is in the philosophy of pastoral counseling psychology on a metaphysical foundation. Metaphysics was the study of the mind and a respected field until mind and body were split to please the church. As science brings us back to solid evidence of the mind-body connection, mainstream researchers are beginning to give metaphysics more attention.

Science fully supports the strategies Dr. Joy teaches using but they are also supported by metaphysical principles, by the texts of many of the world's religions, and by the wisdom of many ancient philosophers. She shares lived experiences that demonstrate the benefits of understanding this information.

She is a sought after keynote speaker and trainer committed to helping people thrive more in every area of life.

PHIL GEISSINGER, *FHFMA, CMPE*

Phil is Senior Vice President, Thrive More Now, LLC, which specializes in providing innovative leadership and operational solutions for healthcare organizations. He guides client management strategies on employee engagement; provider business and performance development, stress management, business acumen, and resilience training; business and practice operations performance improvement; and payer contract management plans, which directly drive economic and operating performance. His extensive background in hospital and physician practice management allows him to bring a broad range of knowledge to each situation. Phil's experience includes financial management of large and mid-sized providers; executive roles in finance and operations, including interim CFO; and, leadership development experience with both public and private organizations.

As a heart-led CFO Phil has always been ahead of his time.

Phil is well-versed on the complexities of the Affordable Care Act, providing thoughtful insights about the implications of the Act and now the AHCA; how organizations should be assessing their situation, developing business strategies in the face of change and accelerating economic demands; and, executing plans of action for organizational sustainability. He has spoken, as a subject matter expert on these topics in many different forums to a broad spectrum of healthcare professionals. He examines both the current state and the future state of the Laws as critical long-term thinking on strategy and operations is explicit in how organizations must take action. He is recognized for his ability to identify and capitalize on business improvement opportunities inherent in new laws and regulations, and provides actionable thinking and strategies for leadership.

He is an accomplished contract negotiator and relationship manager with a keen ability to recognize and evaluate risks associated with organizational, cultural, reputation management, regulatory, and compliance issues. Building organizational value and patient oriented outcomes through our development programs is a hallmark of how Phil works with organizations.

Phil earned Fellowship status in the Healthcare Financial Management Association (FHFMA) and is a Certified Member (CMPE) in the American College of Medical Practice Executives (ACMPE). He received an MBA from Northeastern University and a Bachelor's Degree from Albion College. He has also served as adjunct faculty at Pfeiffer University, North Carolina, the Cabarrus College of Health Sciences in Concord, N.C., Simmons College in Boston, MA. and University of Massachusetts – Lowell, in Lowell, MA.

APPENDIX I – EGSC

Appendix I
Appendix I - Emotional Guidance Scale (EGSc)

In general, emotional states can be defined (broadly) with the following feelings:

Sweet Zone
- Joy
- Empowered
- Passion
- Happy
- Inspired
- Optimism
- Fulfilled
- Appreciation
- Love
- Enthusiasm
- Positive Expectation
- Trust
- Serene
- Secure
- Freedom
- Awe
- Eagerness
- Belief
- Faith
- Satisfied
- At ease

Hopeful Zone
- Hopefulness
- Grateful
- Upbeat

Blah Zone
- Contentment
- Apathy
- Boredom
- Dispirited
- Pessimism
- Empty

Drama Zone
- Frustration
- Overwhelmed
- Irritation
- Disappointment
- Impatience
- Indignant

Give Away Zone
- Doubt
- Guilt
- Cynical
- Worry
- Discouragement
- Blame
- Offended

Hot (Red) Zone
- Anger
- Outraged
- Revenge
- Easily provoked
- Rage
- Furious

Powerless Zone
- Victimized
- Hatred
- Insecure
- Grief
- Powerless
- Hopeless
- Suicidal
- Bullied
- Excessively Detached
- Fear
- Depression
- Learned Helplessness
- Melancholy
- Unimportant
- Jealousy
- Envy
- Unworthiness
- Despair
- Guarded
- Unwanted
- Exploited

APPENDIX II – BURNOUT QUESTIONNAIRE (CLINICAL SUBTYPES)

The Maslach Burnout Inventory Questionnaire (MBI) and other earlier burnout measures treat burnout as the result of one factor. Further research indicates that there is more than one pathway to burnout. This questionnaire identifies the pathway.

Burnout Clinical Subtypes Questionnaire (BCSQ-12)[405] Mark the answers that most closely reflect how you felt most often during the past month. See Scoring Appendix VI to score your answers.	Totally Disagree	Mostly Disagree	Somewhat Disagree	Neither Agree Or Disagree	Somewhat Agree	Mostly Agree	Totally Agree
1. I think the dedication I invest in my work is more than what I should for my health.							
2. I would like to be doing another job that is more challenging for my abilities.							
3. When things at work don't turn out as well as they should, I stop trying.							
4. I neglect my personal life when I pursue important achievements in my work.							
5. I feel that my work is an obstacle to the development of my abilities.							
6. I give up in response to difficulties in my work.							
7. I risk my health when I pursue good results in my work.							
8. I would like to be doing another job where I can better develop my talents.							
9. I give up in the face of any difficulties in my work tasks.							
10. I overlook my own needs to fulfill work demands.							
11. My work doesn't offer me opportunities to develop my abilities.							
12. When the effort I invest in work is not enough, I give up.							

APPENDIX III – BURNOUT QUESTIONNAIRE

There are a variety of validated methods of determining the level of burnout an individual is experiencing. The most commonly used is Maslach Burnout Inventory (MBI) which is available online for a modest fee.

Studies indicate that answering the single question, "I feel emotionally drained from my work" has been a strong indicator of burnout.

If you agree with the statement that you're feeling emotionally drained by your work you may be experiencing burnout. The more emphatic you feel about affirming the statement, the more likely the level of burnout you're experiencing is high and the more important it is to take actions to improve, recover from, and prevent further burnout.

APPENDIX IV - DEPRESSION QUESTIONNAIRE (PHQ-9)

Over the <u>last 2 weeks</u>, how often have you been bothered by any of the following:

Patient Health Questionnaire-9 (PHQ-9) See Appendix VII for scoring	Not at all	Several days	More than half the days	Nearly every day
1. Little interest or pleasure in doing things?				
2. Feeling down, depressed, or hopeless?				
3. Trouble falling or staying asleep, or sleeping too much?				
4. Feeling tired or having little energy?				
5. Poor appetite or overeating?				
6. Feeling bad about yourself—or that you are a failure or have let yourself or your family down?				
7. Trouble concentrating on things, such as reading the newspaper or watching television?				
8. Moving or speaking so slowly that other people could have noticed? Or the opposite—being so fidgety or restless that you have been moving around a lot more than usual?				
9. Thoughts that you would be better off dead or of hurting yourself in some way?				

APPENDIX V - GENERAL ANXIETY QUESTIONNAIRE (GAD-7)

Over the last 2 weeks, how often have you been bothered by the following problems? **GAD-7** See Appendix VIII for scoring	Not at all	Several days	More than half the days	Nearly every day
1. Feeling nervous, anxious, or on edge				
2. Not being able to stop or control worrying				
3. Worrying too much about different things				
4. Trouble relaxing				
5. Being so restless that it is hard to sit still				
6. Becoming easily annoyed or irritable				
7. Feeling afraid as if something awful might happen				

APPENDIX VI - QUESTIONNAIRE SCORING (BCSQ-12)

Scoring **Burnout Clinical Subtypes Questionnaire (BCSQ-12)**[406]	Totally Disagree	Mostly Disagree	Somewhat Disagree	Neither Agree Or Disagree	Somewhat Agree	Mostly Agree	Totally Agree
3) When things at work don't turn out as well as they should, I stop trying.	0	1	2	3	4	5	6
6) I give up in response to difficulties in my work.	0	1	2	3	4	5	6
9) I give up in the face of any difficulties in my work tasks.	0	1	2	3	4	5	6
12) When the effort I invest in work is not enough, I give up.	0	1	2	3	4	5	6
2) I would like to be doing another job that is more challenging for my abilities.	0	1	2	3	4	5	6
5) I feel that my work is an obstacle to the development of my abilities.	0	1	2	3	4	5	6
8) I would like to be doing another job where I can better develop my talents.	0	1	2	3	4	5	6
11) My work doesn't offer me opportunities to develop my abilities.	0	1	2	3	4	5	6
1) I think the dedication I invest in my work is more than what I should for my health.	0	1	2	3	4	5	6
4) I neglect my personal life when I pursue important achievements in my work.	0	1	2	3	4	5	6
7) I risk my health when I pursue good results in my work.	0	1	2	3	4	5	6
10) I overlook my own needs to fulfill work	0	1	2	3	4	5	6

demands.						

Scoring:

Circle the answers that correspond to your answers. Add your scores in each group of four questions:

0 – 12

You seem to be doing fine. If your intuition disagrees with this assessment do not use this assessment as a reason not to seek help.

13 – 24

You are expressing some symptoms of burnout. The higher the number, the more symptoms you are experiencing and the more important it is to take actions to improve, recover and prevent further burnout.

The BCSQ-12 takes the classification of burnout further than the older scale that looked for exhaustion, cynicism, and a lack of accomplishment. The BCSQ-12[407] divides burnout into three types:

- Frenetic (Questions 1, 4, 7, 10)

    "characterized by the investment of a large amount of time to work and is common in highly involved, ambitious and overloaded individuals. 'involvement' is the investment of every effort required to overcome difficulties; 'ambition' is a great need to obtain important success and achievements at work; and 'overload' is risking one's own health and neglecting of one's own personal life in the pursuit of good results."

- Underchallenged (Questions 2, 5, 8, 11)

    "is influenced by occupation type. It appears in indifferent and bored individuals who do not find personal development in their work. 'Indifference' is lack of concern, interest and enthusiasm in work-related tasks; 'boredom' is caused by the understanding of work as a mechanical and routine experience with little variation in activities; and 'lack of development' is the absence of personal growth experiences for individuals together with their desire for taking on other jobs where they can better develop their skills."

- Worn-out (Questions 3, 6, 9, 12)

    "determined by the rigidity of the organizational structure of an individual's workplace and is characterized by a lack of control over results, lack of recognition for efforts and neglect of responsibilities. 'Lack of control' is the feeling of helplessness as a result of dealing with many situations that are beyond their control; 'lack of acknowledgement' is the belief that the organizations those individuals work for fail to take their efforts and dedication into account; and 'neglect' refers to individuals' disregard as a response to any difficulty."

Identifying the sub-classification(s) of burnout an individual is experiencing points us toward possible solutions. For example, an individual in a job that is not challenging who has no apparent opportunities to change jobs should consider self-development to feel more challenged and to prepare for a job that will be more challenging.

This does not have to be through formal education if cost considerations limit access to advanced educational opportunities. There are many online courses that are free or nearly free. Use your search engine and look for "free online college courses." Keep records of the courses you complete and add them to your resume and to your professional online profile (i.e. LinkedIn).

Libraries are also free and offer many books that you can study to expand your skill set. Many highly successful people did not complete a formal university curriculum. The most successful people who completed a formal education continue reading to acquire knowledge after graduation.

This individual who feels unchallenged can also apply The Smart Way™ to his or her perception of the situation. The feeling that one has no options is a perfect example of a situation where it is possible to look for other perspectives that feel better. The sense of being trapped in an unchallenging occupation is usually a construct the individual has created that does not reflect all possible outcomes. An individual who understands negative emotion is a sign that better perspectives could be explored will take action to find better feeling perspectives that will be more empowering. Perceiving more options opens the way for positive changes.

APPENDIX VII - DEPRESSION QUESTIONNAIRE SCORING (PHQ-9)

SCORING **Patient Health Questionnaire-9** **(PHQ-9)**	Not at all	Several days	More than half the days	Nearly every day
1. Little interest or pleasure in doing things?	0	1	2	3
2. Feeling down, depressed, or hopeless?	0	1	2	3
3. Trouble falling or staying asleep, or sleeping too much?	0	1	2	3
4. Feeling tired or having little energy?	0	1	2	3
5. Poor appetite or overeating?	0	1	2	3
6. Feeling bad about yourself—or that you are a failure or have let yourself or your family down?	0	1	2	3
7. Trouble concentrating on things, such as reading the newspaper or watching television?	0	1	2	3
8. Moving or speaking so slowly that other people could have noticed? Or the opposite—being so fidgety or restless that you have been moving around a lot more than usual?	0	1	2	3
9. Thoughts that you would be better off dead or of hurting yourself in some way?	0	1	2	3

Depression is serious but curable. If any of your answers correspond to the boxes (questions 1, 2, and 9) that have a heavier border, you should contact your physician for an appointment or, if you are considering harming yourself, call 911 or go to your local Emergency room for immediate assistance.

Add your total score for questions 1 – 9 and find the category on the following chart that it corresponds to your score.

None - Minimal	Mild	Moderate	Moderately Severe	Severe
0- 4	5-9	10-14	15-19	20-27

The treatments suggested in the literature are (phqscreeners.com):

None-Minimal: None

Mild: Watchful waiting: repeat PHQ-9 at follow-up

Moderate: Treatment plan, consider counseling, follow-up and/or pharmacotherapy

Moderately Severe: Active treatment with pharmacotherapy and/or psychotherapy

Immediate initiation of pharmacotherapy and, if severe impairment or poor response to therapy, referral to a mental health specialist for psychotherapy and/or collaborative management

Personally, I would be more aggressive. The current mental health model has a goal of zero on a scale that goes from -10 to +10. Research has clearly shown that there are significant physical health benefits between 8 and 10. Relationships are also better when we feel better emotionally. The skills and knowledge in this book can help anyone move well beyond zero.

Given the high success rate of Cognitive Behavioral Therapy (CBT) I'd also encourage therapy in addition to any pharmacology that your health care provider deems necessary. Some of the techniques you'll learn in this book are similar to CBT. I am biased toward The Smart Way™ because with The Smart Way™ you know your goal and how to get there. With CBT, the therapist knows the goal (healthy thoughts) and guides you to them but not in as straightforward of a path. That being said, if you have more than moderate symptoms a trained mental health provider should be involved in your care.

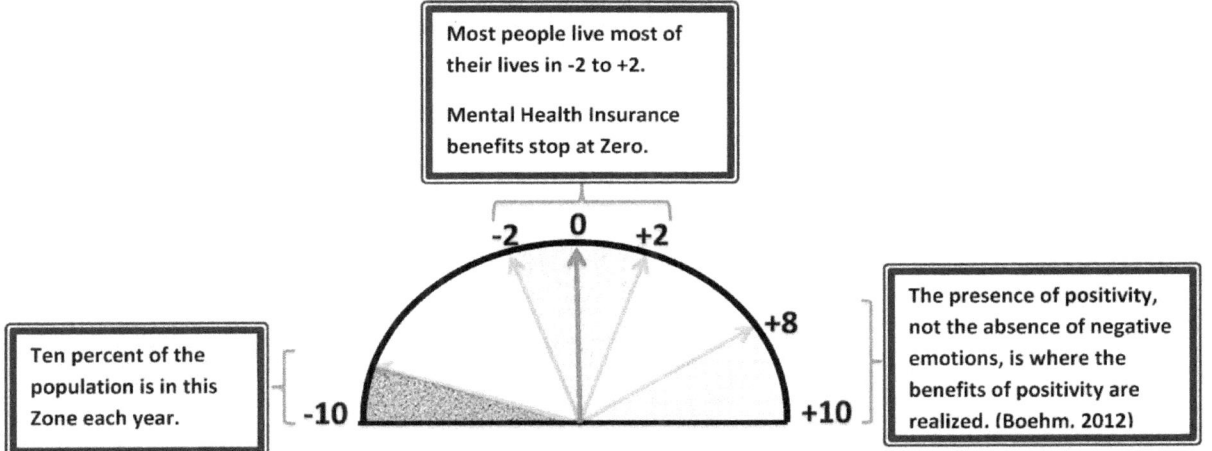

We all have the potential to be happy and given the benefits of being happy and, with the right skills, the ease of being happy often, I don't know why anyone would chose to be satisfied being consistently below +5.

If you are thinking that maybe you'd rather be dead or that those you care about would be better off if you were, call the toll-free, 24-hour hotline of the National Suicide Prevention Lifeline now at 1-800-273-TALK (1-800-273-8255); TTY: 1-800-799-4TTY (4889) to talk to a trained counselor.

Or, **call your doctor**

Dial 911

or go to an emergency room

For a free detailed booklet on depression and its treatment, go to: http://www.nimh.nih.gov/health/publications/depression/complete-index.shtml

International Emergency Numbers

Australia	000	Switzerland	112	UAE	112
New Zealand	111	India	102	Brazil	192
Fiji	000 or 911	Hong Kong	999	Costa Rica	911
United Kingdom	112 or 999	Israel	101 or 112	S. Africa	112, 10 177
Ireland	112 or 999	Japan	119	China	120
Turkey	112	Nepal	102	Philippines	117 or 112

APPENDIX VIII - GENERAL ANXIETY QUESTIONNAIRE (GAD-7) SCORING

SCORING Over the last 2 weeks, how often have you been bothered by the following problems? GAD-7	Not at all	Several days	More than half the days	Nearly every day
1. Feeling nervous, anxious, or on edge	0	1	2	3
2. Not being able to stop or control worrying	0	1	2	3
3. Worrying too much about different things	0	1	2	3
4. Trouble relaxing	0	1	2	3
5. Being so restless that it is hard to sit still	0	1	2	3
6. Becoming easily annoyed or irritable	0	1	2	3
7. Feeling afraid as if something awful might happen	0	1	2	3

Add the score that corresponds to your answers together and get a total score. If your total score is 10 or above you should consult a mental health care professional. Many of the techniques provided in this book will help you ease anxious thoughts. Specifically, going more general will often calm worries. Changing the subject you're thinking about can be effective. *The Smart Way*™ is a very effective method of finding thoughts that feel better. The more you use your emotional guidance the more you will trust it which makes it easier to calm worries and fears. Be sure to apply the techniques in the book, not just read about them. They will begin feeling natural and easy far quicker than you might expect. Anxiety is curable. You don't have to suffer.

APPENDIX IX – BURNOUT QUESTIONNAIRES

A single item burnout questionnaire has consistent reliability with the full MBI scale using either of the following two questions:[408]

- I feel burned out from my work, or
- I have become more callous toward people since I took this job.

If you prefer to explore the subject in more depth, the following questionnaire does that. Note: This questionnaire also appears in the text of the book

Using Yes and No answers, indicate how you've felt during the past month:

1. Have you felt burned out from you work?

2. Have you worried that your work is hardening you emotionally or felt cynical toward your work or patients?

3. Have you often felt down, depressed, hopeless, or wondered what was the point of it all?

4. Have you fallen asleep unexpectedly or when you didn't want to such as when you were driving?

5. Have you felt overwhelmed, as if there is too much to do and that completing all the tasks is impossible?

6. Have you felt anxious, depressed, irritable, or easily angered?

7. Has your physical health declined or have you been ill more frequently?

8. Do you feel your work is important and that it matters?

9. Do you find yourself simply wanting to escape your reality such as by reading a lot of fiction, binge watching shows, surfing the web, alcohol or drugs or other addictive behaviors?

See Appendix X for scoring.

APPENDIX X – BURNOUT QUESTIONNAIRE SCORING

You may be experiencing one or more signs of burnout if you answered yes to questions 1 – 7, and 9. Question 8 is reverse scored because not feeling that your work makes a difference is a sign of burnout.

APPENDIX XI - STRESS SYMPTOM CHART

Warning Signs (Indicators of) Stress

Physical

Muscle tension
Headaches
Exhaustion/fatigue
Weight changes
Sleep disturbances
Teeth grinding
Frequent illnesses
Stomach aches
Hypertension
Sweating or trembling hands
Sexual dysfunction
Diarrhea or constipation
Back pain
Restlessness
Indigestion
Increased pain
Dizziness
Racing heart
Ringing in the ears
Immune function decreases
Digestive function worsens
Central Nervous System issues
More accidents
Increased risk of pre-term births
Increased risk of adverse epigenetic changes
Increased risk of adverse behavior and health outcomes in offspring

Behavioral

Hurrying
Increased accidents
Decreased productivity
Increased use of drugs
Increased use of alcohol
Unhealthy eating patterns
Isolation
Cigarette smoking
Procrastination
Conflicts with others
Restricted breathing
More sedentary
Bossiness
Compulsive gum chewing
Inability to get things done
Increased relationship conflict
Engage in riskier behaviors

Cognitive

Trouble thinking clearly
Lack of creativity
Forgetfulness
Memory Loss
Inability to make decisions
Poor concentration

Psychological

Irritability
Less emotional control
Often worried
Feeling overwhelmed
Easily frustrated
Thoughts of running away
Loss of sense of humor
Difficulty making decisions
Crying spells
Intense bouts of anger
Attitude critical of others
Restlessness
Nervousness
Anxiety
Boredom, no meaning
Edginess, ready to explode
Feeling powerless
Loneliness
Unhappy for no reason
Easily upset
Burnout
Depression
Anxiety
Suicidal Thoughts
Suicide

APPENDIX XII – COPE QUESTIONNAIRE

COPE *(Full Version)*

Respond to each of the following items by blackening one number on your answer sheet for each, using the response choices listed just below. Please try to respond to each item separately in your mind from each other item. Choose your answers thoughtfully, and make your answers as true FOR YOU as you can. Please answer every item. There are no "right" or "wrong" answers, so choose the most accurate answer for YOU--not what you think "most people" would say or do. Indicate what YOU usually do when YOU experience a stressful event.

See Appendix XIII for a Brief Cope Questionnaire

See Appendix XIV for Scoring

	I usually don't do this at al	I usually do this a little bit	I usually do this a medium amount	I usually do this a lot
1. I try to grow as a person as a result of the experience.				
2. I turn to work or other substitute activities to take my mind off things.				
3. I get upset and let my emotions out.				
4. I try to get advice from someone about what to do.				
5. I concentrate my efforts on doing something about it.				
6. I say to myself "this isn't real."				
7. I put my trust in God.				
8. I laugh about the situation.				
9. I admit to myself that I can't deal with it, and quit trying.				
10. I restrain myself from doing anything too quickly.				
11. I discuss my feelings with someone.				
12. I use alcohol or drugs to make myself feel better. .				
13. I get used to the idea that it happened				
14. I talk to someone to find out more about the situation.				
15. I keep myself from getting distracted by other thoughts or activities.				
16. I daydream about things other than this.				
17. I get upset, and am really aware of it.				

18. I seek God's help.				
19. I make a plan of action.				
20. I make jokes about it.				
21. I accept that this has happened and that it can't be changed.				
22. I hold off doing anything about it until the situation permits.				
23. I try to get emotional support from friends or relatives.				
24. I just give up trying to reach my goal.				
25. I take additional action to try to get rid of the problem.				
26. I try to lose myself for a while by drinking alcohol or taking drugs.				
27. I refuse to believe that it has happened.				
28. I let my feelings out.				
29. I try to see it in a different light, to make it seem more positive.				
30. I talk to someone who could do something concrete about the problem.				
31. I sleep more than usual.				
32. I try to come up with a strategy about what to do.				
33. I focus on dealing with this problem, and if necessary let other things slide a little.				
34. I get sympathy and understanding from someone.				
35. I drink alcohol or take drugs, in order to think about it less.				
36. I kid around about it.				
37. I give up the attempt to get what I want.				
38. I look for something good in what is happening.				
39. I think about how I might best handle the problem.				
40. I pretend that it hasn't really happened.				
41. I make sure not to make matters worse by acting too soon.				
42. I try hard to prevent other things from interfering with my efforts at dealing with this.				
43. I go to movies or watch TV, to think about it less.				

44. I accept the reality of the fact that it happened.				
45. I ask people who have had similar experiences what they did.				
46. I feel a lot of emotional distress and I find myself expressing those feelings a lot.				
47. I take direct action to get around the problem.				
48. I try to find comfort in my religion.				
49. I force myself to wait for the right time to do something.				
50. I make fun of the situation.				
51. I reduce the amount of effort I'm putting into solving the problem.				
52. I talk to someone about how I feel.				
53. I use alcohol or drugs to help me get through it.				
54. I learn to live with it.				
55. I put aside other activities in order to concentrate on this.				
56. I think hard about what steps to take.				
57. I act as though it hasn't even happened.				
58. I do what has to be done, one step at a time.				
60. I pray more than usual.				
52. I talk to someone about how I feel.				
53. I use alcohol or drugs to help me get through it.				
54. I learn to live with it.				
55. I put aside other activities in order to concentrate on this.				
56. I think hard about what steps to take.				
57. I act as though it hasn't even happened.				
58. I do what has to be done, one step at a time.				
59. I learn something from the experience.				
60. I pray more than usual.				

Citation to the full COPE: Carver, C. S., Scheier, M. F., & Weintraub, J. K. (1989). Assessing coping strategies: A theoretically based approach. *Journal of Personality and Social Psychology, 56*, 267-283.

APPENDIX XIII - BRIEF COPE

BRIEF COPE	I usually don't do this at al	I usually do this a little bit	I usually do this a medium amount	I usually do this a lot
1. I've been turning to work or other activities to take my mind off things.				
2. I've been concentrating my efforts on doing something about the situation I'm in.				
3. I've been saying to myself "this isn't real.".				
4. I've been using alcohol or other drugs to make myself feel better.				
5. I've been getting emotional support from others.				
6. I've been giving up trying to deal with it.				
7. I've been taking action to try to make the situation better.				
8. I've been refusing to believe that it has happened.				
9. I've been saying things to let my unpleasant feelings escape.				
10. I've been getting help and advice from other people.				
11. I've been using alcohol or other drugs to help me get through it.				
12. I've been trying to see it in a different light, to make it seem more positive.				
13. I've been criticizing myself.				
14. I've been trying to come up with a strategy about what to do.				
15. I've been getting comfort and understanding from someone.				
16. I've been giving up the attempt to cope.				
17. I've been looking for something good in what is happening.				
18. I've been making jokes about it.				
19. I've been doing something to think about it less, such as going to				

movies, watching TV, reading, daydreaming, sleeping, or shopping.				
20. I've been accepting the reality of the fact that it has happened.				
21. I've been expressing my negative feelings.				
22. I've been trying to find comfort in my religion or spiritual beliefs.				
23. I've been trying to get advice or help from other people about what to do.				
24. I've been learning to live with it.				
25. I've been thinking hard about what steps to take.				
26. I've been blaming myself for things that happened.				
27. I've been praying or meditating.				
28. I've been making fun of the situation.				

Brief Cope Citation: Carver, C. S. (1997). You want to measure coping but your protocol's too long: Consider the Brief COPE. *International Journal of Behavioral Medicine*, 4, 92-100. [abstract]

APPENDIX XIV - COPE SCORING

The COPE Inventory was developed to assess a broad range of coping responses, several of which had an explicit basis in theory. The inventory includes some responses that are expected to be dysfunctional, as well as some that are expected to be functional. It also includes at least 2 pairs of polar-opposite tendencies. These were included because each scale is unipolar (the absence of this response does not imply the presence of its opposite), and because people engage in a wide range of coping during a given period, including both of each pair of opposites.

The items have been used in at least 3 formats. One is a "dispositional" or trait-like version in which respondents report the extent to which they usually do the things listed, when they are stressed. A second is a time-limited version in which respondents indicate the degree to which they actually did have each response during a particular period in the past. The third is a time-limited version in which respondents indicate the degree to which they have been having each response during a period up to the present. The formats differ in their verb forms: the dispositional format is present tense, the situational-past format is past tense, the third format is present tense progressive (I am ...) or present perfect (I have been ...).

Scales (sum items listed, with no reversals of coding):

Positive reinterpretation and growth: 1, 29, 38, 59
Mental disengagement: 2, 16, 31, 43
Focus on and venting of emotions: 3, 17, 28, 46
Use of instrumental social support: 4, 14, 30, 45
Active coping: 5, 25, 47, 58
Denial: 6, 27, 40, 57
Religious coping: 7, 18, 48, 60
Humor: 8, 20, 36, 50
Behavioral disengagement: 9, 24, 37, 51
Restraint: 10, 22, 41, 49
Use of emotional social support: 11, 23, 34, 52
Substance use: 12, 26, 35, 53
Acceptance: 13, 21, 44, 54
Suppression of competing activities: 15, 33, 42, 55
Planning: 19, 32, 39, 56

APPENDIX XV - BRIEF COPE SCORING

The brief cope categorizes the coping strategies. Scales are computed as follows (with no reversals of coding):

Self-distraction, items 1 and 19
Active coping, items 2 and 7
Denial, items 3 and 8
Substance use, items 4 and 11 (Dysfunctional)
Use of emotional support, items 5 and 15
Use of instrumental support, items 10 and 23
Behavioral disengagement, items 6 and 16
Venting, items 9 and 21
Positive reframing, items 12 and 17 (Advanced)
Planning, items 14 and 25
Humor, items 18 and 28
Acceptance, items 20 and 24
Religion, items 22 and 27
Self-blame, items 13 and 26

APPENDIX XVI – HIGH LEVEL FACTOR CHART BIBLIO

[1] (Boehm, 2012)
[2] (Danner, 2001)
[3] (Dockray & Steptoe, 2010)
[4] (Khansar, Murgo, & Faith, 1990)
[5] (Lai JC, 2005)
[6] (Ong, Mroczek, & Riffin, 2011)
[7] (Robertson, Stanley, Cully, & Naik, 2012)
[8] (Steptoe, 2005)
[9] (Bhatia & Tandon, 2005)
[10] (Armstrong, Galligan, & Critchley, 2011)
[11] (Baratta, Rozeske, & Maier, 2013)
[12] (Bonanno, 2004)
[13] (Bond & Shapiro, 2014)
[14] (Cohn, 2009)
[15] (Infurna & Luthar, 2016)
[16] (Lyubomirsky & Porta, (in press))
[17] (Catalino & Fredrickson, 2011)
[18] (Boehm, 2012)
[19] (Wingo, Ressler, & Bradley, 2014)
[20] (Boehm, 2012)
[21] (APA, 2013)
[22] (Creswell, et al., 2005)
[23] (Martin & Dahlen, 2005)
[24] (Ong, Bergeman, Bisconti, & Wallace, 2006)
[25] (Steptoe, 2005)
[26] (Nubold, Muck, & Maier, 2013)
[27] (Fredrickson, 2010)
[28] (Larson, Norman, Hughes, & Avey, 2013)
[29] (Dweck, 2008)
[30] (Bryan, 1991)
[31] (Estrada, 1997)
[32] (Fredrickson B. L., 2005)
[33] (Ashby, 1999)
[34] (Johnson, 2010)
[35] (Zimmer-Gembeck & Skinner, 2014)
[36] (Nubold, Muck, & Maier, 2013)
[37] (Larson, Norman, Hughes, & Avey, 2013)
[38] (Dweck, 2008)
[39] (Vaillant, 2012)
[40] (Lyubomirsky, King, & Diener, The Benefits of Frequent Positive Affect: Does Happiness Lead to Success?, 2005)
[41] (Nubold, Muck, & Maier, 2013)
[42] (Larson, Norman, Hughes, & Avey, 2013)
[43] (Larson, Norman, Hughes, & Avey, 2013)
[44] (Nubold, Muck, & Maier, 2013)
[45] (Larson, Norman, Hughes, & Avey, 2013)
[46] (Larson, Norman, Hughes, & Avey, 2013)
[47] (Larson, Norman, Hughes, & Avey, 2013)
[48] (Larson, Norman, Hughes, & Avey, 2013)
[49] (Larson, Norman, Hughes, & Avey, 2013)
[50] (Larson, Norman, Hughes, & Avey, 2013)
[51] (Larson, Norman, Hughes, & Avey, 2013)
[52] (Larson, Norman, Hughes, & Avey, 2013)
[53] (Christian, 2012)
[54] (Voellmin, Entringer, Moog, Wadhwa, & Buss, 2013)
[55] (Liberman, Anderson, & Ross, 2010)
[56] (McCarthy & Casey, 2011)
[57] (Peterson & DeHart, 2013)
[58] (Wong, Tschan, Messerli, & Semmer, 2013)

Citations to this chart not listed elsewhere[409, 410, 411, 412, 413, 414, 415, 416, 417, 418, 419, 420, 421, 422, 423, 424, 425, 426, 427, 428, 429, 430, 431, 432, 433, 434, 435, 436, 437, 438, 439, 440, 441, 442, 443, 444, 445, 446]

APPENDIX XVII - EFFECTS OF A POSITIVE MINDSET

This chart becomes too unwieldly when citations are added. Every box is supported by research, much of which is documented in my first five books. Many of them are documented and cited in Appendix XVI and the related high-level factor chart in this book.

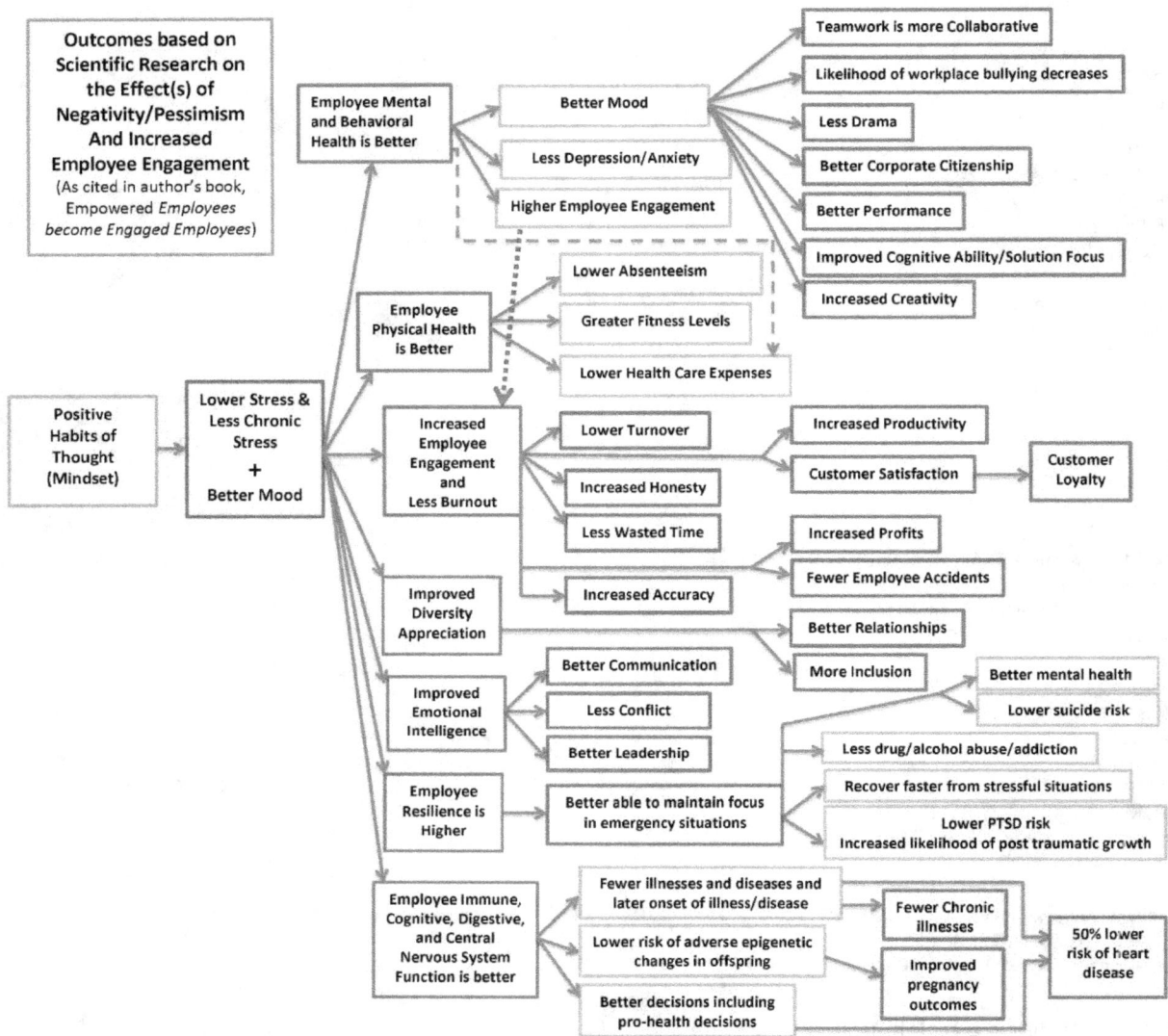

APPENDIX XVIII: SELF-ESTEEM QUESTIONNAIRE

Self-esteem Questionnaire	YES	NO
Mark the 1st answer that comes to your mind. Answer Quickly.		
1. Do you like yourself?		
2. Do you have the right to be happy?		
3. If you're not in a relationship do you feel incomplete?		
4. Do you deflect compliments?		
5. Do you hold back from doing things you want to do out of fear of rejection?		
6. Do you feel like an imposter waiting for people to figure out you don't deserve what you've achieved professionally, in relationships, or financially?		
7. Do you struggle taking criticism?		
8. Do you apologize frequently for things that you don't need to apologize for?		
9. Can you accept a compliment?		
10. Do you make decisions based on what you believe will appeal to others or get their approval instead of what pleases you?		
11. Do you avoid arguments and disagreements by suppressing your needs and feelings?		
12. Can you comfortably walk up to a stranger and introduce yourself?		
13. Do you embellish the truth about yourself in an attempt to project an image you hope others will deem is good enough?		
14. Do you act as if your opinions matter?		
15. Can you choose where you want to eat or do you always defer to others?		
16. Do you seem to need more sleep than others?		
17. Do you take care of your body because you're worth it?		
18. Do you take care of your body because others' opinions of your body matter to you?		
19. Do you share meaningful details of your life with friends?		
20. Do you believe people will like you if they know the real you?		
21. Do you try to make yourself small or wish you could disappear		

or run away when you have a negative emotional experience with someone you care about?		
22. Can you stand in front of a mirror, look yourself in the eyes, and tell yourself:		
I. I am good		
II. I am wise		
III. I love you		
23. Do good things happen in your life because you prepare for opportunities so you're ready when they appear?		

APPENDIX IXX: SELF-ESTEEM QUESTIONNAIRE SCORING

Some comments about this questionnaire before you score it. This is not a validated questionnaire. It is based on scientifically known indicators of low and healthy self-esteem. I couldn't find a validated questionnaire for self-esteem that was not restricted by copyright protections.

The happy faces indicate the answer is associated with healthy self-esteem. If you have answers associated with low self-esteem do your best not to be upset or to beat yourself up for having low self-esteem. Seek professional help from a mental health professional if you feel it is needed. For a long time in my past, my answers to nearly every question would not have had a happy face. Today almost all of them have happy faces. The techniques that worked for me are described in this book. You have the ability to improve your self-esteem. The best way to view results that indicate areas where there is low self-esteem is of having good information on areas you CAN change about your life that will make your life considerably better than it has been in the past. The worst ways to treat the information are 1) another reason to criticize yourself, and 2) anger at yourself for having low self-esteem. It's pretty difficult to fix something you don't know is not working at optimal capacity. You were instructed to answer quickly because someone with low self-esteem tends to second guess their answers and try to answer the way they think will make them look good.

When the check engine light in your vehicle comes on you don't put a piece of paper over it. You get your engine checked. Answering these questions to look good instead of being honest is like covering the check engine light with a piece of paper—eventually it will bite you.

SCORING
Self-esteem Questionnaire

Mark the 1st answer that comes to your mind. Answer Quickly.

	YES	NO
1. Do you like yourself?	☺	
2. Do you have the right to be happy?	☺	
3. If you're not in a relationship do you feel incomplete?		☺
4. Do you deflect compliments?		☺
5. Do you hold back from doing things you want to do out of fear of rejection?		☺
6. Do you feel like an imposter waiting for people to figure out you don't deserve what you've achieved professionally, in relationships, or financially?		☺
7. Do you struggle taking criticism?		☺
8. Do you apologize frequently for things that you don't need to apologize for?		☺
9. Can you accept a compliment?	☺	

10. Do you make decisions based on what you believe will appeal to others or get their approval instead of what pleases you?		☺
11. Do you avoid arguments and disagreements by suppressing your needs and feelings?		☺
12. Can you comfortably walk up to a stranger and introduce yourself?	☺	
13. Do you embellish the truth about yourself in an attempt to project an image you hope others will deem is good enough?		☺
14. Do you act as if your opinions matter?	☺	
15. Can you choose where you want to eat without always deferring to others?	☺	
16. Do you seem to need more sleep than others?		☺
17. Do you take care of your body because you're worth it?	☺	
18. Do you take care of your body because others' opinions of your body matter to you?		☺
19. Do you share meaningful details of your life with friends?	☺	
20. Do you believe people will like you if they know the real you?	☺	
21. Do you try to make yourself small or wish you could disappear or run away when you have a negative emotional experience with someone you care about?		☺
22. Can you stand in front of a mirror, look yourself in the eyes, and tell yourself:		
a. I am good	☺	
b. I am wise	☺	
c. I love you	☺	
23. Do good things happen in your life because you prepare for opportunities so you're ready when they appear?	☺	

Appendix XX: Thriving Questionnaire

Thriving Questionnaire See Appendix XXII for Scoring The purpose of this questionnaire is to see where you are so you can measure your progress as you learn *The Smart Way*™. Indicate the answer that most closely resembles how you usually feel.	Completely Agree	Somewhat Agree	Neither Agree nor Disagree	Somewhat Disagree	Completely Disagree
1. I feel energized					
2. I am looking forward to each new day					
3. I feel so alive I just want to burst					
4. I am failing to progress					
5. I think I am continuing to develop					
6. I am looking forward to each new day					
7. I feel alert and awake					
8. I do not feel very energetic (reverse code)					
9. I have energy and spirit					
10. I feel like I am forgetting things I once knew					
11. I feel alive and vital					
12. I find myself learning often					
13. I continue to learn more as time goes by					
14. I see myself continually improving					
15. I am not learning (reverse code)					
16. I am developing a lot as a person					
17. I am not interested in learning					
18. I am lethargic (reverse score)					
19. I feel depleted (reverse score)					
20. I am finding new ways to develop					
21. I lack energy (reverse score					
22. I am experiencing considerable personal growth					
23. I am growing in positive ways					
24. I have not grown much recently (reverse score)					
25. I am stagnating (reverse score)					
26. I enjoy seeing how my views have progressed					
27. I am not moving forward (reverse score)					
28. I enjoy learning					
29. I feel young when I wake up in the morning					
30. I often have inspired ideas in my mind when I wake up in the morning					
TOTALS					

APPENDIX XXI – STATE OF BURNOUT RESEARCH AND FUTURE DIRECTIONS

It is important to contextualize solutions with an awareness of the research that has been done and what hasn't been studied. A recent Delphi Study[447] to determine the factors that affect burnout that have been studied reveal that many areas of research that hold clues to the solution are not considered in the scientific research on burnout. This is largely due to silo'd research patterns. It is the reason we do not limit our research to specific areas. Despite a panel of 40 experts, there were significant factors that contribute to burnout that were not listed:

- Motivation theory and research
  - Deci and Ryan's body of work provides insights
- Positive Psychology
  - Bodies of work from Seligman, Lyubomirsky, the Diener's, Kashdan, Csikszentmihalyi, Dweck, Achor, and others
- Emotion Regulation
  - Notably, James Gross's work
- Purpose and meaning of emotions
  - Roy F. Baumeister and Katherine Peil's work plus Vohs, DeWall, etc.
- Coping
- Teams, teamwork
- Cognitive Behavioral Therapy (CBT)
- Mindfulness
- Organizational Theory
- Self-control
  - Notably Charles S. Carver's body of work
- Employee engagement research
- Internal locus of control
- Resilience
- Optimism
- Psychological flexibility

There are tremendous bodies of work that can be applied to prevent and recover from burnout that are being ignored because the researchers working on burnout aren't from those silos. There's not much point in having knowledge if we don't apply it to solve problems.

The Smart Way™ includes research from these areas because after decades of studying what makes humans thrive in spite of adversity we understand the most important factors that motivate and de-motivate individuals.

APPENDIX XXII – THRIVING QUESTIONNAIRE SCORING

Thriving questionnaire scoring

SCORING Thriving Questionnaire	Completely Agree	Somewhat Agree	Neither Agree nor Disagree	Somewhat Disagree	Completely Disagree
31. I feel energized	4	3	2	0	0
32. I am looking forward to each new day	4	3	2	0	0
33. I feel so alive I just want to burst	8	6	4	0	0
34. I am failing to progress	0	0	-2	-3	-4
35. I think I am continuing to develop	4	3	2	1	0
36. I am looking forward to each new day	4	3	2	1	0
37. I feel alert and awake	4	3	2	1	0
38. I do not feel very energetic (reverse code)	0	1	-2	-3	-4
39. I have energy and spirit	4	3	2	1	0
40. I feel like I am forgetting things I once knew	0	-1	-4	-6	-8
41. I feel alive and vital	4	3	2	0	0
42. I find myself learning often	4	3	2	0	0
43. I continue to learn more as time goes by	4	3	2	1	0
44. I see myself continually improving	4	3	2	0	0
45. I am not learning (reverse code)	0	1	-2	-3	-4
46. I am developing a lot as a person	4	3	2	0	0
47. I am not interested in learning	0	-1	-4	-6	-8
48. I am lethargic (reverse score)	0	-1	-4	-6	-8
49. I feel depleted (reverse score)	0	-1	-4	-6	-8
50. I am finding new ways to develop	6	4	2	1	0
51. I lack energy (reverse score	0	-1	-4	-6	-8
52. I am experiencing considerable personal growth	6	4	2	1	0
53. I am growing in positive ways	4	3	2	1	0
54. I have not grown much recently (reverse score)	0	-1	-	-6	-8

55. I am stagnating (reverse score)	0	-1	-4	-6	-8
56. I enjoy seeing how my views have progressed	4	3	2	1	0
57. I am not moving forward (reverse score)	0	-1	-4	-6	-8
58. I enjoy learning	4	3	2	1	0
59. I feel young when I wake up in the morning	4	3	2	1	0
. I often have inspired ideas in my mind when I wake up in the morning	4	3	2	1	0
	84	56	2	-45	-76

Before you add up your score, remember that you're only thoughts away from improved vitality and knowledge. You are never too old to learn or improve your vitality. The amount of energy you feel (vitality) is directly proportional to how empowered you feel. If you feel disempowered you won't feel interested in life or learning.

Thriving	Doing pretty well	Normal	Suffering	Miserable
57 to 84	25 to 56	-20 to 24	-24 to -21	-25 to -76

BIBLIOGRAPHY

ACGME. (2011). Updated standards for resident duty hours, education, and supervision. Accreditation Council for Graduate Medical Education .

Alkadhi, K. (2013). Brain Physiology andn pathophysioogy in Mental Stress: A Review Article. *Hindawi Publishing Corporation*, 23.

American Medical Association (AMA). (2016). AMA Principles of Medical Ethics. *9.3.1*.

Antoniou, A.-S. G., Davidson, M. J., & Cooper, C. L. (2003). Occupational stress, job satisfaction and health state in male and female junior hostpial doctors in Greece. *ournal Manag Psychol, 18*, 592-621.

APA. (2013). *Stress in America: Missing the Health Care Connection* .

APA. (2014). *Stress in America: Are Teens Adopting Adults' Stress Habits?* American Psychological Association. American Psychological Association.

APA. (2015). *Stress in America: Paying with our Health.* American Psychological Association.

Argentero, P., Dell'Olivo, B., & Ferretti, M. S. (1, January). Staff burnout and patient satisfaction with the quality of dialysis care. *American Journal Kidney Disease, 51*(1), 80-92.

Armon, G., Shirom, A., Shapira, I., & Melamed, S. (2008). On the nature of burnout-insomnia relationships: a prospective study of employed adults. *Journal of Psychosomatic Research, 65*(1), 5-12.

Armstrong, A. R., Galligan, R. F., & Critchley, C. R. (2011). Emotional Intelligence and psychological resilience to negative life events. *Personalit and Individual Differences, 51*, 331-336.

Ashby, F. G. (1999). A neuropsychological theory of positive affect and its influence on cognition. *Psychological Review*, 106, No. 3: 529-50.

Aspinwall, L. G. (2011). Future oriented Thinking, Proactive Coping, and the Management of Threats to Health and Well-Being. In S. Folkman, *Oxford Handbook of Stress, Health, and Coping* (pp. 334-368). Oxford Handbooks.

Assagioli, R. (1965). *Psychosynthesis: A Collection of Basic Writings.* New York: The Viking Press.

Association of Professors of Medicine: The American Journal of Medicine. (2001). *Predicting and Preventing Physician Burnout: Results from the United States and the Netherlands.* Excerpta Medica, Inc.

Baratta, M. V., Rozeske, R. R., & Maier, S. F. (2013). Understanding Stress Resilience. *Frontiers in Behavioral Neuroscience*, 1-112.

Barnes, C., & Spreitzer, G. (2015, Winter). Why it Pays to Ensure Adequate Sleep for Your Employees. (U. o. Ross School of Business, Ed.) *MIT Sloan Management Review*.

Baumeister, R. F., & Beck, A. (1999). *Evil: Inside Human Violence and Cruelty.* New York: Henry Holt and Co.

Baumeister, R. F., Vohs, K. D., DeWall, C. N., & Zhang, L. (2007, May 16). How Emotion Shapes Behavior: Feedback, Anticipation, and Reflection, Rather Than Direct Causation. *Personality and Social Psychology Review, 11*(2), 167-203.

Bedynsa, S., & Zolnierczyk-Zreda, D. (2015). Stereotype threat as a determinant of burnout or work engagement. Mediating role of positive and negative emotions. *International Journal of Occupational Safety and Ergonomics, 21*(1), 2-8.

Bhatia, V., & Tandon, R. K. (2005, March). Stress and the gastrointestinal tract. *Journal of Gastroenterology and Hepatology, 20*(3), 332-339.

Bigman, Y. E., Mauss, I. B., Gross, J. J., & Tamir, M. (2015, July 29). Yes I can: Expected success promotes actual success in emotion regulation. *Cognition and Emotion, 30*(7), 1380-1387.

Boden, M. T., & Gross, J. J. (2013). An Emotion Regulation Perspective on Belief Change. In D. Reisberg (Ed.), *The Oxford Handbook of Cognitive Psychology* (pp. 585-599). Oxford University Press.

Boden, M. T., Berenbaum, H., & Gross, J. J. (2016). Why Do People Believe What They Do? A Functionalist Perspective. *Review of General Psychology, 20*(4), 399-411.

Boden, M. T., Kulkarni, M., Shurick, A., Bonn-Miller, M. O., & Gross, J. J. (2014). Responding to Trauma and Loss: An Emotion Regulation Perspective. In M. Kent, M. C. Davis, & J. W. Reich (Eds.), *The Resilience Handbook: Approaches to Stress and Trauma* (pp. 86-99). New York, NY, United States of America: Routledge, Taylor & Francis Group.

Boehm, J. K. (2012, July). The heart's content: The association between positive psychological well-being and cardiovascular health. *Psychological Bulletin, Epub April 2012*, 138(4):655-91.

Bonanno, G. (2004). Loss, trauma, and human resilience: Have we underestimated the human capacity to thrive after extremely aversive events? *American Psychologist*, 59: 20-28.

Bond, S., & Shapiro, D. (2014). *Tough AT The Top? New Rules of ResilieNce foR womeN's leAdeRship success.* Research report.

Brandstatter, V., Job, V., & Schulze, B. (2016, August). Motivational Incongruence and Well-Being at the Workplace: Person-Job Fit, Job Burnout, and Physical Symptoms. *frontiers in Psychology*.

Bretland, R. J., & Thorsteinsson, E. B. (n.d.). Reducing workplace burnout: the relative benefits of cardiovascular and resistance exercise. (D. Frydecka, Ed.) *PeerJ*.

Brooks, M. (2015, January 2). Less Money, More Rules for US Physicians in 2015. *Medscape*.

Brownstein, J. (2009, March 26). Do Doctor Dramas Make for Bad Docs? *ABC News*.

Bryan, T. a. (1991). Positive mood and math performance. *Journal of Learning Disabilities*, 24:490-94.

Busis, N. A., Shanafelt, T. D., Keran, C. M., Levin, K. H., Schwarz, H. B., Molano, J. R., et al. (2017, February). Burnout, career satisfaction, and well-being among US neurologists in 2016. *Neurology, 88*(8), 797-808.

Butler, A. C., Chapman, J. E., Forman, E. M., & Beck, A. T. (2006). The empirical status of cognitive-behavioral therapy: A review of meta-analyses. *Clinical Psyhology Review, 26*, 17-31.

Carmona, C., Buunk, A. P., Peiró, J. M., Rodríguez, I., & Bravo, M. J. (2006). Do social comparison and coping styles play a role in the development of burnout? Cross-sectional and longitudinal findings. *Journal of Occupational and Organizational Psychology, 79*(1), 85-99.

Carver, C. S. (2015, July 9). Control Processes, Priority Management, and Affective Dynamics. *Emotion Review, 7*(4), 301-307.

Carver, C. S., & Connor-Smith, J. (2010). Personality and Coping. *Annual Review of Psychology, 61*, 679-704.

Catalino, L. I., & Fredrickson, B. L. (2011). A Tuesday in the Life of a Flourisher: The Role of Positive Emotional Reactivity in Optimal Mental Health. *Emotion, 11*(4), 938-950.

Chana, N., Kennedy, P., & Chessell, Z. J. (2015, October). Nursing staffs' emotional well-being and caring behaviours. *Journal of Clinical Nursing*.

Chang, J. (2011). A Case Study of the "Pygmalion Effect""Teacher Expectations and Student Achievement. *International Education Studies, 4*(1), 198-201.

Cheung, F., Tang, C. S.-k., & Tang, S. (2011). Psychological capital as a moderator between emotional labor, burnout, and job satisfaction among school teachers in China. *International Journal of Stress Management, 18*(4), 348-371.

Chigerwe, M., Boudreaux, K. A., & Ilkiw, J. E. (2014). Assessment of burnout in veterinary medical students using hte Maslach Burnout Inventory-Educational Survey: a survey during two semesters. *BMC Medical Education, 14*, 1-7.

Chin, W., Guo, Y. L., Hung, Y. J., Hsieh, Y. T., Wang, L. J., & Shiao, J. S. (2017, January). Workplace justice and intention to leave the nursing profession. *Nursing Ethics*, ePub.

Christian, L. M. (2012). Psychoneuroimmunology in pregnancy: Immune pathways linking stress with maternal health, adverse birth outcomes, and fetal development. *Neuroscience and Biobehavioral Reviews, 36*, 350-361.

Cisler, J. M., & Olatunji, B. O. (2012). Emotion Regulation and Anxiety Disorders. *Current Psychiatry Reports, 14*(3), 182-187.

Clore, G. L., & Palmer, J. (2009). Affective guidance of intelligent agents: How emotion controls cognition. (J. Gratch, Ed.) *Cognitive Systems Research, 10*, pp. 21-30.

Cohn, M. A. (2009). Happiness unpacked: Positive emotions increase life satisfaction by building resilience. *Emotion*, 9: 361-368.

Consoli, S. M. (2015, July-August). Occupational stress and myocardial infarction. *Presse Medicine, 44*(7-8), 745-751.

Creswell, J. D., Welch, W. T., Taylor, S. E., Sherman, D. K., Gruenewax, T. L., Gruenewald, T. L., et al. (2005). Affirmation of Personal Values Buffers Neuroendocrine and Psychological Stress Responses. *Psychological Science, 16*(11), 847-851.

Cusack, L., Smith, M., Hegney, D., Rees, C. S., Breen, L. J., Witt, R. R., et al. (2016, May 13). Exploring Environmental Factors in Nursing Workplaces That Promote Psychological Resilience: Constructing a Unified Theoretical Model. *frontiers in Psychology, 7*(600), 1-8.

Dan-Glauser, E. S., & Gross, J. J. (2013). Emotion Regulation and Emotion Coherence: Evidence for Strategy-Specific Effects. *Emotion*, 832-842.

Danner, D. D. (2001). Positive Emotions in Early Life and Longevity. Findings from the Nun Study. *Journal of Personality and Social Psychology, 80*, No. 5.804-813.

De Castella, K., Goldin, P., Jazaien, H., Heimberg, R. G., Dweck, C. S., & Gross, J. J. (2015, March 6). Emotion Beliefs and Cognitive Behavioural Therapy for Social Anxiety Disorder. *Cognitive Behavioral Therapy, 44*(2), 128-141.

De Castella, K., Goldin, P., Jazaieri, H., Ziv, M., Dweck, C. S., & Gross, J. J. (2013). Beliefs About Emotion: Links to Emotion Regulation, Well-Being, and Psychological Distress. *Basic and Applied Social Psychology*, 497-505.

Deci, E. L., & Ryan, R. M. (2000). The "What" and "Why" of Goal Pursuits: Human Needs and the Self-Determination of Behavior. *Psychological Inquiry, 11*(4), 227-268.

Dewa, C. S., McDaid, D., & Ettner, S. L. (2007). An International perspective on worker mental health problems: who bears the burden and how are costs addressed? *Canadian Journal of Psychiatry, 52*(6), 346-56.

DiMatteo, M. R., Sherbourne, C. D., Hays, R. D., Ordway, L., Kravitz, R. L., McGlynn, E. A., et al. (1993). Physicians' characteristics influence patients' adherence to medical treatment: results from the Medical Outcomes Study. *Health Psychology, 12*(2), 93-102.

Ding, Y., Yang, Y., Yang, X., Zhang, T., Qiu, X., He, X., et al. (2015, April 21). The Mediating Role of Coping Style in the Relationship between Psychological Capital and Burnout among Chinese Nurses. *PLOSone, 10*(4).

Dockray, S., & Steptoe, A. (2010). Positive Affect and psychobiological processes. *Neuroscience and Biobehavioral Reviews*, 69-75.

Doolittle, B. R., & Windish, D. M. (2015). Correlation of burnout syndrome with specific coping strategies, behaviors, and spiritual attitudes among interns at Yale University, New Haven, USA. *Journal of Educational Evaluation for Health Professions*, 12-41.

Draper, B., Kolves, K., Leo, D. D., & Snowden, J. (2014). The impact of patient suicide and sudden death on health care professionals. *General Hospital Psychiatry: Psychiatry, Medicine and Primary Care, 36*(6), 721-725.

Dweck, C. S. (2008). *Mindset: The New Psychology of Success.* New York: Ballantine Books.

Dyrbye, L. N., & Shanafelt, T. D. (2011). Physician Burnout: a potential threat to successful health care reform. *JAMA, 305*(19), 2009-2010.

Dyrbye, L. N., Shanafelt, T. D., Balch, C. M., Satele, D., Sloan, J., & Freischlag, J. (2011, February). Relationship between work-home conflicts and burnout among American surgeons: a comparison by sex. *Archives of Surgery*, 211-217.

Dyrbye, L. N., Thomas, M. R., Massie, F. S., Power, D. V., Eacker, A., Harper, W., et al. (2008). Burnout and Suicide Ideation among U.S. Medical Students. *Annals of Internal Medicine, 149*(5), 334-331.

Edress, H., Connors, C., Paine, L., Norvell, M., & Taylor, H. (2016). Implementing the RISE second victim support programme at the Johns Hopkins Hospital: a case study. *BMJ Open, 6*, e011708.

Eiser, J. R., & Pahl, S. (2001). Optimism, Pessimism, and the Direction of Self-Other Comparisons. *Journal of Experimental Social Psychology, 37*, 77-84.

Erickson, S. M., Rockwern, B., Koltov, M., & McLean, R. (2017, March 28). Putting Patients First by Reducing Administrative Tasks in Health Care: A Position Paper of the American College of Physicians. *Annals of Internal Medicine*, 1-22.

Estrada, C. I. (1997). Positive affect facilitates integration of information and decreases anchoring in reasoning among physicians. *Organizational Behavior and Human Decision Processes*, 72: 117-135.

Fagley, N. S. (2012). Appreciation uniquely predicts life satisfaction above demographics, the Big 5 personality factors, and gratitude. *Personality and Individual Differences, 53*, 59-63.

Fahrenkopf, A. M., Sectish, T. C., Barger, L. K., Sharek, P. J., Lewin, D., & Chiang, V. W. (2008). Rates of medication errors among depressed and burnt out residents: Prospective chohort study. *British Medical Journal, 336*, 488-491.

Fares, J., Tabosh, H. A., Saadeddin, Z., Mouhayyar, C. E., & Aridi, H. (2016, February). Stress, Burnout and Coping Strategies in Preclinical Medical Students. *North American Journal Medical Science, 75-81*, 75-81.

Feldman, M. S., & Worline, M. (2011). Resourcefulness. In K. S. Cameron, & G. M. Spreitzer (Eds.), *A Path Forward: Assessing Progress and Exploring Core Questions for the Future of Positive Organizational Scholarship* (pp. Chapter 47, 629-641). New York, NY: Oxford University Press.

Folkman, S., & Moskowitzz, J. T. (2004, February). Coping: Pitfalls and Promise. *Annual Review of Psychology, 55*, 745-774.

Fredrickson, B. L. (2005). Positive affect and the complex dynamics of human flourishing. *American Psychologist*, 60(7): 678-686.

Fredrickson, B. L. (2010). *Positivity*. Three Rivers Press.

Freeborn, D. K. (2001). Satisfaction, commitment, and psychological well-being among HMO physicians. *Western Journal of Medicine*, 22-30.

Gandi, J. C., Wai, P. S., Karick, H., & Dagona, Z. K. (2011). The role of stress and level of burnout in job performance among nurses. *Mental Health Family Medicine, 8*(3), 181-194.

Gold, K. J., Sen, A., & Schwenk, T. L. (2013, Jauary - February). Details on suicide among US physicians: data from the National Violent Death Reporting System. *General Hospital Psychiatry: Psychiatry, Medicine and Primary Care, 35*(1), 45-49.

Grant, A. M., & Sonnentag, S. (2010). Doing good buffers against feeling bad: Prosocial impact compensates for negative task and self-evaluations. *Organizational Behavior and Human Decision Processes, 111*, 13-22.

Gross, J. J. (2015). The Extended Process Model of Emotion Regulation: Elaborations, Applications, and Future Directions. *Psychological Inquiry, 26*, 130-137.

Gross, J. J., & John, O. P. (2003, August). Individual differences in two emotion regulation processes: implications for affect, relationships, and well-being. *Journal Personal Sociology and Psychology, 85*(2), 348-362.

Haggerty, T. S., Fields, S. A., Selby-Nelson, E. M., Foley, K. P., & Shrader, C. D. (2013). Physician wellness in rural America: a review. *International Journal Psychiatry Medicine, 46*(3), 303-313.

Haidt, J. (2013). *The Righeeous Mind: Why Good People Are Divided by Politics and Religion.* New York: First Vintage Books.

Hamilton, J. (2010). *Work Related Stress: What the Law Says.* London: CIPD.

Hampton, T. (2005). Experts Address Risk of Physician Suicide. *JAMA,* 1189-1191.

Handbook, O. H. (2013, September). Guidelines for Physician Well-Being Committees: Policies and Procedures. *CMA Legal Counsel and California Public Protection and Physician Health.* CA.

Hein, I. (2017, March 27). Relieve Overloaded Physicians by Overhauling Health IT. *Medscape Medical News> Conference News,* p. ePub.

Heller, A. S., van Reekum, C. M., Schaefer, S. M., Lapate, R. C., Radler, B. T., Ryff, C. D., et al. (2013). Sustained Striatal Activity Predicts Eudaimonic Well-Being and Cortisol Output. *Psychological Science, 24*(11), 2191-2200.

Hofmann, S. G., Asnaani, A., Vonk, I. J., Sawyer, A. T., & Fang, A. (2012, October 1). The Efficacy of Cognitive Behavioral Therapy: A Review of Meta-analyses. *Cognitive Therapy and Research, 36*(5), 427-440.

Honkonen, T., Ahola, K., Pertovaara, M., Isometsä, E., Kalimo, R., Nykyri, E., et al. (2006, Jul). The association between burnout and physical illness in the general population--results from the Finnish Health 2000 Study. *Journal of Psychosomatic Research, 61*(1), 59-66.

Hopp, H., Troy, A. S., & Mauss, I. B. (2011). The unconscious pursuit of emotion regulation: Implications for psychological health. *Cognitive Emoiton,* 532-545.

Houkes, I., Winants, Y., Twellaar, M., & Verdonk, P. (2011). Development of burnout over time and the causal order of the three dimensions of burnout among male and female GPs. A three-wave panel study. *BMC Pubic Health, 11*, 1-13.

Hu, T., Zhang, D., Wang, J.-L., Mistry, R., Ran, G., & Wang, X. (2014, April). Relation between emotion regulation and mental health: A meta-analysis-review. *Psychological Reports, 114*(2), 341-362.

Huby, G., Gerry, M., McKinstry, B., Porter, M., Shaw, J., & Wrate, R. (2002, July 20). Morale among general practitioners: qualitative study exploring relations between partnership arrangements, personal style, and workload. *The BMJ, 325,* .

Hunsaker, S., Chen, H. C., Maughan, D., & Heaston, S. (2015, March). Factors that influence the development of compassion fatigue, burnout, and compassion satisfaction in emergency department nurses. *Journal Nursing Scholarship, 47*(1), 186-94.

Infurna, F. J., & Luthar, S. S. (2016, March). Resilience to Major Life Stressors Is Not as Common as Thought. *Perspectives in Psychological Science, 11*, 175-194.

Jackson, D., Firtko, A., & Edenborough, M. (2007, October). Personal resilience as a strategy for surviving and thriving in the face of workplace adversity: a literature review. *Journal Advances in Nursing, 60*(1), 1-9.

Jensen, RN PhD, P. M., Trollope-Kumar, MD PhD, K., Waters, MD CCFP, H., & Everson, MD CCFP FCFP, J. (2008, May). Building Physician Resilience. *Canadian Family Physician, 54*(5), 722-729.

John, O. P., & Gross, J. J. (2004). Healthy and Unhealthy Emotion Regulation: Personality Processes, Individual Differences, and Life Span Development. *Journal of Personality, 72*(6), 1301-1335.

Johnson, K. J., Waugh, C. E., & Fredrickson, B. L. (2010). Smile to see the forest: Facially expressed positive emotions broaden cognition. *COGNITION AND EMOTION,* 24(2): 299-321.

Joy, J. (2017, January 25). Floridas suicide ruling puts physicians at risk. *Medical Economics.*

Keeney, J., & Ilies, R. (2011). Positive Work--Family Dynamics. In K. S. Cameron, & G. M. Spreitzer (Eds.), *A Path Forward: Assessing Progress and Exploring Core Questions for the Future of Positive Organizational Scholarship* (pp. Chapter 45, 601-616). New York, NY: Oxford University Press.

Khamisa, N., peltzer, K., & Oldenburg, B. (2013, May). Burnout in Relation to Specific Contributing Factors and Health Outcomes among Nurses: A Systematic Review. *International Journal of Environmental Research and Public Health, 10*, 2214-2240.

Khansar, D. N., Murgo, A. J., & Faith, R. E. (1990). Effects of Stress on the Immune System. *Immunology Today, 11*, 170-176.

King, R. B., McInerney, D. M., & Watkins, D. A. (2012). How you think about your intelligence determines how you feel in school: The role of theories of intelligence on academic emotions. *Learning and Individual Differences*(22), 814-819.

Kobylinska, D., & Karwowska, D. (2015, October 27). How automatic activation of emotion regulation influences experiencing negative emotins. (P. Kusev, Ed.) *Frontiers in psychology*, 1-4.

Koole, S. L. (2009). The psychology of emotion regulation: An integrative review. *Cognition and Emotion, 23*(1), 4-41.

Korownyk, C., Kolber, M. R., McCormack, J., Lam, V., Overbo, K., Cotton, C., et al. (2014). Televised medical talk shows—what they recommend and the evidence to support their recommendations: a prospective observational study. *British Medical Journal (BMJ), 349*(g7346).

Kubicek, B., & Korunka, C. (2015, October 2). Does job complexity mitigate the negative effect of emotion-rule dissonance on employee burnout? *Work Stress, 29*(4), 379-400.

Kudinova, A. Y., Owens, M., Burkhouse, K. L., Barretto, K. M., Bonanno, G. A., & Gibb, B. E. (2015, May). Differences in emotion modulation using cognitive reappraisal in individuals with and without suicidal ideation: An ERP study. *Cognitive Emotion, 15*, 1-9.

Kumar, S. (2016). Burnout and Doctors: Prevalence, Prevention, and Intervention. (P. A. Leggat, & D. R. Smith, Eds.) *Healthcare, 4*(37).

Kutluturkan, S., Sozeri, E., Uysal, N., & Bay, F. (2016). Resilience and burnout status among nurses working in oncology. *Anals of General Psychiatry, 15*(33), 1-9.

Kwong, J. Y., Wong, K. F., & Tang, S. K. (2013). Comparing predicted and actual affective responses to process versus outcome: An Emotion-as-feedback perspective. *Cognition, 129*, 42-50.

Lai JC, E. P. (2005). Optimism, positive affectivity, and salivary cortisol. *British Journal of Health Psychology*, 4:467-84.

Landrum, B., Knight, D. K., & Flynn, P. M. (2012, March). The Impact of Organizational Stress and Burnout on Client Engagement. *Journal of Substance Abuse Treatment, 42*(2), 222-230.

Langer, E. J. (2009). *Counterclockwise: Mindful Health and the Power of Possibility.* New York: Random House.

Larson, M. D., Norman, S. M., Hughes, L. W., & Avey, J. B. (2013). Psychological Capital: A New Lens for Understanding Employee Fit and Attitudes. *Internal Journal of Leadership Studies, 8*(1), 28-43.

Lashinger, H. K., Borgogni, L., Consiglio, C., & Read, E. (2015, June). The effects of authentic leadership, six areas of worklife, and occupational coping self-efficacy on new graduate nurses' burnout and mental health: A cross-sectional study. *international Journal Nursing Studies, 52*(6), 1080-1089.

Lashinger, H. S., & Grau, A. L. (2012, March). The influence of personal dispositional factors and organizational resources on workplace violence, burnout, and health outcomes in new graduate nurses: A cross-sectional study. *Journal of Nursing Studis, 49*(3), 282-291.

Lazarus. (1991). *Cognition and Emotion.*

Lee, MD, F. J., Brown, PhD, J. B., & Stewart, PhD, M. (2009). Exploring Family Physician Stress. *Canada Family Physician, 55*(3), 280-289.

Lemelle, C. J., & Seielzo, S. A. (2012). How You Feel About Yourself Can Affect How You Feel About Your Job: A Meta-Analysis Examing the Relationship of Core Self-Evaluations and Job Satisfaction. *Journal of Business Diversity, 12*(3), 116-133.

Leung, J., & Rioseco, P. (2017). Burnout, stress and satisfaction among Australian and New Zealand radiation oncology trainees. *Journal of Medical Imaging and Radiation Oncology, 61*, 146-155.

Li, X., Guan, L., Chang, H., & Zhang, B. (2014, December 26). Core Self-Evaluation and Burnout among Nurses: The Mediating Role of Coping Styles. *PLoS One*, 1-12.

Lian, P., Sun, Y., Ji, Z., Li, H., & Peng, J. (2014). Moving Away from Exhaustion: How Core Self-Evaluations Inflluence Academic Burnout. *PLoS ONE, 9*(1).

Liberman, V., Anderson, N. R., & Ross, L. (2010). Achieving difficult agreements: Effects of Positive Expectations on negotiation processes and outcomes. *Journal of Experimental Social Psychology, 46*, 494-504.

Linzer, MD, M., Levine, MD, MPH, R., Melter, MD, D., Poplau, S., Warde, MD, C., & West, MD, PhD, C. P. (2013). 10 Bold Steps to Prevent Burnout in General Internal Medicine. *Society of General Internal Medicine, 29*, pp. 18-20. Denver, CO.

Livingston, J. S. (2003, January 1). Pygmalion in Management (HBR Classic). *Harvard Business Review*.

Lopez, A., Sanderman, R., Smink, A., Zhang, Y., van Sonderen, E., Ranchor, A., et al. (2015). A Reconsideration of the Self-Compassion Scale's Total Score: Self-Compassion Versus Self-Criticism. *PLoS One*, 1-12.

Luken, M., & Sammons, A. (2016). Systematic Review of Mindfulness Practice for Reducing Job Burnout. *The American Journal of Occupational Therapy, 70*.

Luthans, F., & Youssef, C. M. (2004). Human, Social, and Now Positive Psychological Capital Management: Investing in People for Competitive Advantage. *Occupational Dynamics, 33*(2), 143-160.

Luthans, F., Luthans, K. W., & Luthans, B. C. (2004, January-February). Positive psychological capital: Beyond human and social capital. *Business Horizons*, pp. 45-50.

Lyubomirsky, S., & Porta, M. D. ((in press)). Boosting Happiness and Buttressing Resilience: Results from Cognitive and Behavioral Interventions. In J. W. Reich, A. J. Zautra, & J. Hall (Eds.), *Handbook of adult resilience: Concepts, methods, and application.* New York, NY, USA: Guilford Press.

Lyubomirsky, S., King, L., & Diener, E. (2005). The Benefits of Frequent Positive Affect: Does Happiness Lead to Success? *Psychological Bulletin, 131*(6), 803-855.

Manzano-García, G., & Ayala, J.-C. (2017, April 7). Insufficiently studied factors related to burnout in nursing: Results from an e-Delphi study. *PLoS ONE, 12*(4).

Martin, R. C., & Dahlen, E. R. (2005). Cognitive emotion regulation in the prediction of depression, anxiety, stress, and anger. *Personality and Individual Differences*, 1249-1260.

Maslach, C., & Leiter, M. P. (2016, June). Understanding the burnout experience: recent research and its implications for psychiatry. *World Psychiatry, 15*(2), 103-111.

Mauss, I. B., & Gross, J. J. (2004). Emotional Suppression and cardiovascular disease Is hiding feelings bad for your heart? In I. Nyklíček, L. Temoshok, & A. Vingerhoets (Eds.), *Emotional Expression and Health* (pp. 62-81). New York, NY, United States of America: Brunner-Routledge, Taylor & Francis Group.

Mauss, I. B., Bunge, S. A., & Gross, J. J. (2007). Automatic Emotion Regulation. *Social and Personality Psychology Compass*, 146-167.

Mauss, I. B., Shallcross, A. J., Troy, A. S., John, O. P., Ferrer, E., Wilhelm, F. H., et al. (2011). Don't Hide Your Happiness! Positive Emotion Dissociation, Social Connectedness, and Psychological Functioning. *ournal of Personality and Social Psychology, 100*(4), 738-748.

McCarthy, B., & Casey, T. (2011). Get Happy! Positive Emotion, Depression and Juvenile Crime. *American Sociological Associaion Annual Meeting.* Las Vegas: UC Davis.

McDonald, MD, J. V. (2001). Letters from the Northwest: Promoting personal growth: The Role of the workplace. *Western Journal of Medicine*, 76-77.

McLeod, S. A. (2009). *Emotion Focused Coping.* Retrieved 2017, from Simple Psychology: https://www.simplypsychology.org/stress-management.html

McManus, I. C., Keeling, A., & Paice, E. (2004). Stress, burnout and doctors' attitudes to work are determined by personality and learning style: A twelve year longitudinal study of UK medical graduates. *MBC Medicine*, 2-29.

Melamed, S., Shirom, A., Toker, S., & Shapira, I. (2006). Burnout and risk of type 2 diabetes: a prospective study of apparently healthy employed persons. *Psychosomatic Medicine, 68*(6), 863-969.

Merrit Hawkins, an AMN Healthcare company. (2011). *2011 Survey of Final-Year Medical Residents: Examining the Career Preferences, Plans and Expectations of Physicians Completing Their Residency Training.* Irving, TX: Merritt Hawkins.

Metlaine, A., Sauvet, F., Gomez-Merino, D., Elbaz, M., Delafosse, J. Y., Leger, D., et al. (2017). Association between insomnia symptoms, job strain and burnout syndrome: a cross-sectional survey of 1300 financial workers. *BMJ Open, 13*(7).

Miller, F. E. (2001). Challenging and changing stress-producing thinking. *Western Journal of Medicine, 174*(1), 49-50.

Miller, G. E., Chen, E., & Zhou, E. S. (2007). If it Goes Up, Must it Come Down? chronic Stress and the Hypothalamic Pituitary-Adrenocortical Axis in Humans. *Psychological Bulletin, 133*(1), 25-35.

Montague, MD (neurologist), J. (n.d.). Why is the brain prone to florid forms of confabulation?

Montero-Marin, J., Demarzo, M. M., Stepinski, L., Gill, M., & Garcia-Campayo, J. (2014, June). Perceived Stress Latent Factors and the Burnout Subtypes: A Structural Model in Dental Students. *PLoS One, 9*(6).

Montero-Marin, J., Prado-Abril, J., Demarzo, M. M., Gascon, S., & Garcı́a-Campayo, J. (2014, February). Coping with Stress and Types of Burnout: Explanatory. *PLoS ONE, 9*(2).

Montero-Marin, J., Skapinakis, P., Araya, R., Gili, M., & Garcia-Campayo, J. (2011). Towards a brief definition of burnout syndrome by subtypes: Development of the "Burnout Clinical Subtypes Questionnarire" (BSCQ-12). *Health and Quality of Life Outcomes, 9*(74), 1-12.

Montero-Marin, J., Zubiaga, F., Cereceda, M., Demarzo, M. M., Trenc, P., & Garcia-Campayo, J. (2016, June 16). Burnout Subtypes and Absence of Self-Compassion in Primary Healthcare Professionals: A Cross-Sectional Study. *PLoS ONE*, 1-17.

Montgomery, A., Spanu, F., Baban, A., & Panagopoulou, E. (2015, September). Job demands, burnout, and engagement among nurses: A multi-level analysis of ORCAB data investigating the moderating effect of teamwork. *Burnout Research, 2*(2-3), 71-79.

Muris, P., & Petrocchi, N. (2016, February 19). Protection or Vulnerability? A Meta-Analysis of the Relations Between the Positive and Negative components of SElf-Compassion and Psychopathology. *Clinical Psychology Psychotherapy*, ePub.

Murphy, E. R., Barch, D. M., Pagliaccio, D., Luby, J. L., & Belden, A. C. (2015 (in press)). Functional connectivity of the amygdala and subgenual cingulate during cognitive reappraisal of emotions in children with MDD history is associated with rumination. *Developmental Cognitive Neuroscience.*

Neff, K. D., & Vonk, R. (2009, February). Self-compassion versus global self-esteem: two different ways of relating to oneself. *ournal of Personality, 77*(1), 23-50.

Nettles, R., & Balter, R. (Eds.). (2011). *Multiple Minority Identities.* New York, NY, USA: Springer Publishing Company.

Nubold, A., Muck, P. M., & Maier, G. W. (2013). A new substitute for leadership? Followers state core self-evaluations. *The Leadership Quarterly, 24*, 29-44.

October, T. W. (2015). Work-life balance is an illusion: replace guilt with acceptance. *frontiers in Pediatrics, 3*(76), ePub.

Ong, A. D., Bergeman, C. S., Bisconti, T. L., & Wallace, K. A. (2006). Psychological Resilience, Postive Emotions, and Successful Adaptation to Stress in Later Life. *Journal of Personaltiy and Social Psychology 91*, 730-49.

Ong, A. D., Mroczek, D. K., & Riffin, C. (2011, August 1). The Health Significance of Positive Emotions in Adulthood and Later Life. *Social and Personality Psychology Compass, 5*(8), 538-551.

Orri, M., Revah-Levy, A., & Farges, O. (2015, November 24). Surgeons' Emotional Experience of Their Everyday Practice - A Qualitative Study. *PLoS ONE*, 1-15.

Papathanasiou, I. V. (2015). Work-related Mental Consequences: Implications of Burnout on Mental Health Status Among Health Care Providers. *ACTA Inform Med*, 22-28.

Papathanasiou, I. V., Fradelos, E. C., Kleisiaris, C. F., Tsaras, K., Kalota, M. A., & Kourkouta, L. (2014, December 14). Motivation, Leadership, Empowerment and Confidence: Their relation with Nurses' Burnout. *Avicena, 26*, 405-410.

Parrott, W. G. (2001, September). Implications of dysfunctional emotions for understanding how emotions function. *Review of General Psychology, 5*(3), 180-186.

Peckham, C. (2015). *Burnout and Happiness in Physicians: 2013 vs 2015: Physician Burnout: It Just Keeps Getting Worse.*

Peckham, C. (2015, January 26). *Physician Burnout: It Just Keeps Getting Worse.* Retrieved 2017, from Medscape: http://www.medscape.com/viewarticle/838437

Peckham, C. (2016). *Medscape Lifestyle Report 2016: Bias and Burnout.* Medcape.

Peckham, H. (2013). Epigenetics: The Dogma-Defying Discovery That Genes Learn from Experience. *Journal of Neuropsyhotherapy, 1*, 9-20.

Peil, K. T. (2014). Emotion: The Self-regulatory Sense. *Global Advances in Health and Medicine*, 80-108.

Penalba, V., McGuire, H., & Leite, J. R. (2008, July). Psychosocial interventions for prevention of psychological disorders in law enforcement officers. *Cochrane Database System Review, 3*.

Peña-Sarrionandia, A., Mikolajczak, M., & Gross, J. J. (2015, February 24). Integrating emotion regulation and emotional intelligence traditions: a meta-analysis. *Frontiers in Psychology, 6*(160).

Pereira, S. M., Teixeira, C. M., Cavalho, A. S., & Hernandez-Marrero, P. (2016, September 9). Compared to Palliative Care, Working in Intensive Care More than Doubles the Chances of Burnout: Results from a Nationwide Comparative Study. *PLoS One*.

Peschke, I. (2015, 3 31). *Career Burnout? How to Relight Your Candle.* Retrieved 2017, from http://www.huffingtonpost.com/ingrid-peschke/career-burnout-how-to-relight-your-candle_b_6968966.html

Peterson, J. L., & DeHart, T. (2013). Regulating connection: Implicit self-esteem predicts positive non-verbal behavior. *Journal of Experimental Social Psychology*, 99-105.

Pfeffer, J. (1998). *The Human Equation: Building Profits by Putting People First.* Boston: the President and Fellows of Harvard College.

Profit, J., Sharek, P. J., Amspoker, A. B., Kowalkowski, M. A., Nisbet, C. C., Thomas, E. J., et al. (2014, October). Burnout in the NICU setting and its relation to safety culture. *BMJ Quality and Safety, 23*(10), 806-813.

Pugh, S. D., Groth, M., & Hennig-Thurau, T. (2011, March). Willing and able to fake emotions: a closer examination of the link between emotion. *Joural Applied Psychology, 96*(2), 377-390.

Rabin, R. C. (2014, July 21). Docs Slam Recertification Rules They Call A Waste of Time. *Kaiser Health News*.

Rasmussen, V., Turnell, A., Butow, P., Juraskova, I., Kirsten, L., Wiener, L., et al. (2016, February). Burnout among psychosocial oncologists: an application and extension of the effort-reward imbalance model. *Psychoncology, 25*(2), 194-202.

Rees, C. S., Breen, L. J., Cusack, L., & Hegney, D. (2015, February 4). Understanding individual resilience in the workplace: the internal collaboration of workforce resilience model. *frontiers in Psychology, 6*(73), 1-7.

Rees, C. S., Heritage, B., Osseriran-Moisson, R., Chamberlain, D., Cusack, L., Anderson, J., et al. (2016, July 19). Can We Predict Burnout among Student Nurses? An Explorationof the ICWR-1 Model of Individual Psychological Resilience. *Frontiers in Psychology, 7*(1072), 1-11.

Resident Duty Hours: Enhancing Sleep, Supervision, and Safety. (2008). *Resident Duty Hours: Enhancing Sleep, Supervision, and Safety.* Institute of Medicine.

Ricard, M. (2003). *Happiness: A Guide to Developing Life's Most Important Skill.* Little, Brown and Company.

Richards, J. M., & Gross, J. J. (1999). Composure at Any Cost? The Cognitive Consequences of Emotional Suppression. *Personality and Social Psychology Bulletin*, 1033-1044.

Richards, J. M., & Gross, J. J. (2005). Personality and emotional memory: How regulating emotion impairs memory for emotional events. *Journal of Research in Personality*, xxx-xxx (in press).

Robertson, S. M., Stanley, M. A., Cully, J. A., & Naik, A. D. (2012). Positive Emotional Health and Diabetes Care: Concepts, Measurement, and Clinical Implications. *Psychosomatics, 53*, 1-12.

Rogala, A., Shoji, K., Luszczynska, A., Kuna, A., Yeager, C., Benight, C. C., et al. (2016, January 8). From Exhaustion to Disengagement via Self-Efficacy Change: Findings from Two Longitudinal Studies among Human Service Workers. *Frontiers in Psychology, 6*.

Rogers, A. E. (2008). Chapter 40: The Effects of Fatigue and Sleepiness on Nurse Performance and Patient Safety. In R. G. Hughes (Ed.), *Patient Safety and Quality: An Evidence-Based Handbook for Nurses.* Ageny for Healthcare Research and Quality (US).

Romani, M., & Ashkar, K. (2014). Burnout among physicians. *Libyan Journal of Medicine*, 1-6.

Roskam, I., Raes, M.-E., & Mikolajczak, M. (2017, February 9). Exhausted Parents: Development and Preliminary Validation of the Parental Burnout Inventory. *Frontiers in Psychology*, 1-12.

Rubenstein, E. (1999). *An Awakening from the Trances of Everyday Life: A Journey to Empowerment.* Sages Way Press.

Rubin, M. (1987). *The Boiled Frog Syndrome.* New York: Alyson Press.

Rublee, MD, C. (2017). Comment (with permission).

Ruotsalainen, J. H., Verbeek, J. H., Marine, A., & Serra, C. (2015, April 7). Preventing Occupational Stress in healthcare workers. *Cochrane Database of Systematic Reviews.*

Sabaté, E. (2003). *Adherence to Long-Term Therapies: Evidence for Action.* WHO. Geneva: World Health Organization.

Samson, A. C., & Gross, J. J. (2014). The Dark and Light Sides of Humor. In J. Gruber, & J. T. Moskowitz (Eds.), *Positive Emotion: Integrating the Light Sides and Dark Sides* (pp. 169-184). Oxford Scholarship Online.

Sbarra, , D. A., Smith, H. L., & Mehl, M. R. (2001, September 21). Advice to divorcees: Go easy on yourself. *Association for Psychological Science.*

Schrijver, MD, I. (2016, September). Pathology in the Medical Profession? Taking the Pulse of Physician Wellness and Burnout. *Archives pathology Lab Medicine, 140*, 976-982.

Schwarzer, R., & Knoll, N. (2003). Positive Coping: Mastering demands and searching for meaning. In S. J. Lopez, & C. R. Snyder (Eds.), *Positive Psychological Assessment: Handbook of Models and Measures.* Washington, D.C., USA.

Schwingshackl, A. (2014). The fallacy of chasing after work-life balance. *frontiers in Pediatrics, 2*(26), ePub.

Scoglio, A. A., Rudat, D. A., Garvert, D., Jarmolowski, M., Jackson, C., & Herman, J. L. (2015, December 16). Self-Compassion and Responses to Trauma: The Role of Emotion Regulation. *Journal Interpersonal Violence*, Epub.

Segerstrom, S. C., & Miller, G. E. (2004, July). Psychological Stress and the Human Immune System: A MetaAnalytic Study of 30 Years of Inquiry. *Psychological Bulletin, 130*(4), 601-630.

Seligman,, M. (2006). *Learned Optimism* (Originally published 1991 ed.). New York: Simon & Schuster.

Seppala, E. M., Hutcherson, C. A., Nguyen, D. T., Doty, J. R., & Gross, J. J. (2014). Loving-Kindness meditation: a tool to improve healthcare provider compassion, resilience, and patient care. *Journal of Compassionate Health Care, 1*(5).

Shad, R., Thawani, R., & Goel, A. (2015). Burnout and Sleepp Quality: A Cross-Sectional Questionnaire-Based Study of Medical and Non-Medical Students in India. *Cureus, 7*(10).

Shanafelt, M.D., T. D., Boone, M.D., S., Tan, PhD, L., Dyrbye, MD, MHPE, L. N., Sotile, PhD, W., Satele, BS, D., et al. (2012, October 8). Burnout and Satisfaction With Work-Life Balance Among US Physicians Relative to the General US Population. *Archives of Internal Medicine, 172*(18), 1377-1385.

Shanafelt, MD, T. D., Kaups, MD, K. L., Nelson, MD, H., Saele, D. V., Sloan, PhD, J. A., Oreskovich, MD, M. R., et al. (2014, January). An Interactive Individualized Intervention to Promote Behavioral Change to Increase Personal Well-Being in US Surgeons. *Anual Surgery, 259*(1), 82-88.

Shanafelt, T. D., Boone, S., Tan, L., Dyrbye, L. N., Sotile, W., Satele, D., et al. (2012, October 8). Burnout and Satisfaction With Work-Life Balance Among US Physicians Relative to the General US Population. *Archieves Internal Medicine, 172*(18).

Shanafelt, T. D., Oreskovich, M. R., Dyrbye, L. N., Sataele, D. V., Hanks, J. B., Sloan, J. A., et al. (2012, April). Avoiding burnout: the personal health habits and wellness practices of US surgeons. *Annals of Surgery, 255*(4), 625-633.

Shanafelt, T., & Dyrbye, L. (2012). Oncologist burnout: causes, consequences, and responses. *Clinical Oncology, 30*(11), 1235-1241.

Shapiro, J., Zhang, B., & Warm, E. J. (2015, December). Residency as a Social Network: Burnout, Loneliness, and Social Network Centrality. *Journal of Graduate Medical Education*, 617-623.

Shatté, A., Perlman, A., Smith, B., & Lynch, W. D. (2017, February). The Positive Effect of Resilience on Stress and Business Outcomes in Difficult Work Environments. *JOEM, 59*(2).

Shenk, D. (2010). *The Genius in All of Us.* Doubleday.

Sheppes, G., & Gross, J. J. (2014). Emotion Generation and Emotion Regulaton: Moving Beyond Traditional Duel-Process Accounts. In J. W. Sherman, PhD, & B. Gawronski, PhD (Eds.), *Dual-Process Theories of the Social Mind* (pp. 483-496). New York, NY, United States of America: The Guilford Press, A Division of Guilford Publications, Inc.

Siemer, M. (2001). Mood-specific effects on appraisal and emotion judgements. *Cognition and Emotion, 15*(4), 453-485.

Siemer, M. (2005, Sept). Mood-congruent cognitions constitute mood experience. *Emotion, 5*(3), 296-308.

Siemer, M., Mauss, I., & Gross, J. J. (2007). Same Situation—Different Emotions: How Appraisals Shape Our Emotions. *Emotion, 7*(3), 592-600.

Smith, T. M. (2017). Surgeon general: Med students can drive solutions to burnout. Washington D.C.: AMA Wire.

Spreitzer, G. M., & Porath, C. (2014). Self-Determination as a Nutriment for Thriving: Building an Integrative Model of Human Growth at Work. In M. Gagne (Ed.), *Oxford Handbook of*

Work Engagement, Motivation, and Self-Determination Theory (pp. 245-258). New York, NY: Oxford University Press.

Spreitzer, G., Porath, C. L., & Gibson, C. B. (2012). Toward human sustainability: How to enable more thriving at work. *Organizational Dynamics, 41*, 155-162.

Srivastava, S., McGonigal, K. M., Richards, J. M., Butler, E. A., & Gross, J. J. (2006). Optimism in Close Relationships: How Seeing Things in a Positive Light Makes Them So. *Personality Processes and Individual Differences, 91*(1), 143-153.

Steptoe, A. W. (2005). Positive affect and health-related neuroendocrine, cardiovascular, and inflammatory responses. *Proceedings of the National Academy of Sciences.*

Strengths. (n.d.). Retrieved from https://en.wikipedia.org/wiki/Values_in_Action_Inventory_of_Strengths#cite_note-3

Suchman, A. L. (2001). The influence of health care organizations on well-being. *Western Journal of Medicine*, 43-47.

Sullivan, P., & Buske, L. (1998). Results from CMA's huge 1998 physician survey point to a dispirited profession. *Canadian Medical Association, 159*(5), 525-528.

Suri, G., Whittaker, K., & Gross, J. J. (2015). Launching Reappraisal: It's Less Common Than You Might Think. *Emotion, 15*(1), 73-77.

Szymczak, J. E., Smathers, S., Hoegg, C., Klieger, S., Coffin, S. E., & Sammons, J. S. (2015). Reasons Why Physicians and Advanced Practice Clinicians Work While Sick: A Mixed Methods Analysis. *JAMA original investigation, 69*(9), 815-821.

Talbot, M. (1991). *The Holographic Universe.* New York: Harper Collins.

Tawfik, D. S., Sexon, J. B., Kan, P., Sharek, P. J., Nisbet, C. C., Rigdon, J., et al. (2017). Burnout in the neonatal intensive ca2017re unit and its relation to healthcare-associated infections. *Journal of Perinatology, 37*, 315-320.

Ter Hoeven, C. L., van Zoonen, W., & Fonner, K. (2016). The practical paradox of technology: The influence of communication technology use on employee burnout and engagement. *Communication Monographs, 83*(2), 244-259.

The Physicians Foundation. (2010). *In Their Own Words: 12,000 Physicians Reveal Their Thoughts on Medical Practice in America.* Garden City, NY: Morgan James.

The Physicians Foundation. (2014). *2014 Survey of America's Physicians: Practice Patterns & Perspectives: an Examination of the Professional Morale, Practice Patterns, Career Plans, and Perspectives of Today's Physicians Based on over 20,000 Surey Responses.* www.physiciansfoundation.org. Merritt Hawkins.

Toker, S., Melamed, S., Berliner, S., Zeltser, D., & Shapira, I. (2012, October). Burnout and risk of coronary heart disease: a prospective study of 8838 employees. *Psychosomatic Medicine, 74*(8), 840-847.

Treglown, L., Palaiou, K., Zarola, A., & Furnham, A. (2016, June 23). The Dark Side of Resilience and Burnout: A Moderation-Meditation Model. *PLOSone, 11*(6).

Troy, A. S., Shallcross, A. J., Davis, T. S., & Mauss, I. B. (2013, September 1). History of Mindfulness-Based Cognitive Therapy is Associated with Increased Cognitive Reappraisal Ability. *Mindfulness, 4*(3), 213-222.

Tsai, F. J., Huang, W. L., & Chan, C. C. (2009). Occupational stress and burnout of lawyers. *Journal of Occupational Health, 51*(5), 443-450.

Ulwelling, J. J., & Christensen, J. F. (2001, January). Northwest Center for Physician Well-Being. *Western Journal of Medicine, 174*(1), 70-73.

Upper Peninsula Community Health Needs Assessments. (2016). *Phase II: Lessons Learned & Summary of Findings.* CHNA.

Vaillant, G. E. (2012). *Triumphs of Experience: The Men of the Harvard Grant Study.*

van Dam, A. (2016, February 4). Subgroup Analysis in Burnout: Relations Between Fatigue, Anxiety, and Depression. *frontiers in Psychology*, 1-9.

van der Wal, R. A., Bucx, M. J., Hendriks, J. C., Scheffer, G. J., & Prins, J. B. (2016, March). Psychological distress, burnout and personality traits in Dutch anaesthesiologists: A survey. *European Journal of Anaesthesiology, 33*(3), 179-186.

van Mol, M. M., Kompanje, E. J., Benoit, D. D., Bakker, J., & Nijkamp, M. D. (2015). The Prevalence of Compassion Fatigue and Burnout among Healthcare Professionals in Intensive Care Units: A Systematic Review. *PLoS ONE*.

Vantiborgh, T., Bidee, J., Pepermans, R., Griep, Y., & Hofmans, J. (2016, May 12). Antecedents of Psychological Contract Breach: the Role of Job Demands, Job Resources, and Affect. *PLoS One*.

Voellmin, A., Entringer, S., Moog, N., Wadhwa, P. D., & Buss, C. (2013). Maternal positive affect over the course of pregnancy is associated with the length of gestation and reduced risk of preterm delivery. *Journal of Psychosomatic Research, 75*, 336-340.

Waddimba, A. C., Scribani, M., Hasbrouch, M. A., Krupa, N., Jenkins, P., & May, J. J. (2016, October). Resilience among Employed Physicians and Mid-Level Practitiners in Upstate New York. *Health Services Research, 51*(5), 706-734.

Wang, X., & Zhen, M. (2012). Research on the Relationship between Psychological Capital and Job Burnout. *Proceedings of the First International Symposium on Public Human Resource Management* (pp. 33-39). Marietta: American Scholars.

Wang, Y., Chang, Y., Fu, J., & Wang, L. (2012). Work-family conflict and burnout among Chinese female nurses: the mediating effect of psychological capital. *BMC Public Health, 12*, 915-922.

Weiner, E. L., Swain, G. R., Wolf, B., & Gottlieb, M. (2001). A qualitative study of physicians' own wellness-promotion practices. *Western Journal of Medicine, 174*(1), 19-23.

Werner, K. H., Jazaieri, H., Goldin, P. R., Ziv, M., Heimberg, R. G., & Gross, J. J. (2012). Self-Compassion and Social Anxiety Disorder. *Anxiety Stress Coping, 25*(5), 543-558.

West, C. P., Dyrbye, L. N., Satele, D. V., Sloan, J. A., & Shanafelt, T. D. (2012, November). Concurrent Validity of Single-Item Measures of Emotional Exhaustion and Depersonalization in Burnout Assessment. *Journal of General Internal Medicine, 27*(11), 1445-1452.

Westermann, S., Boden, M. T., Gross, J. J., & Lincoln, T. M. (2013). Maladaptive Cognitive Emotion Regulation Prospectively Predicts. *Cognitive Therapy Resarch, 37*, 881-885.

Western North Carolina Medical Society. (2017). Retrieved from http://mywcms.org/news-and-events/newsroom/a-change-in-policy-regarding-physician-burnout-by

Whitney, D., & Trosten-Bloom, A. (2010). *The Power of Appreciative Inquiry: A Practical Guide to Positive Change* (2 ed.). NY: McGraw-Hill.

Wingo, A. P., Ressler, K. J., & Bradley, B. (2014). Resilience characteristics mitigate tendency for harmful alcohol and illicit drug use in adults wiht a history of childhood abuse: A Cross-sectional study of 2024 inner-city men and women. *Journal of Psychiatric Research*.

Wong, E., Tschan, F., Messerli, L., & Semmer, N. K. (2013). Expressing and Amplifying Positive Emotions Facilitate Goal Attainment in Workplace Interactions. *Frontiers in Psychology*, 188.

Wurm, W., Vogel, K., Holl, A., Ebner, C., Bayer, D., Morkl, S., et al. (2016, March 1). Depression-Burnout Overlap in Physicians. *PLoS One*.

Yamaguchi, Y., Inoue, T., Harada, H., & Oike, M. (2016, December). Job control, work-family balance and nurses' intention to leave their profession and organization: A Comparative cross-sectional survey. *Internal Journal of Nursing Studies*, 52-62.

Zambrano, S. C., Chur-Hansen, A., & Crawford, G. B. (2012, September). On the emotional connection of medical specialists dealing with death and dying: a qualitative study of oncologists, surgeons, intensive care specialists and palliative medicine specialists. *BMJ Support Pallative Care, 2*(3), 270-275.

Zambrano, S. C., Chur-Hansen, A., & Crawford, G. B. (2014, August). The experiences, coping mechanisms, and impact of death and dying on palliative medicine specialists. *Palliative Support Care, 12*(4), 209316.

Zencirci, A. D., & Arslan, S. (2011, July 6). Morning-evening type and burnout levels as factors influencing sleep quality of shift nurses: a questionnaire study. *Croatian Medical Journal: Public Health*, 527-537.

Zimmer-Gembeck, M. J., & Skinner, E. A. (2014). The Development of Coping: Implications for Psychopathology and Resilience. In D. Cicchetti (Ed.), *Developmental Psychopathology* (Vol. Resubmission #2, pp. 1-117). Oxford, England: Wiley & Sons.

Zyromski, B., & Joseph, A. E. (n.d.). *Utilizing Cognitive Behavioral Interventions to Positively Impact Achievement in Middle School Students*.

CITATIONS

[1] (Chana, Kennedy, & Chessell, 2015)
[2] (Rees, et al., 2016)
[3] (Baumeister, Vohs, DeWall, & Zhang, 2007)
[4] (Clore & Palmer, 2009)
[5] (King, McInerney, & Watkins, 2012)
[6] (Dan-Glauser & Gross, 2013)
[7] (Kwong, Wong, & Tang, 2013)
[8] (Wong, Tschan, Messerli, & Semmer, 2013)
[9] (Peil, 2014)
[10] (Carver, Control Processes, Priority Management, and Affective Dynamics, 2015)
[11] (Gandi, Wai, Karick, & Dagona, 2011)
[12] (Bretland & Thorsteinsson)
[13] (Papathanasiou, Work-related Mental Consequences: Implications of Burnout on Mental Health Status Among Health Care Providers, 2015)
[14] (Montero-Marin, Skapinakis, Araya, Gili, & Garcia-Campayo, 2011)
[15] (Profit, et al., 2014)
[16] (Shanafelt & Dyrbye, 2012)
[17] (Doolittle & Windish, 2015)
[18] (Doolittle & Windish, 2015)
[19] (Fahrenkopf, Sectish, Barger, Sharek, Lewin, & Chiang, 2008)
[20] (Tawfik, et al., 2017)
[21] (Haggerty, Fields, Selby-Nelson, Foley, & Shrader, 2013)
[22] (Profit, et al., 2014)
[23] (Schrijver, MD, 2016)
[24] (Haggerty, Fields, Selby-Nelson, Foley, & Shrader, 2013)
[25] (Shanafelt, M.D., et al., 2012)
[26] (Freeborn, 2001)
[27] (Argentero, Dell'Olivo, & Ferretti, 1)
[28] (Profit, et al., 2014)
[29] (Gandi, Wai, Karick, & Dagona, 2011, p. 3)
[30] (Freeborn, 2001)
[31] (DiMatteo, et al., 1993)
[32] (Haggerty, Fields, Selby-Nelson, Foley, & Shrader, 2013)
[33] (Rees, Breen, Cusack, & Hegney, 2015)
[34] (Landrum, Knight, & Flynn, 2012)
[35] (Montero-Marin, Skapinakis, Araya, Gili, & Garcia-Campayo, 2011)
[36] (Shanafelt, M.D., et al., 2012)
[37] (Peckham C. , Burnout and Happiness in Physicians: 2013 vs 2015: Physician Burnout: It Just Keeps Getting Worse, 2015)
[38] (Hamilton, 2010)
[39] Burnout is not recognized as a mental illness in the DSM and we don't advocate for its inclusion, we see burnout as evidence of unhealthy habits of thought that lead to poor mental health outcomes.
[40] (Peckham C. , Physician Burnout: It Just Keeps Getting Worse, 2015)

[41] (Ulwelling & Christensen, 2001)
[42] (McManus, Keeling, & Paice, 2004)
[43] (Doolittle & Windish, 2015)
[44] (Leung & Rioseco, 2017)
[45] (Chigerwe, Boudreaux, & Ilkiw, 2014)
[46] (Fares, Tabosh, Saadeddin, Mouhayyar, & Aridi, 2016)
[47] (Shanafelt, MD, et al., 2014)
[48] (Pereira, Teixeira, Cavalho, & Hernandez-Marrero, 2016)
[49] (van Mol, Kompanje, Benoit, Bakker, & Nijkamp, 2015)
[50] (Wurm, et al., 2016)
[51] (Schrijver, MD, 2016)
[52] (Rublee, MD, 2017)
[53] (Peckham C. , Burnout and Happiness in Physicians: 2013 vs 2015: Physician Burnout: It Just Keeps Getting Worse, 2015)
[54] (Shanafelt, et al., 2012)
[55] (Hampton, 2005)
[56] (Gold, Sen, & Schwenk, 2013)
[57] (Gold, Sen, & Schwenk, 2013)
[58] (Dyrbye, et al., 2008)
[59] (Dyrbye, et al., 2008)
[60] (Dyrbye, et al., 2008)
[61] (Western North Carolina Medical Society, 2017)
[62] (Western North Carolina Medical Society, 2017)
[63] (American Medical Association (AMA), 2016)
[64] (Jensen, RN PhD, Trollope-Kumar, MD PhD, Waters, MD CCFP, & Everson, MD CCFP FCFP, 2008)
[65] (Suchman, 2001)
[66] (Peckham C. , Physician Burnout: It Just Keeps Getting Worse, 2015)
[67] (The Physicians Foundation, 2014)
[68] (The Physicians Foundation, 2010, p. 79)
[69] (Gandi, Wai, Karick, & Dagona, 2011, p. 3)
[70] (Bedynsa & Zolnierczyk-Zreda, 2015)
[71] (Rasmussen, et al., 2016)
[72] (Shanafelt, et al., 2012)
[73] (Busis, et al., 2017)
[74] (Tsai, Huang, & Chan, 2009)
[75] (Montgomery, Spanu, Baban, & Panagopoulou, 2015)
[76] (van Mol, Kompanje, Benoit, Bakker, & Nijkamp, 2015)
[77] (Zambrano, Chur-Hansen, & Crawford, On the emotional connection of medical specialists dealing with death and dying: a qualitative study of oncologists, surgeons, intensive care specialists and palliative medicine specialists, 2012)
[78] (van Mol, Kompanje, Benoit, Bakker, & Nijkamp, 2015)
[79] (Merrit Hawkins, an AMN Healthcare company, 2011)
[80] (Merrit Hawkins, an AMN Healthcare company, 2011, p. 8)
[81] (Merrit Hawkins, an AMN Healthcare company, 2011, p. 8)
[82] (Lee, MD, Brown, PhD, & Stewart, PhD, 2009)
[83] (Sabaté, 2003)
[84] (Honkonen, et al., 2006)
[85] (Toker, Melamed, Berliner, Zeltser, & Shapira, 2012)
[86] (Consoli, 2015)
[87] (Toker, Melamed, Berliner, Zeltser, & Shapira, 2012)
[88] (Melamed, Shirom, Toker, & Shapira, 2006)
[89] (Armon, Shirom, Shapira, & Melamed, 2008)
[90] (Metlaine, et al., 2017)
[91] (Boehm, 2012)
[92] (Boehm, 2012)
[93] (Boden, Berenbaum, & Gross, Why Do People Believe What They Do? A Functionalist Perspective, 2016)
[94] (McManus, Keeling, & Paice, 2004)
[95] (McManus, Keeling, & Paice, 2004)
[96] (Antoniou, Davidson, & Cooper, 2003)
[97] (van Dam, 2016)
[98] (Smith, 2017)

[99] (Smith, 2017)
[100] (Gross, The Extended Process Model of Emotion Regulation: Elaborations, Applications, and Future Directions, 2015)
[101] (Baumeister, Vohs, DeWall, & Zhang, 2007)
[102] (Kwong, Wong, & Tang, 2013)
[103] (Peil, 2014)
[104] (Carver, Control Processes, Priority Management, and Affective Dynamics, 2015)
[105] (Spreitzer & Porath, 2014)
[106] (Spreitzer & Porath, 2014)
[107] (Peil, 2014)
[108] (Peckham C. , Medscape Lifestyle Report 2016: Bias and Burnout, 2016)
[109] (Seligman,, 2006)
[110] (Seligman,, 2006)
[111] (Montague, MD (neurologist))
[112] (Sheppes & Gross, 2014)
[113] (Baumeister, Vohs, DeWall, & Zhang, 2007)
[114] (Peil, 2014)
[115] (Kwong, Wong, & Tang, 2013)
[116] (Carver, Control Processes, Priority Management, and Affective Dynamics, 2015)
[117] (Hopp, Troy, & Mauss, 2011)
[118] (Peil, 2014)
[119] (Peil, 2014)
[120] (Peil, 2014)
[121] (Mauss, Bunge, & Gross, Automatic Emotion Regulation, 2007)
[122] (Siemer, Mauss, & Gross, Same Situation—Different Emotions: How Appraisals Shape Our Emotions, 2007)
[123] The EGSc is a compilation of scales used by a variety of teachers including David Hawkins, L. Ron Hubbard, and Abraham-Hicks. The Zones are my addition. The science supporting the Emotional Guidance Scale, or that emotions provide guidance, did not exist when the earlier scales were created. All emotions could be placed on the scale. It is simplified to reflect emotions that are similar in degrees of empowerment in each Zone. The higher the Zone, the greater the sense of empowerment the person feels.
[124] (Montero-Marin, Prado-Abril, Demarzo, Gascon, & García-Campayo, 2014)
[125] (Montero-Marin, Prado-Abril, Demarzo, Gascon, & García-Campayo, 2014)
[126] (Aspinwall, 2011)
[127] (APA, 2015)
[128] (van der Wal, Bucx, Hendriks, Scheffer, & Prins, 2016)
[129] (Rees, et al., 2016)
[130] (Houkes, Winants, Twellaar, & Verdonk, 2011)
[131] (Carmona, Buunk, Peiró, Rodríguez, & Bravo, 2006)
[132] (Rees, et al., 2016)
[133] (Lee, MD, Brown, PhD, & Stewart, PhD, 2009)
[134] (McLeod, 2009)
[135] (Peil, 2014)
[136] (Siemer, Mood-congruent cognitions constitute mood experience, 2005)
[137] (Luthans, Luthans, & Luthans, Positive psychological capital: Beyond human and social capital, 2004)
[138] (Kutluturkan, Sozeri, Uysal, & Bay, 2016)
[139] (van der Wal, Bucx, Hendriks, Scheffer, & Prins, 2016)
[140] (Treglown, Palaiou, Zarola, & Furnham, 2016)
[141] (Waddimba, Scribani, Hasbrouch, Krupa, Jenkins, & May, 2016)
[142] (Jackson, Firtko, & Edenborough, 2007)
[143] (Profit, et al., 2014)
[144] (Srivastava, McGonigal, Richards, Butler, & Gross, 2006)
[145] (Shatté, Perlman, Smith, & Lynch, 2017, p. 139)
[146] (Jensen, RN PhD, Trollope-Kumar, MD PhD, Waters, MD CCFP, & Everson, MD CCFP FCFP, 2008)
[147] (Luthans, Luthans, & Luthans, Positive psychological capital: Beyond human and social capital, 2004)
[148] (Ding, et al., 2015)
[149] (Lashinger & Grau, 2012)
[150] (Carver, Control Processes, Priority Management, and Affective Dynamics, 2015)
[151] (Baumeister & Beck, Evil: Inside Human Violence and Cruelty, 1999)
[152] (Manzano-García & Ayala, 2017)

[153] (Baumeister, Vohs, DeWall, & Zhang, 2007)
[154] (Peil, 2014)
[155] (Carver, Control Processes, Priority Management, and Affective Dynamics, 2015)
[156] (Baumeister, Vohs, DeWall, & Zhang, 2007)
[157] (Rubenstein, 1999)
[158] (Talbot, 1991)
[159] (Ricard, 2003)
[160] (Eiser & Pahl, 2001)
[161] (Treglown, Palaiou, Zarola, & Furnham, 2016)
[162] (Treglown, Palaiou, Zarola, & Furnham, 2016)
[163] (Treglown, Palaiou, Zarola, & Furnham, 2016)
[164] (Danner, 2001)
[165] (Vaillant, 2012)
[166] (Papathanasiou, Work-related Mental Consequences: Implications of Burnout on Mental Health Status Among Health Care Providers, 2015)
[167] (Assagioli, 1965)
[168] (Siemer, Mood-specific effects on appraisal and emotion judgements, 2001)
[169] (Folkman & Moskowitzz, 2004)
[170] (Schwarzer & Knoll, 2003)
[171] (Peña-Sarrionandia, Mikolajczak, & Gross, 2015)
[172] (Mauss & Gross, Emotional Suppression and cardiovascular disease Is hiding feelings bad for your heart?, 2004)
[173] (Koole, 2009)
[174] (Suri, Whittaker, & Gross, 2015)
[175] (Nettles & Balter, 2011)
[176] (Orri, Revah-Levy, & Farges, 2015)
[177] (Orri, Revah-Levy, & Farges, 2015)
[178] (Alkadhi, 2013)
[179] (Orri, Revah-Levy, & Farges, 2015)
[180] (Westermann, Boden, Gross, & Lincoln, 2013)
[181] (Seligman,, 2006)
[182] (Langer, 2009)
[183] (Chang, 2011)
[184] (Gross & John, Individual differences in two emotion regulation processes: implications for affect, relationships, and well-being, 2003)
[185] (Richards & Gross, Personality and emotional memory: How regulating emotion impairs memory for emotional events, 2005)
[186] (Parrott, 2001)
[187] (Lazarus, 1991)
[188] (Rogala, et al., 2016)
[189] (Lemelle & Seielzo, 2012)
[190] (Grant & Sonnentag, 2010)
[191] (Rogala, et al., 2016)
[192] (Rogala, et al., 2016)
[193] (Doolittle & Windish, 2015)
[194] (McManus, Keeling, & Paice, 2004)
[195] (Huby, Gerry, McKinstry, Porter, Shaw, & Wrate, 2002)
[196] (Doolittle & Windish, 2015)
[197] (Treglown, Palaiou, Zarola, & Furnham, 2016)
[198] (Doolittle & Windish, 2015)
[199] (Doolittle & Windish, 2015)
[200] (Hopp, Troy, & Mauss, 2011)
[201] (Shanafelt, et al., 2012)
[202] (John & Gross, 2004)
[203] (Montero-Marin, Demarzo, Stepinski, Gill, & Garcia-Campayo, 2014)
[204] (Samson & Gross, 2014)
[205] (Miller F. E., 2001)
[206] (Weiner, Swain, Wolf, & Gottlieb, 2001)
[207] (Carver & Connor-Smith, Personality and Coping, 2010)
[208] (Kumar, 2016)

[209] (Bedynsa & Zolnierczyk-Zreda, 2015)
[210] (Heller, et al., 2013)
[211] (Li, Guan, Chang, & Zhang, 2014)
[212] (Strengths)
[213] (Pugh, Groth, & Hennig-Thurau, 2011)
[214] (Carmona, Buunk, Peiró, Rodríguez, & Bravo, 2006)
[215] (Neff & Vonk, 2009)
[216] (Montero-Marin, Zubiaga, Cereceda, Demarzo, Trenc, & Garcia-Campayo, 2016)
[217] (Muris & Petrocchi, 2016)
[218] (Werner, Jazaieri, Goldin, Ziv, Heimberg, & Gross, 2012)
[219] (Lopez, et al., 2015)
[220] (Neff & Vonk, 2009)
[221] (Scoglio, Rudat, Garvert, Jarmolowski, Jackson, & Herman, 2015)
[222] (Sbarra, , Smith, & Mehl, 2001)
[223] (De Castella, Goldin, Jazaieri, Ziv, Dweck, & Gross, 2013)
[224] (Seligman,, 2006)
[225] 1925 January 28, The Marcellus Observer, Stick to the Finish, (Acknowledgement to Exchange), Quote Page 1, Column 7, Marcellus, New York. (Old Fulton)
[226] (Chang, 2011)
[227] (Livingston, 2003)
[228] (Bigman, Mauss, Gross, & Tamir, 2015)
[229] (Keeney & Ilies, 2011)
[230] (Romani & Ashkar, 2014)
[231] (Shanafelt, et al., 2012)
[232] (Boden & Gross, An Emotion Regulation Perspective on Belief Change, 2013)
[233] (Boden & Gross, An Emotion Regulation Perspective on Belief Change, 2013)
[234] (Hopp, Troy, & Mauss, 2011)
[235] (Hopp, Troy, & Mauss, 2011)
[236] (Hopp, Troy, & Mauss, 2011)
[237] (Hu, Zhang, Wang, Mistry, Ran, & Wang, 2014)
[238] (Troy, Shallcross, Davis, & Mauss, 2013)
[239] (Cisler & Olatunji, 2012)
[240] (Armstrong, Galligan, & Critchley, 2011)
[241] (Kobylinska & Karwowska, 2015)
[242] (APA, 2014)
[243] (Murphy, Barch, Pagliaccio, Luby, & Belden, 2015 (in press))
[244] (Kudinova, Owens, Burkhouse, Barretto, Bonanno, & Gibb, 2015)
[245] (Zyromski & Joseph)
[246] (Butler, Chapman, Forman, & Beck, 2006)
[247] (Hofmann, Asnaani, Vonk, Sawyer, & Fang, 2012)
[248] (Hu, Zhang, Wang, Mistry, Ran, & Wang, 2014)
[249] (Nettles & Balter, 2011)
[250] (Nettles & Balter, 2011)
[251] (Nettles & Balter, 2011)
[252] (Nettles & Balter, 2011)
[253] (Nettles & Balter, 2011)
[254] (Nettles & Balter, 2011)
[255] (Nettles & Balter, 2011)
[256] (Nettles & Balter, 2011)
[257] (Fagley, 2012)
[258] (Gross & John, Individual differences in two emotion regulation processes: implications for affect, relationships, and well-being, 2003)
[259] (Jensen, RN PhD, Trollope-Kumar, MD PhD, Waters, MD CCFP, & Everson, MD CCFP FCFP, 2008)
[260] (Peckham C. , Burnout and Happiness in Physicians: 2013 vs 2015: Physician Burnout: It Just Keeps Getting Worse, 2015)
[261] (Luken & Sammons, 2016)
[262] (Peschke, 2015)
[263] (Luken & Sammons, 2016)
[264] (Seppala, Hutcherson, Nguyen, Doty, & Gross, 2014)
[265] (Doolittle & Windish, 2015)
[266] (Whitney & Trosten-Bloom, 2010)

[267] (Romani & Ashkar, 2014)
[268] (Rubin, 1987)
[269] (Cusack, et al., 2016)
[270] (Shanafelt, M.D., et al., 2012)
[271] (Schrijver, MD, 2016)
[272] (Linzer, MD, Levine, MD, MPH, Melter, MD, Poplau, Warde, MD, & West, MD, PhD, 2013)
[273] (Shanafelt, et al., 2012)
[274] (Zencirci & Arslan, 2011)
[275] (Papathanasiou, Fradelos, Kleisiaris, Tsaras, Kalota, & Kourkouta, 2014)
[276] (Vantiborgh, Bidee, Pepermans, Griep, & Hofmans, 2016)
[277] (Sullivan & Buske, 1998)
[278] (Shanafelt, MD, et al., 2014)
[279] (The Physicians Foundation, 2010, p. 84)
[280] (The Physicians Foundation, 2014)
[281] (The Physicians Foundation, 2014)
[282] (October, 2015)
[283] (October, 2015)
[284] (Schwingshackl, 2014)
[285] (Kubicek & Korunka, 2015)
[286] (Orri, Revah-Levy, & Farges, 2015)
[287] (Brandstatter, Job, & Schulze, 2016)
[288] (Barnes & Spreitzer, 2015)
[289] (Rogers, 2008)
[290] (Resident Duty Hours: Enhancing Sleep, Supervision, and Safety, 2008)
[291] (ACGME, 2011)
[292] (Association of Professors of Medicine: The American Journal of Medicine, 2001)
[293] (Yamaguchi, Inoue, Harada, & Oike, 2016)
[294] (Huby, Gerry, McKinstry, Porter, Shaw, & Wrate, 2002)
[295] (Freeborn, 2001)
[296] (Deci & Ryan, 2000)
[297] (Mauss, et al., 2011)
[298] (Richards & Gross, Composure at Any Cost? The Cognitive Consequences of Emotional Suppression, 1999)
[299] (Cheung, Tang, & Tang, 2011)
[300] (The Physicians Foundation, 2014)
[301] (Erickson, Rockwern, Koltov, & McLean, 2017)
[302] (The Physicians Foundation, 2014)
[303] (The Physicians Foundation, 2014)
[304] (Hein, 2017)
[305] (Dyrbye & Shanafelt, Physician Burnout: a potential threat to successful health care reform, 2011)
[306] (Rabin, 2014)
[307] (Peckham C. , Medscape Lifestyle Report 2016: Bias and Burnout, 2016)
[308] (The Physicians Foundation, 2014)
[309] (The Physicians Foundation, 2014)
[310] (Joy, 2017)
[311] (The Physicians Foundation, 2014)
[312] (The Physicians Foundation, 2014)
[313] (Peckham C. , Burnout and Happiness in Physicians: 2013 vs 2015: Physician Burnout: It Just Keeps Getting Worse, 2015)
[314] (McDonald, MD, 2001)
[315] (Shad, Thawani, & Goel, 2015)
[316] (Ruotsalainen, Verbeek, Marine, & Serra, 2015)
[317] (Rogers, 2008)
[318] (Rogers, 2008)
[319] (DiMatteo, et al., 1993)
[320] (Ter Hoeven, van Zoonen, & Fonner, 2016)
[321] (Maslach & Leiter, 2016)
[322] (Treglown, Palaiou, Zarola, & Furnham, 2016)
[323] (Shapiro, Zhang, & Warm, 2015)
[324] (Hamilton, 2010)
[325] (Lashinger, Borgogni, Consiglio, & Read, 2015)

[326] (Lian, Sun, Ji, Li, & Peng, 2014)
[327] (Orri, Revah-Levy, & Farges, 2015)
[328] (Luthans & Youssef, Human, Social, and Now Positive Psychological Capital Management: Investing in People for Competitive Advantage, 2004)
[329] (Pfeffer, 1998)
[330] (Ter Hoeven, van Zoonen, & Fonner, 2016)
[331] (Maslach & Leiter, 2016)
[332] (Handbook, 2013)
[333] (De Castella, Goldin, Jazaien, Heimberg, Dweck, & Gross, 2015)
[334] (Bretland & Thorsteinsson)
[335] (APA, 2015)
[336] (Upper Peninsula Community Health Needs Assessments, 2016)
[337] (Penalba, McGuire, & Leite, 2008)
[338] (Miller, Chen, & Zhou, 2007)
[339] (Szymczak, Smathers, Hoegg, Klieger, Coffin, & Sammons, 2015)
[340] (Korownyk, et al., 2014)
[341] (Korownyk, et al., 2014)
[342] (Brownstein, 2009)
[343] (Kumar, 2016)
[344] (The Physicians Foundation, 2014)
[345] (Haidt, 2013)
[346] (Chin, Guo, Hung, Hsieh, Wang, & Shiao, 2017)
[347] (Chin, Guo, Hung, Hsieh, Wang, & Shiao, 2017)
[348] (Maslach & Leiter, 2016)
[349] (The Physicians Foundation, 2010, p. 87)
[350] (Hamilton, 2010)
[351] (Brooks, 2015)
[352] (The Physicians Foundation, 2010)
[353] (The Physicians Foundation, 2014)
[354] (The Physicians Foundation, 2014)
[355] (Gandi, Wai, Karick, & Dagona, 2011)
[356] (Association of Professors of Medicine: The American Journal of Medicine, 2001)
[357] (Wang, Chang, Fu, & Wang, 2012)
[358] (Keeney & Ilies, 2011)
[359] (Feldman & Worline, 2011)
[360] (Wang & Zhen, 2012)
[361] (Linzer, MD, Levine, MD, MPH, Melter, MD, Poplau, Warde, MD, & West, MD, PhD, 2013)
[362] (Roskam, Raes, & Mikolajczak, 2017)
[363] (Dyrbye, Shanafelt, Balch, Satele, Sloan, & Freischlag, 2011)
[364] (Yamaguchi, Inoue, Harada, & Oike, 2016)
[365] (Draper, Kolves, Leo, & Snowden, 2014)
[366] (Zambrano, Chur-Hansen, & Crawford, The experiences, coping mechanisms, and impact of death and dying on palliative medicine specialists, 2014)
[367] (Edress, Connors, Paine, Norvell, & Taylor, 2016)
[368] (Edress, Connors, Paine, Norvell, & Taylor, 2016)
[369] (Edress, Connors, Paine, Norvell, & Taylor, 2016)
[370] (van Mol, Kompanje, Benoit, Bakker, & Nijkamp, 2015)
[371] (Hunsaker, Chen, Maughan, & Heaston, 2015)
[372] (Boden, Kulkarni, Shurick, Bonn-Miller, & Gross, 2014)
[373] (Dewa, McDaid, & Ettner, 2007)
[374] (Gandi, Wai, Karick, & Dagona, 2011)
[375] (Association of Professors of Medicine: The American Journal of Medicine, 2001)
[376] (Gandi, Wai, Karick, & Dagona, 2011)
[377] (Gandi, Wai, Karick, & Dagona, 2011)
[378] (Gandi, Wai, Karick, & Dagona, 2011)
[379] (Gandi, Wai, Karick, & Dagona, 2011)
[380] (Linzer, MD, Levine, MD, MPH, Melter, MD, Poplau, Warde, MD, & West, MD, PhD, 2013)
[381] (Gandi, Wai, Karick, & Dagona, 2011)
[382] (Gandi, Wai, Karick, & Dagona, 2011)
[383] (Gandi, Wai, Karick, & Dagona, 2011)
[384] (Association of Professors of Medicine: The American Journal of Medicine, 2001)

[385] (Gandi, Wai, Karick, & Dagona, 2011)
[386] (Association of Professors of Medicine: The American Journal of Medicine, 2001)
[387] (Association of Professors of Medicine: The American Journal of Medicine, 2001)
[388] (Association of Professors of Medicine: The American Journal of Medicine, 2001)
[389] (Linzer, MD, Levine, MD, MPH, Melter, MD, Poplau, Warde, MD, & West, MD, PhD, 2013)
[390] (Gandi, Wai, Karick, & Dagona, 2011, p. 3)
[391] (Gandi, Wai, Karick, & Dagona, 2011, p. 3)
[392] (Association of Professors of Medicine: The American Journal of Medicine, 2001)
[393] (Gandi, Wai, Karick, & Dagona, 2011, p. 3)
[394] (Gandi, Wai, Karick, & Dagona, 2011, p. 3)
[395] (Association of Professors of Medicine: The American Journal of Medicine, 2001, p. 173)
[396] (Gandi, Wai, Karick, & Dagona, 2011, p. 3)
[397] (Gandi, Wai, Karick, & Dagona, 2011, p. 3)
[398] (Khamisa, peltzer, & Oldenburg, 2013)
[399] (Segerstrom & Miller, 2004)
[400] (Miller, Chen, & Zhou, 2007)
[401] (Shatté, Perlman, Smith, & Lynch, 2017)
[402] (Shatté, Perlman, Smith, & Lynch, 2017)
[403] (Peckham H. , 2013)
[404] (Spreitzer, Porath, & Gibson, 2012)
[405] (Montero-Marin, Skapinakis, Araya, Gili, & Garcia-Campayo, 2011)
[406] (Montero-Marin, Skapinakis, Araya, Gili, & Garcia-Campayo, 2011)
[407] (Montero-Marin, Skapinakis, Araya, Gili, & Garcia-Campayo, 2011)
[408] (West, Dyrbye, Satele, Sloan, & Shanafelt, 2012)
[409] (Danner, 2001)
[410] (Dockray & Steptoe, 2010)
[411] (Khansar, Murgo, & Faith, 1990)
[412] (Lai JC, 2005)
[413] (Ong, Mroczek, & Riffin, 2011)
[414] (Robertson, Stanley, Cully, & Naik, 2012)
[415] (Steptoe, 2005)
[416] (Bhatia & Tandon, 2005)
[417] (Armstrong, Galligan, & Critchley, 2011)
[418] (Baratta, Rozeske, & Maier, 2013)
[419] (Bonanno, 2004)
[420] (Bond & Shapiro, 2014)
[421] (Cohn, 2009)
[422] (Infurna & Luthar, 2016)
[423] (Lyubomirsky & Porta, Boosting Happiness and Buttressing Resilience: Results from Cognitive and Behavioral Interventions, (in press))
[424] (Catalino & Fredrickson, 2011)
[425] (Wingo, Ressler, & Bradley, 2014)
[426] (APA, 2013)
[427] (Creswell, et al., 2005)
[428] (Martin & Dahlen, 2005)
[429] (Ong, Bergeman, Bisconti, & Wallace, 2006)
[430] (Steptoe, 2005)
[431] (Nubold, Muck, & Maier, 2013)
[432] (Fredrickson B. L., 2010)
[433] (Larson, Norman, Hughes, & Avey, 2013)
[434] (Dweck, 2008)
[435] (Bryan, 1991)
[436] (Estrada, 1997)
[437] (Fredrickson B. L., 2005)
[438] (Ashby, 1999)
[439] (Johnson, Waugh, & Fredrickson, 2010)
[440] (Zimmer-Gembeck & Skinner, 2014)

[441] (Lyubomirsky, King, & Diener, The Benefits of Frequent Positive Affect: Does Happiness Lead to Success?, 2005)
[442] (Christian, 2012)
[443] (Voellmin, Entringer, Moog, Wadhwa, & Buss, 2013)
[444] (Liberman, Anderson, & Ross, 2010)
[445] (McCarthy & Casey, 2011)
[446] (Peterson & DeHart, 2013)
[447] (Manzano-García & Ayala, 2017)